MOSBY'S

MEDICAL SURFARI

A GUIDE TO
EXPLORING THE
INTERNET AND
DISCOVERING
THE TOP
HEALTH CARE
RESOURCES

MOSBY'S

MEDICAL SURFARI

A GUIDE TO

EXPLORING THE

INTERNET AND

DISCOVERING THE

TOP HEALTH CARE

RESOURCES

Scott R. Gibbs, M.D., M.A.

Micaela Sullivan-Fowler, M.S., M.A.

Nigel W. Rowe

M Mosby

St. Louis Baltimore Boston Carlsbad Chicago Naples New York Philadelphia Portland
London Madrid Mexico City Singapore Sydney Tokyo Toronto Wiesbaden

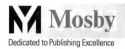

Mosby
Dedicated to Publishing Excellence

A Times Mirror
Company

Vice President and Publisher, Continuity Publishing: Kenneth Killion
Director, Editorial Development: Gretchen C. Murphy
Developmental Editor: Kelly Poirier
Editorial Assistant: Suchitra Gururaj
Acquisitions Editor: Li Wen Huang
Director, Continuity EDP: Maria Nevinger
Project Manager: Jill C. Waite
Assistant Project Supervisor: Laura Higgins
Freelance Staff Supervisor: Barbara M. Kelly
Vice President, Medical Direct Response and Continuity Marketing: Bruce A. F. Polsky

Printed in the United States of America
Design by Angela Moody
Illustrations by Dan Steffan
Composition by Andrea Field
Disk development by MWP Software
Printed by Malloy Lithographing, Inc.

Mosby–Year Book, Inc.
11830 Westline Industrial Drive
St. Louis, MO 63146

Editorial Office:
Mosby–Year Book, Inc.
161 N. Clark St.
Chicago, IL 60601

EDITOR-IN-CHIEF

Scott R. Gibbs, M.D., M.A.

Scott Gibbs is a neurosurgeon, writer, and editor with more than 20 years combined experience in business and medical education. He is dedicated to excellence and committed to sharing knowledge. These ideals, combined with recognizing the impact of converging information, communication, and medical technologies stimulated his particular interest in the Internet and its applications to health care.

EDITORS

Micaela Sullivan-Fowler, M.S., M.A.

Micaela Sullivan-Fowler, a medical historian and medical librarian, has published articles on the history of 17th and 19th century medicine, as well as on historical and contemporary aspects of alternative medicine. She is a contributing editor to *JAMA's* "One Hundred Years Ago" column. Initially honing her searching skills at the American Medical Association library, she is now an independent researcher who spends her time thinking of ways to successfully navigate the Internet and help healthcare professionals and the public find "the perfect review article."

Nigel W. Rowe

Nigel Rowe is a senior marketing specialist at Mosby–Year Book, Inc. Since 1983, when he purchased his first computer (48K of RAM!), he has been getting overly excited about computers. His main area of interest is in designing information systems and helping friends and colleagues to get more mileage from their computers. Although originally from New Zealand, he moved twice in 1992, each time to a new country, in a complicated maneuver to obtain cheaper Internet access.

DISCLAIMER

The resources listed within this publication and accompanying diskette must be used cautiously because unsupported information about medical research and products can be rapidly disseminated on the Internet without the traditional process of peer review. This information is no substitute for clinical judgment and common sense.

This information is only a summary of resources available for those interested in health care. No attempt has been made to furnish an actual teaching text or a guide for therapy. These resources are neither intended nor properly used as a substitute for clinical experience, certified professional training, or therapeutic treatment. Please direct your medical questions to your physician or health care provider.

The medical information available on the World Wide Web comes from many sources. Every effort has been made to ensure the accuracy of the information presented in these pages. Additionally, the pricing and terms of services listed may change without notice. No effort has been made to update this material after the publication date reflected herein. Neither Mosby–Year Book, Inc., its editors, nor its contributors can be responsible for any errors or omissions.

Of necessity, this book uses certain product and brand names which may be trade names or trademarks and which appear in capitalized form. We take no responsibility for and express no opinion as to the validity of any such trade name or trademark claims.

The "Information Superhighway" is a marvelous thing to behold, even if it remains under construction, is pocked by more than a few potholes, and is often overhyped.

The Internet and especially its user friendly subset, the World Wide Web, offer a nearly limitless supply of information—there were an estimated 500,000-plus Web sites alone at last count, with scores of new entries being added every day. Almost all of this information is free and available to anyone with the right equipment and know-how. If, as the old saying goes, "knowledge is power," then there may be no more empowering piece of technology than the Internet.

Medical information is available in particular abundance on the Net; health and medical sites are already among the more popular destinations and promise to become even more so. There seems to be a site for every condition and concern, every medical center, and commercial health interest.

However, despite the proliferation of on-line health and medical information and the availability of ever more sophisticated search services, it's not always easy to find what you want or need. The Net has been described as the world's largest library, but one in which all the books are on the floor. Even as users pick their way through sites seemingly of interest or relevance, it is quickly apparent that information quality is uneven at best. In a world where anyone can be a "publisher," uninitiated users have few clues to help them determine whether what they're viewing hews to any particular standard. So far, the Web has few rules, which is a source of both the excitement and the frustration that seems to strike Internet surfers in equal amounts.

These dilemmas undeniably are among the reasons that physicians and other health care professionals have begun slowly and cautiously to use computers as everyday clinical, management, and communication tools. Vast improvements in computer technology have led many to expect that health care professionals would embrace the appeal of this nearly instantaneous information resource. But this hasn't happened as quickly and broadly as forecasted. Many remain wary of the Net, hobbled by their lack of surfing experience and the unprecedented volume of information.

This will change. The Net is becoming more appealing and even indispensable to health care professionals as awareness of its usefulness grows, as computer systems become a common part of professional training, and as improvements in technology make accessing the electronic information easier and faster. Professional imperatives, economics, and questions from patients are all inducing clinicians to explore and use digital technology. Health care organizations are increasingly looking to these technologies to reduce costs and provide more efficient and effective service. From medical records to prescription tracking to Web sites developed for consumers, health care organizations recognize the utility of this electronic information resource. Patients also are becoming highly informed health care consumers. Many patients, their families, and caregivers increasingly use the Web to gather information and exchange experiences via chat groups and other on-line communication forums. Patients may access drug information, clinical trials protocols, the latest reports from leading medical journals, and physician search services and profiles, all by using their personal computers. Information is not the same as knowledge, however, nor should either be confused with wisdom. Knowledge combined with experience is what health care professionals can contribute to their patients' quest to be medically informed.

Consequently, it is essential to know where and how to help patients locate high-quality and timely information resources, as well as to help them sift and interpret what they find. To that end, health care professionals who are Internet savvy can be exceptionally valuable resources for patients. Indeed, health care professionals must become far better acquainted with this new medium, because it holds so much potential to teach and inform.

So how can budding Net surfers best get on the "Infobahn" and pick their way through the jungle of medical information available? One good approach is to use a text written with the health care professional in mind, a road map for navigating the intricacies of getting connected and then more easily finding valuable Web sites.

This text does that; it provides useful guidance for health care professionals regardless of their level of Net skill. For the novice, it offers practical tips on how to get on the Net in the first place and on the basics of surfing. For the novice and the expert, it provides targeted, timely guidance on the unique challenge of cruising the electronic superhighway for reliable, useful health and medical information.

Of particular note is the fact that the authors and editors of this book have worked with numerous practicing physicians, nurses, and other providers to review a diverse set of sites, using specific criteria such as usefulness, credibility, uniqueness, and the authority of the information source. These reviewed sites as well as more than 1,200 others are bookmarked on the disk that accompanies this book. The review process offers a useful set of baseline criteria for surfers to judge the quality and utility of sites they find on their own. For after all, it is through repeated sojourns in cyberspace that health care professionals will gain the knowledge and experience needed to truly embrace the vast medical resources of the electronic frontier.

Bonnie Chi-Lum, M.D., M.P.H.
Assistant Professor,
Schools of Medicine and Public Health,
Loma Linda University
National Project Coordinator
AMA Physicians Accessing the Internet (PAI) Initiative
Loma Linda, California

William Silberg
Editorial Director, New Media Office
AMA Scientific Information and Multimedia Group
Chicago, Illinois

INTRODUCTION

We are in the first age since the dawn of civilization in which people have dared to think it practicable to make the benefits of civilization available to the human race.
Arnold J. Toynbee (1889–1975)
English historian and internationalist

One of the richest benefits of civilization is the attainment of knowledge—knowledge embraced is information. The human race clearly distinguishes itself from the rest of the animal kingdom by deliberately striving to record, comprehend, and retrieve meaningful information. Initially we shared information with those around us, and later, with scholars in other lands. With the advent of the printing press, we began distributing it to a target audience, and now, through the Internet, information is fast becoming ubiquitous.

Our information resources are burgeoning and in many ways are like none before. They are born of collective, cumulative, and collaborative scholarship through the Internet, and they will ultimately be accessed and transmitted by fiberoptics at the speed of light, to you, your patients, and your peers.

Multiauthored, multidisciplinary information resources may sound like a novel, computer-age concept—a product of advances in telecommunications technology. However, the concept of a cumulative scholarly work dates to the middle ages. The *Glossa Ordinaria,* the origins of which are still shrouded in mystery, is a collective book of biblical commentary that circulated among writers and grew for centuries. During that period of western European history, the doubling time for world knowledge was more than 400 years, and hand-written books were slow to develop and be distributed. Consequently, the global dissemination of information was exceedingly slow and generally only available to scholars. In contrast, the current doubling time of world knowledge is estimated to be a mere 18 months, and the Internet transmission time is measured in seconds.

We are living in a time of profound change and interconnection. The Internet's World Wide Web is a brilliant example, and, if current trends persist, we most surely will witness its evolution into something monumental with arresting combinations of text, sound, and video. The Internet clearly looms as the dominant forum for rapid global communication and dissemination of information. Already, some health professionals commonly access and use a variety of medical knowledge bases, continuing education services, electronic journals, health forums, referral services, and practice guidelines. The importance of having the skills to readily use these resources becomes increasingly evident and was the impetus for this guide.

This book was originally intended for those within the health and health-related professions, but it may also serve anyone with a particular interest in health care. It certainly will serve as an indispensable guide for beginners and experienced Internet users. It is not intended to be an exhaustive instructional guide but, rather, it is designed to shepherd you through the boggy aspects of getting connected directly to valuable health information resources.

It offers an introduction to the basic equipment, software, and services necessary to get connected. The sites reviewed were assessed based on content and quality. Only those that met the standards of our review criteria are featured in the book. The enclosed diskette contains bookmarks for more than 1,600 health information resources!

If we should accomplish our objective with this book, that is, reducing the barriers of entry into the information resources on the Internet, and consequently enlist the participation of more health care professionals, we will create a ripple of influence in health care that may likely be felt at the change of the next millennium.

Scott R. Gibbs, M.D., M.A.

ACKNOWLEDGMENTS

EDITORS' ACKNOWLEDGMENTS

Much time, thought, energy and patience went into producing this book as well as some less conspicuous but essential contributions. To my partner in life, Barbara and our children, Carol, Alex, and Eric, who bring us great joy, I thank you for your unflagging love and understanding. To Nigel and Micaela, I applaud your knowledge and endurance and I pay you my highest compliment——I have learned from you. I'm especially grateful to Dr. John Oró for introducing me to the bounty of the WWW and to Kelly Poirier, who truly deserves the highest plaudits for her quiet-confidence development style and her ability to artfully catalyze all that is necessary to successfully complete a project of this enormity.

Scott R. Gibbs, M.D., M.A.

I'd like to thank my husband, Peter, without whom this "write a book about the Internet in 12 weeks" project would not have gone so smoothly and my children, Alex and Drake, who unendingly allowed Mom "to work on the computer." Thank you also to my knowledgeable co-editors Nigel and Scott, and Mosby's Li Wen Huang and Ken Killion for their initial enthusiasm. Special kudos to our Developmental Editor, Kelly Poirier, for her unerring attention to detail, and singular devotion to keeping her editors and reviewers on track.

Micaela Sullivan-Fowler, M.S., M.A.

My participation in this book would not have been possible without the support and help of my partner, Karen, who had to put up with me being preoccupied for 5 long months.

Nigel W. Rowe

PUBLISHER'S ACKNOWLEDGMENTS

Special thanks to our reviewers and scanners who generously gave their time to help make this publication possible: Blake Alexander, M.D. (diabetes, general medicine, nutrition); Michael Anderson (scanner); Stephen Aronoff, M.D. (infectious diseases); Karen Babich (CompuServe); William Bales (toxicology); Alfred Berg, M.D. (family practice); Chuck Biddle, C.R.N.A. (nursing); Marion Broome, R.N. (nursing, pain and pain management); Kevin Clyne (America Online); Katie DiPrima (medical law and ethics); Maria Evans, M.D. (pathology); Randall Floyd, M.D. (obstetrics and gynecology); Joel Goldwein, M.D. (oncology); Martha Guerrero (scanner); Suchi Gururaj (osteopathy, scanner); Xavier Harel (scanner); Steven Hata, M.D. (pulmonary, anesthesiology); Timothy Herr, M.D. (otolaryngology); Andrew James, R.N. (nursing); Ramesh Khanna, M.D. (nephrology); Edward Kim, M.D. (urology); Paul King, M.D. (gastroenterology); Dana Lawrence, D.C. (chiropractic); Jhemon Lee, M.D. (radiology, scanner); Sharon Lee, R.N. (midwifery); Lorna Lippes (scanner); Larry Lipshultz, M.D. (urology); Judith Miles, M.D. (genetics); Jonathan Panush (rheumatology, scanner); Richard Panush, M.D. (rheumatology, scanner); Faith Reidenbach (Alzheimer's disease, allied health); Jean Sax, R.N. (midwifery); Joseph Scherger, M.D. (medical education, continuing medical education, business and politics); John Schowalter, M.D. (psychiatry and mental health); Tom Selva, M.D. (pediatrics); Dina Shriver, R.N. (scanner); Donna Steinhagen (orthopedics, plastic surgery); Shanker Sundrani, M.D. (neurology); Richard Teff, M.D. (neurology, allergy, and immunology, physician assistants, drugs, diagnostics, and devices, societies and agencies); Kevin Toller, M.D. (ophthalmology); Eileen Trigoboff, R.N. (nursing); Sarah Vogel, M.D. (emergency medical services, emergency medicine); Sharon Watling, Pharm.D. (pharmacy); Peter Whitehouse, M.D. (Alzheimer's disease); Lionel Young, M.D. (radiology); Karen Zanol, M.D. (dermatology); John Zimmerman, D.D.S. (dentistry).

We also thank those individuals who reviewed our manuscript and provided invaluable guidance: Pete Abrahams, Michael Bentley, E. Diane Johnson, Christina Khojasteh, and Bruce Polsky.

Finally, we thank John Oró, M.D., founder, editor, and webmaster of NeuroSource, for providing the Appendix, "Building a Web Site."

CONTENTS

Foreword   *vii*
Introduction   *ix*
Acknowledgments   *xi*

PART 1: GETTING CONNECTED

1 / Equipment, *by Nigel W. Rowe*   **3**

Selecting the Right Computer   3
Operating Systems   6
Other Operating Systems   7
MAC vs. PC   8
What Else Do I Need?   10
Considerations When Buying a Computer   11

2 / Communications, *by Nigel W. Rowe*   **13**

Connecting to the Internet   13
Selecting a Modem   18
How Does It Actually Work   22

3 / Getting Started on the Infobahn:
Internet Basics, *by Nigel W. Rowe*   **25**

E-mail   26
World Wide Web (WWW)   36
USENET   45
TELNET   51
Internet Mailing Lists   52
File Transfer Protocol   55
Gopher   55
Veronica and Jughead   56
Archie   57
WAIS   57
Internet Relay Chat (IRC)   58

4 / Choosing an On-line Service, *by Nigel W. Rowe* **59**

Internet Service Providers and On-line Services   59
Other On-line Services   66
Conclusion   67

5 / Optimizing Internet Software, *by Nigel W. Rowe* **69**

WWW Browsers   70
USENET Newsgroups   78
Setting Up Multiple Winsock Connections   80
Dealing With Compressed Files   83
Transferring Files Between a PC and a Mac   84

6 / Searching: "I Know It's Got to Be Here Somewhere,"
        by Micaela Sullivan-Fowler, M.S., M.A. **85**

A Little Introduction   85
Using the Search Engines   86
Search Strategies   87
Construction of a Search   87
Know Your Search Engine!   88
The Search   91
Two Problems   91
Eleven Search Engines   95
Once the Result Is Available   98
Getting Sophisticated   99
The Dream Search Machine   100

7 / Rules of the Road, *by Nigel W. Rowe* **101**

Netiquette, Security, and Viruses   101
Security on the Internet   103
Viruses   108

PART 2: INTERNET MEDICAL RESOURCES

8 / Medical Networks:
    Where Only Librarians Dared to Tread
        by Micaela Sullivan-Fowler, M.S., M.A. **111**

The Networks   112
Conclusion   125

9 / General Health Care Resources   127

Allied Health and Nursing   127
Alternative and Complementary Therapies   141
     (Introduction *by Micaela Sullivan-Fowler, M.S., M.A.)*
Business and Politics of Health Care   152
Diagnostics, Drugs, and Devices   154
Diseases, Disorders, and Disabilities   156
Diverse Health Disciplines   218
Health-related Information   231
Medical Law and Ethics   247
Medical Education   249
Professional Associations and Societies   252
Governmental and International Societies and Agencies   259

10 / Other Health Care Resources   263

CompuServe   263
America Online (AOL)   273

Appendixes   279

Building a Website, *by John Oró, M.D.*   281
Internet Providers and Obtaining Internet Software   289
Fun Internet Resources   295
Health Care Newsgroups   301
Further Reading   305

Index   307

Part 1

Getting Connected

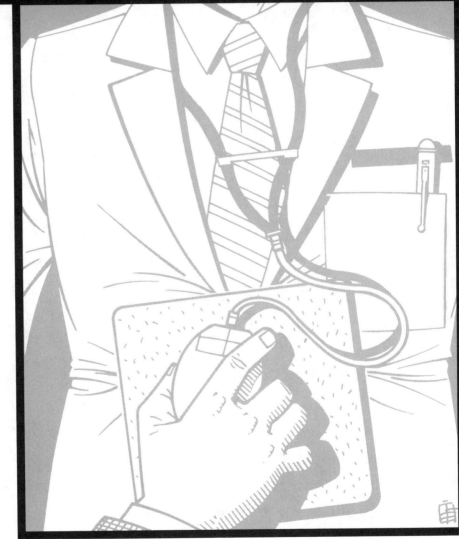

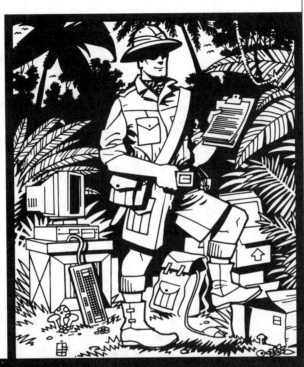

Chapter 1

Equipment

SELECTING THE RIGHT COMPUTER

If the Internet has achieved only one thing, surely this is to bridge the gulf between disparate computer hardware and different operating systems. More recently, the Web browser (first Mosaic and lately its more formidable successor, Netscape Navigator) has appeared as the Rosetta stone of computer communication. Seemingly overnight, huge electronic libraries have sprung up around the globe covering every conceivable area of knowledge, both practical and esoteric. Whereas only a few short years ago one would have had few choices as to which computer hardware and software could be used to access this material, this is no longer the case.

From its first appearance in 1993, the Web browser has provided a simple interface that functions the same way whether it is run on a high-powered UNIX workstation, a Macintosh, or an IBM-compatible PC. With plug-in software accessories being developed as a standard feature of the Web browser package, it has never been easier to access material written for widely varying software programs and computer platforms. The most amazing thing is that this is all available with just a few clicks of the mouse, a modem, and a phone line, no matter where in the world the original document is located.

Glossary Terms A–B

Access speed
The speed at which an Internet connection is maintained.

3

Unfortunately, as with all simple scenarios, a fair amount of behind-the-scenes work must be done to ensure all goes smoothly.

Computer equipment must be purchased, set up, and tested. Communications software needs to be installed, and last, but not least, everything needs to be connected to the outside world via the phone line or direct dedicated connection. Each one of these steps can be a painless exercise requiring little extra effort other than unpacking a box and connecting a few wires, or it can be fraught with frantic nail-biting sessions lasting hours, if not days. As with everything, a little advance planning and patience go a long way toward alleviating anxiety later on.

It is not the purpose of this chapter to tell how to install a computer system. Hopefully, you would have received several instruction manuals detailing these procedures. If you didn't get any manuals and are presently reading this book while staring at a heap of cables, assorted pieces of equipment, and various unlabeled floppy disks, then I would recommend sorting out this problem first, before we start telling you how easy it all is.

And it is easy. Perhaps the hardest part about getting onto the "Information Super Highway" is in first buying the computer, or at least getting your job redefined so someone else is paying for that sleek, fast, powerful beast on your desk.

During the '80s, many widely incompatible computer systems came and went. During the '90s personal computers are essentially of two kinds, IBM compatibles (or PCs) and Apple Macintoshes (Macs). Computers used in business are a different story altogether; there are mainframes (which surprisingly are as much in demand today as 30 years ago), minicomputers, powerful workstations, and PCs and Macs. Actually, when you get down to it, there are more differences at the operating system level than there are between different computer hardware setups.

For the purposes of this discussion we'll stick to PCs and Macs, although the basics can be applied toward most other computer setups. At the time this book was written (mid 1996), a system consisting of the following basic configurations could be purchased for between $1,500 and $2,500 (recommended options).

An entry-level personal computer should be one of the following:

PC (IBM compatible)
- 486 DX4 75 MHz processor or better (Pentium recommended)
- SVGA 15" color monitor
- 8 megabytes (MB) of random access memory (RAM) (16 MB is recommended)
- Windows 3.1 or Windows 95 operating system
- 14.4 baud modem (28.8 baud recommended)
- 2 button mouse
- 540 MB hard drive (1.2 gigabytes (GBs) recommended)

Note: Windows 95 requires a 486 or better, equipped with at least 8 MB of RAM.

Address
This can be one of two things: "an electronic mail address" and "an Internet address." An electronic mail address identifies a particular person at a specific Internet location. An Internet address is a unique code that identifies a specific computer in a system or network.

To make use of multimedia software and to experience the World Wide Web at its best, your PC should be equipped with these additional items:

- Soundblaster compatible soundcard with external speakers
- High resolution SVGA monitor (1024 x 768 at 256 colors)
- Quad speed compact disk-read only memory (CD-ROM) drive

Mac

- 75 MHz PowerPC 601 RISC Processor (or better)
- 8 MB of RAM (16 MB recommended)
- 15" color monitor (either Apple Multiple Scan or equivalent PC monitor)
- 700 MB hard drive
- Mouse
- 16-bit stereo sound
- System 7 operating system (System 7.5 recommended)
- 14.4 baud modem (28.8 baud recommended)

Note: Most Mac Internet applications require a version of System 6 (often 6.07 or better); many expect System 7.

The addition of a high resolution SVGA monitor (1024 x 768 at 256 colors), CD-ROM, and external speakers is recommended.

Most computer stores sell a basic package of multimedia items (sound card, speakers, microphone, software, and other extras) for about $250. These are perfect for upgrading an existing system.

Laptops Versus Desktop Computers

This is really a matter of deciding where the computer will principally be used. If you travel and require constant access to important files or need to be able to access on-line services or e-mail while on the road, then a laptop, or notebook computer, as the even smaller models are called, is the best choice. However, if all your work is done in one place, then a desk-bound computer may be more appropriate. The golden rule is, the smaller the computer the more expensive it will be. Laptop and notebook computers typically are as powerful as full-sized systems and contain a hard drive, a floppy drive, a modem, some form of mouse or other pointing device, and sometimes a CD-ROM. But be warned—all this miniaturization is expensive.

It is an easy matter to convert a laptop computer into a full-sized system simply by plugging in an external keyboard, an external color display monitor, and a mouse. All of which can be purchased for less than $500. Similarly, some computers are packaged as *dockable* meaning that the laptop slides into a base station, which is connected to all the other full-sized components. When you are at your desk, you have a "real" computer; when you travel, you just take the laptop.

Archie
A program used to locate files at FTP sites.

Article
The original journal piece to which a citation refers. The article itself is generally not retrieved, unless a system offers full text or document delivery.

OPERATING SYSTEMS

At the heart of every computer, big or small, is an operating system. Essentially this is a collection of computer programs that control all aspects of the computer operation, from starting the computer, to writing and reading files, sending documents to a printer, displaying text and graphics on the screen, and everything else that is not so noticeable underneath the hood.

ASCII
American Standard Code for Information Interchange. A standard code for representing characters and symbols as numbers.

Windows and DOS are the operating systems found on most PCs, whereas System 6, or System 7 or 7.5 are present on Macs, often referred to as the Mac OS. For much of its life, the Mac had a head start over the PC in ease of use. This advantage was provided by its operating system, which is intuitive, flexible, and user friendly. Unfortunately, the PC has been hampered with a succession of varying operating systems, beginning with DOS, then Windows, and now, Windows 95. Each PC operating system has become better with time, but only with the advent of Windows 95 can it be said that the PC is finally user friendly. This change is winning favor with a large number of Mac users, who are slowly being won over to the Windows world.

At a bare minimum, a PC needs to be running Windows 3.1 for you to partake of any of the graphic delights of the Internet. A computer equipped with DOS alone is certainly not at a disadvantage when it comes to going on-line; until recently all on-line materials were purely text, but an increasing amount of Internet and on-line resources can only be accessed from a GUI (pronounced "gooey" for graphical user interface) like Windows.

Windows 95 speeds things up considerably and also introduces multitasking to the Windows environment; this allows several programs to be running simultaneously without getting in each other's way. Windows 3.1 allows for multitasking, albeit at a slower pace and at a greater risk of something going wrong.

On board the Mac, System 7.5 is the major operating system, and whereas earlier versions will suffice for a number of on-line activities, System 7.5 has a number of communications programs built-in that previously had to be acquired and configured separately.

The biggest difference between PCs and Macs is that Macs have always had a graphic operating system, whereas the plain, unadorned DOS command line was about as sophisticated as things got on PCs until the late eighties. Things have changed however, and the PC and Windows reign as the computer system of choice. Apple is fighting back, however, with a new operating system ("ahh, let's see, that would be System 8?") due in early 1997 and promising more functionality than either operating system offers at present.

With the advent of the PowerPC chip installed in all new Macs since early 1996, DOS and Windows software can now be run reliably with the help of emulation software. This software emulates the hardware of the PC system, fooling the PC programs into thinking they are operating on a real PC. SoftWindows is the most popular of these versatile packages (version 3 is now 100% compatible with Windows 95 software).

Emulation software is also available for Macs not equipped with the PowerPC chip, but generally they don't provide satisfactory performance, especially with Windows programs.

Emulation software does not exist to run modern Mac programs on the PC, but this is a reflection of the much wider range of PC software than Mac software. With the notable exception of desktop publishing, the Mac has generally had fewer software packages available for users to choose from.

OTHER OPERATING SYSTEMS

Besides DOS/Windows and the Mac OS, there are a number of other operating systems available. IBM itself offers OS/2, which, in its present incarnation of OS/2 Warp 4, is often cited as better and easier to use than Windows 95. However true this may be, OS/2 is at its best only when working with software purposely configured to take advantage of its many features. So although most DOS and Windows applications will run fine under OS/2, separate OS/2 versions need to be purchased to really see a difference.

The reverse is not true; OS/2 programs will not run under Windows. However, OS/2 Warp 4 and Windows can be used side-by-side on the same PC, with the ability to swap between the two environments. OS/2 is best suited for an intermediate to an advanced computer user who wants to make full use of the powerful OS/2 abilities for their own sake, rather than using it as just an operating system.

Various versions of UNIX can be run on PCs. Probably the most common variant is Linux, which has the added advantage of being available free. UNIX however, like DOS, is primarily a command line operating system. Unlike DOS, it is also a powerful multi-user, multitasking operating system. UNIX is best suited to multiuser networked environments, most commonly found in university settings. When UNIX is used in conjunction with another suite of programs called X-Windows, it becomes a GUI that is similar to Windows and the Mac OS. However, running UNIX on a PC is not for the faint of heart and cannot be recommended unless you *know* what you are doing.

Windows for Workgroups and Windows NT are the high-end business environment versions of Windows, typically loaded on computers running as part of larger connected networks. Windows for Workgroups is still principally a 16-bit operating system (like Windows 3.1), although it can be configured to take advantage of 32-bit file access for increased speed and reliability.

Windows NT Workstation is Microsoft's top-of-the line 32-bit operating system. Version 4.0, released in late 1996, brings NT up to date with many of the improvements first introduced to the PC environment with Windows 95. NT is Windows exemplified. It is an industrial strength operating system with high performance multitasking and the ability to run on a multitude of high-end computer processors, including the PowerPC.

Backup
The process of making a copy of important programs and files, which can be used to restore lost or damaged programs and files. The backups should be stored in a secure place, preferably away from the originals.

Windows NT will not run all Windows and DOS programs, but this stems from the way it has been built to provide a secure operating environment. Most computer crashes derive from "buggy" software, and Windows NT will not run the types of software with recognized problems.

Unlike Windows 95, which was designed to be compatible with software created for earlier versions of Windows and DOS, NT was designed to work only with software written to exacting standards. It is because of this reliability that NT is becoming more common in the business environment and is seen by many as a possible replacement for Unix.

Bandwidth
This describes the transmission capacity of a communications channel, like a telephone line. High bandwidth means more data can be sent and at a faster rate than low bandwidth.

MAC vs. PC

One could be forgiven for thinking, given the foregoing discussion, that a person buying a Mac was getting a better deal than a person choosing a PC. After all, the Mac remains more user friendly, is easier to get running right out of the box, and can also run DOS and Windows in addition to its own software. So why is there such disparity in PCs being king of the heap and Macs languishing near the bottom with less than 10% of computer market share?

There are many answers to this question. Principally, it comes down to how the two systems have been marketed. From the very beginning, IBM, after developing the PC, allowed other computer manufacturers to licence the technology and build their own versions, hence the term *IBM compatible*. More computer makers equaled competitive pressures, which in turn drove prices down, and made PCs much cheaper than Macs.

Apple on the other hand, wanted to control both the manufacture and selling of what it had positioned as a high-end product and refused (until the early nineties) to licence this technology to other companies. This policy ensured that all Macs and their associated peripherals (e.g., disk drives, display monitors, and printers) were principally manufactured (or repackaged) by Apple and priced substantially higher than their PC counterparts. PCs became a standard simply because they were cheaper to buy, and there was a greater degree of freedom when it came time to add other peripherals and in selecting software.

With Apple's about-face around 1994, the price of most Macs fell, substantially more models were produced, and Mac users were finally able to exercise freedom in putting together a computer system made up of components from various manufacturers.

Now, the only real difference between PCs and Macs is one of perception. Macs are seen as the systems of choice for anyone serious about graphic design and publishing, whereas PCs are firmly rooted in the business and home environments. Both systems serve equally well for exploring the Internet and the on-line community (Tables 1–1 and 1–2).

TABLE 1–1.—KEY FEATURES OF PC OPERATING SYSTEMS

Feature	DOS 5 * (1991)	Windows 3.1 (1993)	Windows 95 (1995)
DOS programs	X	X	X
Graphics	X	X	X
CD-ROM capability	X	X	X
Built-in Internet connectivity		Available separately	X
32-bit OS		Only with additional OS extensions	X
Plug and play			X
Trash can for deleted files			X
Program shortcuts			X
Multitasking			X
Desktop objects			X
Quick-start menu			X
Menu selection of recent documents			X

*And later versions (e.g., DOS 6 and 7).

TABLE 1–2.—KEY FEATURES OF MAC OPERATING SYSTEMS

Feature	System 6 (1989)	System 7 (1991)	System 7.5 (1995)	PowerPC (1995)
Run multiple programs	X (with Multifinder)	X	X	X
Automatic read/write PC disks		X	X	X
Customizable Apple menu		X	X	X
True Type fonts		X	X	X
Aliases		X	X	
Help menu		X	X	X
32 bit OS		X	X	X
Built-in Internet connectivity			X	X
Menu selection of recent documents			X	
Quick launcher			X	X
QuickDraw GX			X	X
Apple help guide			X	X
MacLink Plus file converters		available separately	X	X
DOS/Windows programs		With a DOS card	DOS, with emulation software or a DOS card	DOS/Windows with emulation software

BAUD
Also known as bits per second (BPS). A measure of how fast information is transmitted. A 9600 baud modem is a modem that transmits at 9,600 bits per second. Divide the baud rate by 10 to see roughly how many characters of information are being sent.

Software Differences Between Macs and PCs

As more software packages have been converted to the other respective platform, compatibility between files on a Mac or PC has been largely resolved. A WordPerfect file created on a PC can be opened on a Mac equipped with the Mac version of WordPerfect. And the reverse is true. Opening the same WordPerfect file within another software program on the Mac, say Microsoft Word, will also work. This rule holds true for most standard software packages, including database, spreadsheet, and graphic file types.

Conversion problems could still arise with less common programs, especially shareware, or documents that use style sheets or other types of specialized formatting. Customized programs developed for medical practices or laboratories will only run on the computer system they were originally designed for.

Files can also be converted for use on the Mac by using one of the many PC to Mac conversion programs. A typical package offers more than 100 different file type conversions, and the conversion process runs automatically as these programs are accessed. Unfortunately, the reverse is not true; most Mac files do not convert easily to run on the PC. Chapter 5, "Optimizing Internet Software," has more information about overcoming specific problems with sharing files between different computers.

WHAT ELSE DO I NEED?

Give some thought to purchasing a backup device. These can be external or internal tape drives, recordable CD-ROMs, Zip or Syquest drives, or an additional plug-in hard drive. A good backup device can offset a hard drive that has become quickly filled with application software and downloaded files. This is almost a necessity, given the large size of most multimedia and Internet files. Backing up essential files then becomes an easy and convenient option, usually on just a couple of disks or tape cartridges, which can then be stored elsewhere.

Iomega Zip drives, with a disk capacity of 100 MB, have become very popular, and the Iomega disk standard has been embraced by many leading manufacturers. The disks themselves are not much bigger than a standard high-density floppy (1.4 MB) and are inexpensive, especially when compared with other backup media. The Zip drive itself is small and portable and lends itself perfectly to being used for several computers at different locations. The slower Parallel version of the Zip drive can backup files at around 5 MB a minute, with higher speeds available using the faster SCSI version. The main difference between the Parallel and SCSI versions, besides speed, is that additional hardware is required for the SCSI drive. The Zip drive can also be used as an alternate hard-disk drive.

Syquest cartridges are common in desktop publishing and the graphic arts industry, especially when supplying files to service bureaus. Tape drives have the advantage of holding gigabytes of information on a small tape cartridge; but the rate of transfer is much slower than that of other backup options.

BBS
Bulletin Board Service. A dial-up computer system in which users can post messages and download computer programs. A BBS can be operated from any standard PC or Macintosh computer using just a modem and an ordinary phone line. Unfortunately, BBSs are being supplanted by on line services and the Internet.

Of course, there are a lot of other accessories that make life easier, including CD-ROM drives, laser printers, cordless mice, and scanners. But these are all a matter of individual preference rather than "must haves."

CONSIDERATIONS WHEN BUYING A COMPUTER

Selecting and buying the most appropriate computer is an important decision and should not be rushed. What is hot today, is not going to be hot in a year or even 6 months from now. The all-important rule is to look a year ahead, the time when most warranties expire, and examine closely how difficult it will be to get repairs.

This selection process should involve all or most of the following points:
- After sales support and service
- Research all similar products
- Ask about key features
- Bundled software and hardware
- Purchase with a credit card
- Arrange insurance coverage

After Sales Support
Most major brand-name computers (e.g., IBM, Apple, Compaq, Hewlett Packard, and Dell) are supported by a large infrastructure of licensed service providers. So even if your particular model is not being sold or supported directly by the manufacturer, it should not be too difficult to find someone who does support it. This level of *official* support is important, not just because it means certain guarantees about quality, original parts, and reliable prices, but also because other minor computer brands (mostly no-name PCs) offer little or no guarantee of after sales support.

Within a certain time frame, you can usually get the problem fixed through the place of purchase; but after this period, it usually falls on the buyer to find someone who is able to fix the problem. And it is here that another important rule comes into play. If a computer fails within a year or so, then the problem is usually major, i.e., expensive to fix. Typically, major problems occur within the first few months, and minor glitches only become noticeable over longer periods. Generally, once computers get through the initial breaking-in period, they are reliable. Of course, there are exceptions to every rule, but who wants to have the computer that proves the exception?

Buying from mail-order merchants is no better or worse than walking into a major computer or home electronics showroom and often offers the opportunity to make additional savings, especially if the merchant is located out of state and does not charge sales tax. So shop around and ask questions. Don't be intimidated into buying something that you don't need. More often than not, salespersons know no more about computers or particular models than you do, despite their fluent command of the jargon and apparent ease with displaying features.

Boolean operators/Boolean logic
The terms *AND, OR, NOT* (and with some systems *ADJ, WITHIN,* etc.) that are placed between terms to create a specific search strategy. Either the user enters the Boolean operators or it is assumed within the search engine.

BPS:
Bits Per Second. See BAUD.

Research All Similar Products

Get familiar with their key features and the other items that come bundled with the machine. Selling computers is a very competitive business, and many sellers are prepared to sell a customized system for the same price as an off-the-shelf standard system. Be wary of too-good-to-be-true special offers. The small print usually says that the price does not include a monitor or keyboard, which could add another $300 to $400 to the "special" price.

Purchase with a Credit Card

Even if you prefer to pay cash up front, using a credit card extends several free or inexpensive benefits such as insurance against loss or damage for the first 90 days, extended warranties, air miles, guarantees against cheaper prices, and often, support against a seller who refuses to correct defects.

Bug
An error in a software program that causes it to stop working or behave in an unexpected fashion. New software programs are "beta-tested" before general release so any bugs can be discovered and corrected.

⚡ **POWER TIP**

Don't forget to increase your home or renter's insurance coverage to include your new purchase. Typically an inexpensive additional rider to a standard policy is required for items in excess of $1,000.

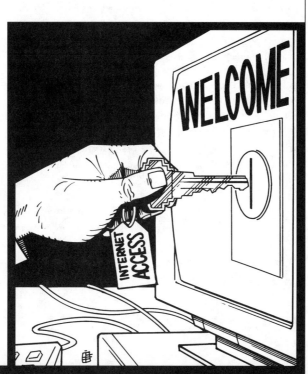

Chapter 2

Communications

CONNECTING TO THE INTERNET

Okay, by now the computer is sitting on your desk and staring back with a high degree of purposefulness. The next step is to actually hook it up to the outside world. Without sounding too alarmist, this is probably the one part of the entire on-line experience that causes the most headaches. But, if it is approached with a clear idea of what to expect, the whole experience will be relatively straightforward.

This is where a degree of familiarity with computer jargon comes in handy. Most of the jargon consists of acronyms and abbreviations, many of which are not self-explanatory and require an amount of patience to understand what they mean. Unfortunately, there is no way to avoid this, so be prepared to flick through the glossary from time to time.

Connecting to the Internet requires two things: (1) either a modem attached to your computer or a direct connection via ISDN (Integrated Services Digital Network) or a computer network and (2) a relationship with an Internet Services Provider (ISP). If you are already connected via a computer network, then you would not normally need the services of an ISP, unless you require more specialized access.

Glossary Terms C–D

CGI
Common Gateway Interface. A software script that runs behind the scenes on Web servers, translating user requests into a format that other programs, typically databases, can understand.

ISPs consist of three types: (1) on-line services, such as CompuServe or America Online (AOL), which offer additional services other than just an Internet connection, (2) telephone companies, such as MCI, AT&T, and Sprint, and (3) national and regional providers, which are "true" ISPs providing only an Internet connection.

Each type of provider offers widely varying services. For the most part, telephone companies are new to the business of offering data connections to the public at large and are still behind everyone else in terms of customer service and software support. A common complaint of national and regional ISPs is that they are more suited to those computer users who are already technically proficient and know exactly what they want. Indirect and direct connections to the Internet are shown in Figure 2-1.

Chat
A term used to describe interactive conversation through the means of sequential typed messages. Many on-line services feature chat areas where groups of people can gather and talk about specific topics.

Connecting to the Internet

INDIRECT   Computer and Modem

Online Service   Internet Service
                                                  Provider

                          Internet

DIRECT   Computer and LAN
                            Internet Gateway

Online Service   Internet Service
                                                  Provider

                          Internet

FIGURE 2-1.—*Connecting to the Internet.*

For much of this chapter, we assume that you are accessing the Internet using the indirect methods of some form of ISP or on-line service.

Although the Internet has been in existence for almost 3 decades, the level of access to it has been limited historically to those who could demonstrate a reasonable case for their connection. Until the early 1980s, this meant that you were either a part of the U.S. Department of Defense or an affiliated scientist. It was only later that people in the academic and wider scientific communities gained access, followed by people in other government agencies and big business. But, you still had to be either a student or an employee at one of these places to take advantage of their connections.

With the advent of cheaper modems and powerful desktop computers in the late 1980s, more people gained limited Internet access through companies offering on-line services, such as CompuServe, AOL, and Delphi. Eventually, this groundswell of interest turned into a flood, and, to remain competitive, the on-line companies offered complete Internet access to their subscribers.

The explosive growth of the World Wide Web since 1993 has ensured that the Internet can no longer be accessible only to those in privileged positions. It is pretty incredible that as few as three years ago, the only part of the Internet that was accessible to the average computer user was that of sending and receiving e-mail.

So far, the general means of access have been discussed, but a more in-depth look at what actually happens makes the process easier to understand and definitely easier to troubleshoot.

Using an On-line Service

CompuServe and AOL are the two best-known and long-established on-line companies providing access within the United States and internationally. Several other providers are discussed in Chapter 4, but this discussion concentrates on the two "Big Boys."

In the United States, AOL has attached a free disk to major magazines, and these have become so ubiquitous that you may feel a sense of disappointment if you buy a magazine and it does not contain a free disk. The point being that AOL has gone out of its way to make it easy to connect your computer to its system. "Just install our software and press connect!"

Undoubtedly, AOL has done much to simplify the process of getting connected, and, after a few years, even CompuServe uses this advertising method to put its software in the hands of prospective new users. If you have a computer and a modem, then one of their free disks is all it takes to connect.

Once the software is installed on your computer, you just make the initial call to establish your local access number. With AOL, a toll-free number is automatically dialed by the software and then you search for access numbers in your area code. With CompuServe, you physically dial a CompuServe toll-free number and follow the voice prompts to choose your local access number. You then set up a default login using this number.

When initiating a CompuServe or AOL connection using a modem, you open what is called a "modem port" on the respective computer network. This port is then kept "alive" for the duration of the connection and all subsequent transactions pass through this point. CompuServe and AOL maintain networks of thousands of these access ports around the world (AOL has 100,000, primarily in the United States, and CompuServe has 60,000 worldwide), although these numbers are steadily increasing. These ports are set to various access speeds. Currently, CompuServe and AOL provide connections of up to 28.8K, and only CompuServe additionally supports faster ISDN connections.

Citation
A bibliographic record of an article. It can include author, title, institutional affiliation, volume and pages, published abstract, MeSH terms that were used in the indexing, and a number of other NLM identifying terms. Networks sometimes allow for customization of the citation.

Once your computer is connected to these services, you have full access to the content they offer and to their Internet services.

If you have a direct connection courtesy of your LAN, you can use this to access CompuServe and AOL directly, bypassing the busy modem ports and gaining a much faster connection. AOL can be accessed as fast as your Internet connection can handle, whereas CompuServe is limited to a speed of approximately 28.8K, although this will be changing soon.

Note: You still need to be a subscriber to these services to access them using this method.

National and Regional Internet Service Providers

There is an important distinction to be made here. Commercial on-line services such as CompuServe and AOL offer an extensive array of services that cannot be found anywhere else on the Internet. These range from searchable databases of business and financial information, including archives of newspapers and magazines, to comprehensive customer service forums for all the major computer hardware and software manufacturers. They also enable participation in thousands of specialized interest groups that have not only a common messaging area but also libraries of related files and conference rooms.

On the other hand, an ordinary ISP, generally for about two thirds of the price, provides only the necessary software and a modicum of support to get you up and running with Internet access. This access comes in two forms: permanent and dial-up.

Typically, a permanent connection is a T1 or T3 telephone line leased from your telephone company and linking it to your LAN. (A T1 telephone line is used for high-speed access. A T3 line provides even faster access.) This type of connection is permanent in that it is connected to the Internet all the time, providing immediate access for you and to your LAN or World Wide Web site. A permanent connection is usually only needed when you run your own Web site, or you have a large number of users needing access to the Internet.

Dial-up connections are made only on demand, usually when you want to send or read e-mail, or embark on other Internet activities. You only pay for the time connected, and typically you receive so many hours a month or unlimited access. Permanent connections are usually prohibitively expensive, whereas dial-up access costs are reasonably priced. Usually, there is a variety of pricing plans that balance dial-up speed, number of paid hours, and site location.

All ISPs provide you with a unique e-mail address and disk space to manage your e-mail mailbox. Otherwise, you are pretty much left to your own devices. To a newcomer, this can seem bewildering. Many people use the commercial on-line services as a training ground, and then switch to an ISP when they feel more comfortable. Appendix 3 lists the major national and international ISPs, along with sample costs and contact information.

Compression
The means by which large files are converted into smaller files, or multiple files are compressed and combined into a single file. File compression can reduce the time if takes to download and transmit files via modem.

Once you have set up an account with an ISP, you will be provided with either a local access number or, depending on where you live, a long distance number to use. Unless you live in a remote part of the country, you should choose an ISP that can provide you with a local access number. This local access number is usually referred to as a POP, or Point Of Presence. An ISP based in San Francisco, for example, could have POPs around the country.

The following checklist summarizes the most important questions to ask when inquiring about ISP connections:

Connection
An active link between two computers. *Direct:* A live-wired connection to the Internet 24 hours a day. *Dial-up:* A modem is used to connect to the Internet as required.

- Can you provide SLIP (Serial Line Internet Protocol) or PPP (Point to Point Protocol) access?
- Do you provide technical support?
- Do you provide SLIP/PPP software for Windows 3.1 or Mac users?
- How many hours of connect time are included in the monthly fee?
- How much do additional hours cost?
- Do you have a POP near me?
- What other services (e.g., Web sites, e-mail forwarding) do you provide?

Also, you should investigate only those companies that have well-established reputations and have been in existence for longer than a few years. Setting up as an ISP has become a popular business in the 1990s and many companies have already foundered amidst all the unregulated competition. If you choose an ISP that later goes out of business, you will not only have to change your e-mail address in a hurry but also, more often than not, all your present e-mail will bounce back to the sender or, worse, just disappear.

As with on-line services, when you make a dial-up connection using an ISP, until you disconnect, you accrue connect time at whatever rate is applicable. Many ISPs have unlimited use plans, which means that, theoretically, you could stay connected 24 hours a day at no extra cost. Although your telephone company and your ISP would probably notice after a while and request a change in habits.

⚡ **POWER TIP**
Unlimited access may sound like a great deal, but the reality is that these types of plans attract far too many users, with the result that, at peak times, it may be impossible to connect to your ISP. This is as much a problem with smaller ISPs as it is with the biggest national providers. Several ISPs offer free trial periods and you can use this time to evaluate access and service.

Direct Access Through a Network Connection

If your computer is being used in a business or academic environment, then it is likely that you are a part of a LAN, which could already be connected to the Internet. The easiest way to determine whether this is the case is to contact the person in charge of your network or, failing that, to contact your Management Information Systems (MIS) or computer services department.

Connecting through a LAN provides a faster connection than using a modem, but often this cannot be used to also access on-line providers such as CompuServe or AOL. Usually, this means your company or institution has decided to limit the degree of contact with the Internet and uses a firewall to restrict access. For the most part, firewalls provide a means of securing computer networks from unauthorized outside access, but they can also be used to prevent employees inside the company from inadvertently providing other means of gaining access.

If your network administrator cannot be persuaded to allow Internet access, then a modem can be connected to your computer and plugged into an outside telephone line.

If you have a standard telephone system, then you simply plug the telephone cable into your modem and make a connection using the software provided by your on-line provider.

Note: Some modern digital telephone systems do not allow a modem to be plugged directly into the telephone system. If so, you will need to arrange an additional dedicated line that is not routed through the main telephone Private Branch Exchange (PBX).

Other than the speed of access, which can be impressive compared with the fastest modems, the biggest advantage to a direct Internet connection is that actual connect time is minimal. Your software only makes a connection when it is necessary to send or receive information, unlike other methods whereby you need to remain connected for long periods of time. It is also possible to initiate several Internet sessions at the same time. You can download a large file from one place and send e-mail somewhere else, without running out of transmission bandwidth. Modems allow only one thing to be done at a time.

SELECTING A MODEM

There is a vast selection of modems available. Features include being internal or external models, being slow or fast, or having compression or no compression capabilities. Seemingly, there is an endless variety to choose from. The key item to focus on is speed. This speed is measured in bits per second (bps) or kilobytes per second (Kbps). The larger the number, the more bits of data a modem can transmit. Baud is a term commonly used in place of bps, so a 9600 baud analogue modem is a modem that transmits at 9,600 bits per second. Faster modem speeds (e.g., 14,400 bps) are

Controlled language
Terms or words that collectively create a vocabulary related to a particular subject, like medicine. MeSH is a controlled language. Retrieval rates tend to be greater and more specific when you use (or can map to) the same terms used by the indexer.

expressed in Kbps (e.g., 14.4 Kbps or 14.4K). And, the faster the modem, the less time is spent waiting for data to be sent or received.

Most new computer systems are sold with modems already assembled as part of the package. This can be a mixed blessing. Often, these modems are slower and inferior to those that can be bought off the shelf in any computer store, and, if something goes wrong, the only recourse is to discard it and purchase a replacement. On the plus side, however, these modems come preinstalled and generally work right away with no further tinkering.

Internal Modems

Internal modems are about $30 cheaper than external models and usually require nothing more than a screwdriver to install. However, you will need to unplug your computer and open the computer casing to get at the expansion slot where you will install the modem board. Take care not to touch any other part of the interior.

PC card modems (PCMCIA) are credit card-sized plug-in cards. These are usually plugged into a special slot in the rear or side of the computer and can be easily removed. Because of their size, however, they are several times the cost of ordinary modems and are usually sold for use with notebook or laptop computers.

Note: You cannot easily use your internal modem on another computer. And, if anything goes wrong, you will have to open the computer casing to remove the modem.

External Modems

External modems can be easily replaced and swapped from computer to computer. Installation is simply a matter of connecting the various cables. The first is cable from your telephone jack to the modem slot labeled "line in." The second cable is from the modem to the serial port at the back of the computer. The third is the power cable to the modem.

Note: Many modems require some cables to be purchased separately. External versions also require a separate power source.

ISDN (Integrated Services Digital Network)

If using a modem costs only pennies per call, then, when using the high-speed alternative of ISDN, you could say "I'm Spending Dollars Now." An ISDN connection provides a fast and reliable connection to the Internet; however, there are a lot more hoops to jump through before being connected. First, you need to lease an ISDN line from your local telephone company and to have this line running between your computer and your ISP.

Second, ISDN removes the need for a modem; unfortunately, it requires a more expensive device called an ISDN adapter, sometimes called a digital modem. These adapters can cost more than $500, but, in return, they contain all the bells and whistles to actually handle the higher connection speed, removing the need for any other specialized software on your computer.

Crash
The sudden complete failure of a computer caused by a hardware or software error. Usually the computer will need to be restarted; any work in progress at the time of the crash will be lost.

An ISDN also introduces the ability to have a permanent fast connection to the Internet. And, although you can use a 28.8K modem connection for permanent access, it is not really recommended. ISDN comes at two speeds, 56.8K and 128K.

Cable Modems

A new technology being tried is the delivery of Internet access through a permanent digital connection similar to that used to supply cable television. The idea is that these

Cyberspace
Coined by William Gibson in his groundbreaking book, *Neuromancer* (1984), which postulated a near future of hightech computer skullduggery. Cyberspace is the non-physical location where all networked computer activity exists.

TABLE 2–1.—COMMUNICATIONS OPTIONS

Features	Modem 14.4 Kbps	Modem 28.8 Kbps	ISDN 56.6 Kbps	ISDN 128 Kbps	T1 line	T3 line	Cable box
Max. speed (Kbps)	19.2	32	64	128	1.544 Mps	44.8 Mps	10 Mps
Initial setup cost	$100	$200	$300+	$300+	$300+	$300+	$50 (est.)
Monthly cost dial-up ISP (20 hrs)	$20–$30	$20–$30	$60	$60+	NA	NA	$30 (est.)
Permanent leased line (24 h access) per month	Not available	>$100	$1,000+	$1,500+	>$2,000	>$10,000	$30 (est.)
Download 1 meg file	10 min	5 min	2.5 min	1 min	5 sec	1 sec	3 sec
Real-time video	No	No	No	No	Yes	Yes	Yes

Note: A permanent leased line can be more expensive than this, especially the further you are located from your ISP service.
Abbreviation: Mps, *million bits per second.*

cable modems will be supplied as an addition to an existing cable service, for a fraction of the cost of alternative high-speed access. Because the service would take advantage of existing connections to the home and office, it is assumed that a large number of consumers will be willing to pay for the convenience of this faster service.

There are still technical problems to be overcome before cable modems become commonplace. However, this type of connection would provide a level of Internet access that would be superior to that presently available and at a price that would be affordable to the average consumer or small business. See Table 2–1 for a comparison of access methods.

Troubleshooting Modem Problems

The following procedure outlines how to troubleshoot modem problems by testing your modem:

- Open the Windows terminal program. (On a MAC, start your modern software.)
- Type AT.
- If you get a message saying "OK," then your modem is properly connected.
- Typing ATDT should produce a dial tone, which is another indicator that all is well.

If you get no response, determine the following:

- Is the modem turned on?
- Is the telephone line connected?
- Are all the cables correctly connected?
- Are the software settings in your communications program set correctly (COM1 should be the correct modem port)?

If problems persist, then you need to refer to the manual supplied with your modem or contact your ISP.

Communications Software

Whichever modem you choose, you will need to install any necessary communications software. Windows 3.1 and Windows 95 come equipped with a simple communications program called Terminal (HyperTerminal on Win 95), which is located in the Accessories folder. Sometimes, the software accompanying a modem has more features. Currently, a popular feature is fax software, which enables your modem to send and receive faxes.

Most of this software is generic with similar key features. To use the software effectively, you should be aware of how to perform at least the following functions:

- Set the volume of the modem speaker.
- Disable the call-waiting feature of your telephone, which is important because, otherwise, incoming calls will disrupt a communications session. (Usually "*70" is placed before the telephone number.)
- Store regularly called numbers in an "electronic" address book or directory.
- Use the on/off logging feature. This captures a complete record of all text appearing on the screen and saves it to a file.

It is also worthwhile to spend some time experimenting with the various software features. Taking the time to learn how to perform the following important functions will save a lot of effort later:

- Reviewing material that has scrolled out of sight.
- Determining what settings are best for sending and receiving files from other computers.
- Customizing parts of the program (e.g., passwords and repetitive login commands) and running this as a login script.

All of these functions can be learned by either experimenting with the software or by reading the accompanying instruction manuals.

For the most part, the communications software that comes with your modem or operating system is best used for communicating with computer systems that are predominantly textual. These can be bulletin boards, text-based on-line services, or ISP shell accounts, or the software may be used for sending and receiving faxes. Other software is more appropriate for more extensive Internet access, especially when graphics or multimedia elements are involved (see Chapter 3).

Database
A collection of on-line bibliographic citations produced from a body of work with the aid of a printed thesaurus and its "controlled language." MEDLINE is a database as are ERIC, PsycINFO, and CINAHL.

CompuServe is the only major on-line service that maintains a text-only interface in addition to a graphical environment. But, this service is rumored to be closing down in late 1996. The biggest advantage of a text-only connection is that you can access CompuServe from any computer with a modem and simple communications software. This is advantageous for travelers.

HOW DOES IT ACTUALLY WORK?

Document
The article, or information, that appears after hyperlinking from a Web page.

Transport Control Protocol/Internet Protocol

Everything traveling through the Internet has to operate under a system called Transport Control Protocol/Internet Protocol (TCP/IP). Essentially, these two standards dictate how data get from point A to point B. When you consider that data on the Internet can consist of simple e-mail messages, graphical images, sound, or even video footage, it is very important that what is received is the same as what was originally sent. For this reason TCP/IP is often called "the language of the Internet."

The TCP puts together "packets" of data, and the IP sends these packets between computers. Typically, an e-mail message is broken up into several data packets, which then travel independently to the same final destination. Upon arrival, each packet is checked to ensure that all the packets arrived safely and that nothing got lost along the way. These are then reassembled into their original order and distributed to the correct mailbox.

This protocol aptly demonstrates the original purpose of the Internet, which was to ensure that, in case of nuclear war or some other major catastrophe, messages and other data could still be sent using whatever pieces remained of the communications system. The intent was that, if parts of the message ran into problems, they would automatically be redirected onto other systems and, ultimately, enough of the original message would get through to be useful.

There is TCP/IP software built into Windows 95 and System 7.5 on the Macintosh; it is commonly referred to as a TCP/IP stack. With Windows software, the file winsock.DLL is the interface to TCP/IP and can be found in the main Windows directory. On the Mac, the interface is known as MacTCP and should be in the system folder. If you are using Windows 3.1 or an earlier version of the Mac operating system, then you will need to obtain this software separately and install it on your system (see Appendix 2).

The Winsock (or MacTCP) acts as a "layer" between Internet software and your TCP/IP stack. Your Internet software, for example, the Netscape Browser, tells Winsock what it wants to do ("request a document"). Winsock translates these commands to the TCP/IP stack and then your TCP/IP stack passes them out to the Internet. When the document is returned, the TCP/IP stack processes it (it is arriving as several disordered packets of data) and then passes it back through the Winsock for your use.

Unfortunately, there are many variants of Winsock available, and many Internet applications frequently come bundled with their own versions, most of which only operate using the software they originated with. The only way to easily tell which version is installed on your computer is to open up File Manager or Windows Explorer, select the winsock.DLL file in the Windows directory, and then inspect its properties (File/Properties).

MacTCP does not have this problem because it is a generic software application produced by Apple, around which all Macintosh Internet software works. The most common Winsock software is produced by Microsoft, which is distributed with Windows 95, and Trumpet Winsock, which is a shareware package out of Australia.

There can only be one winsock.DLL file located in the Windows directory, and this should be the version that you use most of the time. If you need to operate a different piece of Internet software that requires its own winsock.DLL file to be used, then you need to swap these files around. The best way to do this is to rename the file that you will not be using (e.g., naming the Microsoft Winsock file as winsock.ms or the CompuServe Winsock file as winsock.cis). It is then an easy matter to swap the files later by simply renaming the appropriate files.

Note: Chapter 5 details a process that enables this to be performed more quickly and conveniently.

Serial Line Internet Protocol/Point to Point Protocol (SLIP/PPP)

The SLIP and PPP are the means by which you can actually run Internet software over a serial connection, such as a telephone line. The PPP is the newest protocol and is a more efficient connection method, because of its robustness and its ability to correct errors caused by noisy telephone lines. With these protocols, your computer becomes a part of the Internet while it is connected via a dial-up SLIP/PPP connection to an ISP or on-line service.

Without a SLIP/PPP connection, it is impossible to be directly connected to the Internet. This means that, to use any Internet resource, you would first have to connect to an Internet host that is directly connected to the Internet and then run the appropriate software on the host's computer. This type of access is called a shell account or a menu-based service, and it is the traditional means of accessing the Internet.

For instance, to download a file, you would have to first copy it to the host's computer and then download it to your own computer. These extra steps add a lot of time to the process and you are restricted as to what software can be used. Only text-based programs can be run over this type of connection, so many recent software advances, especially those transmitted over the Web, cannot be used.

Document delivery
The delivery, either by FAX, e-mail, or mail, of an article, the citation of which you have retrieved in a MEDLINE or other database search. Usually the network or service facilitates the ordering through an independent source.

As with TCP/IP software, SLIP/PPP software comes bundled with Windows 95, and the Macintosh version (MacPPP) is freely available (see Appendix 2). The Trumpet Winsock package contains the appropriate SLIP/PPP drivers for Windows 3.1.

When starting an account with an ISP, always request a SLIP or PPP connection.

Download
To transfer files from one computer to another.

> ⚡ **POWER TIP**
>
> If you find access to AOL erratic or even unavailable at peak times and you have an account with CompuServe or another ISP, you can use this other account to establish a direct TCP/IP connection to AOL. If your AOL settings have been configured with TCP/IP access, then this direct connection bypasses the bottlenecks (which only occur when all the AOL modem ports are being used) and lets you in the back door, so to speak (see Chapter 4).
>
> *Note: You will effectively be paying double access fees while connected this way.*

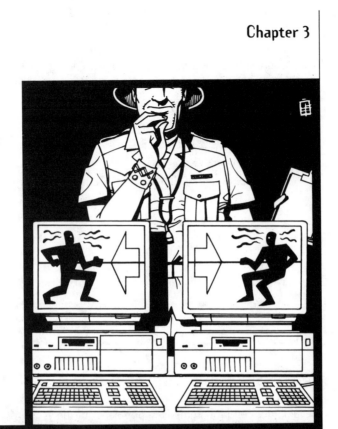

Chapter 3

Getting Started on the Infobahn

Internet Basics

In Chapter 1 we introduced the idea of the Web browser as the Rosetta stone of the Internet. A browser enables anyone throughout the world to access the Internet, using a wide variety of computers, operating systems, and even languages. Mosaic was the first Web browser, and when it appeared in late 1993, it provided a tantalizing glimpse of the Internet of the future. Its ease of use captured the media's attention, increased the popularity of the Internet, and ushered in millions of new users within a few short years.

The Web browser has come a long way since then, and by using the latest versions of Netscape or Microsoft Internet Explorer, it is now possible for you to access every part of the Internet armed with just a browser and no other Internet software. This is the on-line equivalent of going from the invention of the wheel directly to the invention of the jet engine.

However, as multifunctional as it seems, the Web browser is but part of a suite of software tools that enhances and makes it easier to access on-line resources. This

Glossary Terms E–N

E-mail
Electronic mail.

chapter provides an overview of the tools you need for specific tasks and the information required to understand how each component of the Internet works to make the whole system function.

Emulation
A software or hardware device that enables software to be run in a totally different environment from what was intended. The device mimics the original process, delivering the same results as if nothing had been changed. For example, emulation software allows the use of DOS programs on Macs.

TABLE 3–1.—BASIC INTERNET FUNCTIONS

Traditional functions include the following:

- Conversation, knowledge sharing (via e-mail, USENET, and mailing lists)
- Sharing files (FTP)
- Remote access to computers (via Telnet)

Expanded functions include the following:

- Collaboration (via video conferencing and e-mail)
- Information retrieval (WAIS, Gopher, and the WWW)
- Business promotion (via e-mail, USENET, WWW, and mailing lists)

Abbreviations: FTP, file transfer protocol; *WAIS,* wide-area information server; *WWW,* World Wide Web.

Before 1993, use of the Internet was limited to the options outlined under traditional in Table 3–1 and was mostly related to users based in the United States. With the development and the immediate popularity of the World Wide Web in 1993, the Internet took on a much more international context. Business use has increased dramatically. In 1994, there was no discernible commercial advertising on the Internet, but 2 years later, most major advertising agencies perceived the Internet as an important adjunct to traditional advertising methods, albeit a flashier and more hip form of advertising.

All this attention has made those involved in traditional Internet activities work that much harder to be visible above the hype and noise of the glamorous newcomers. Although it is true that the Web is fast becoming a much larger component of the Internet, there is still a lot of growth, information, and excitement to be found in the other areas, some of which have been in operation for several decades.

E-MAIL

The bedrock of the Internet, electronic mail (e-mail) is what started it all. Since the first message was sent in the late 1960s, e-mail is probably still the first part of the Internet most newcomers experience, usually through an affiliation with a university or a business, but increasingly via on-line services such as CompuServe or America Online (AOL).

Electronic mail at its most basic is a simple text message sent from one Internet address (Nigel.Rowe@Mosby.com) to another Internet address (Tom.Cardy @Kosmos.wcc.govt.nz).

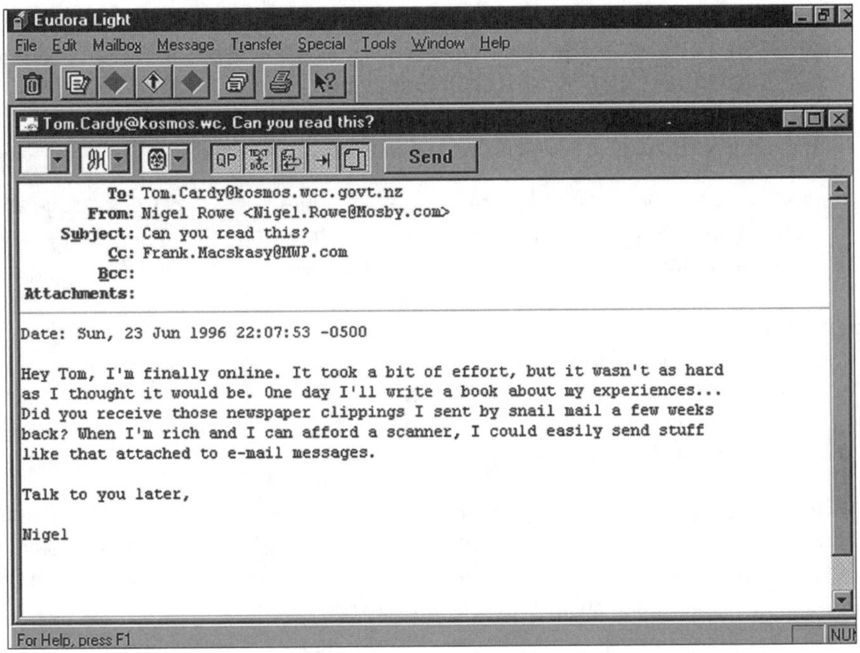

FAQ
Frequently Asked Question. Lists of FAQs are posted on Usenet Newsgroups and on many WWW pages.

Firewall
Special computers or software that are set up on a network to prevent unauthorized access to a computer system or computer files.

FIGURE 3–1.—*Example of e-mail message (before sending).*

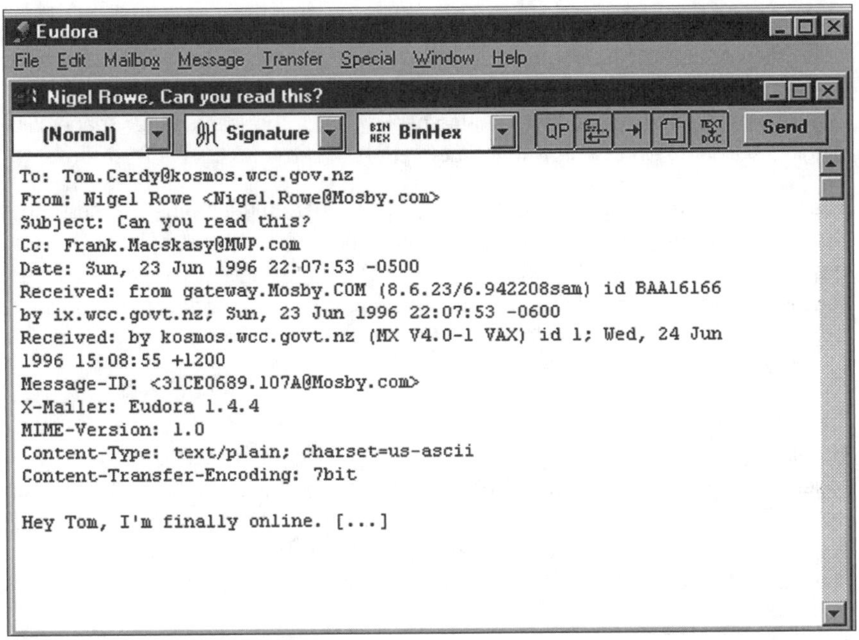

FIGURE 3–2.—*Example of e-mail message (as received).*

Flame
A heated and emotional response to some on-line activity. Usually expressed in an e-mail or Usenet message. Politeness is not usually a factor. Two or more people engaging in flaming each other is called a flame war. This term is especially applicable to situations in which people other than the original participants have become involved.

As shown in Figure 3–1, the layout of a message is fairly straightforward. The *subject* and *recipient's address* along with any recipients of a *carbon-copy,* are typed in by the sender. Most of the other information, including the *sender's name,* return address, and the date, is supplied by the e-mail software, usually from information set up as default settings.

Figure 3–1 shows the message before it was sent. Figure 3–2 shows the message as received on Tom's computer, after it has been passed from computer network to computer network, finally arriving in Wellington, New Zealand.

Let's look at the anatomy of an e-mail message. The first thing you'll notice is all the extra information added to the message header. Some of these fields were generated automatically when the message was sent: *MessageID* (a unique message identifier), *ContentType* (identifies the message as text or an attached file); and *X-Mailer* displays the name of the e-mail software used (Eudora).

A *Received* tag was inserted at each point on the Internet that the message passed through. This message passed through two Internet "gateways," although sometimes the message may be routed through more connections. This information is used to help understand any delivery problems encountered.

Several e-mail programs strip this header, presenting just the standard *Date, Subject, To,* and *From* fields along with the message. Programs like cc:Mail present the header as a separate accompanying file.

Most modern e-mail software comes with a standard set of features including special formatting options such as bold, italic, and underlined type, and provisions to attach graphics, spreadsheet files, and computer programs, as well as sound and video images. For instance, we could have attached copies of the scanned newspaper clippings to our sample message with no more effort than a few clicks of the mouse.

The beauty of e-mail is that it is fast, cheap, and easy. From the moment a message is sent, it is on its way, often arriving at its destination within minutes, irrespective of the distance traveled. Most of the delays in receiving messages occur while the message is waiting in the recipient's computer system to be read. And replying to a message couldn't be simpler; just select the *Reply* button, type your response, and click on *Send.*

The costs of sending e-mail vary from free at one extreme to inexpensive at the other. Usually any per-message costs relate to the cost of the phone call to send the message, but if you pay a monthly Internet subscription fee, then this should be included as well. By any reckoning, it will always be cheaper than sending the equivalent message via the U.S. Postal Service or via fax, especially when the time taken to purchase stamps, envelopes, and other materials is considered.

E-mail is easy. After composing the message and making the connection to your e-mail provider, clicking the *Send* button is all that remains. It sure beats finding an envelope, trudging to the post office, standing in line to buy a stamp, and then dropping the letter in a mailbox where it could sit for up to a day before being collected and sent on its way. And if you want to send copies of the letter to others, then it's simply a matter of identifying them in the *CC* (carbon copy) field. Most software also allows you to send *BCCs* (blind carbon copies), in which the original recipient's message includes no indication that a copy has been sent to someone else.

FTP
File Transfer Protocol. The most common method used to transfer files through the Internet.

> ⚡ **POWER TIP**
>
> If your e-mail software does not have a blind carbon copy feature, then *forward* a copy of the original message instead. This feature has the added advantage of allowing additional comments to be inserted.
>
> *Note: Make sure this message is only sent to the BCC person and not the original recipient.*

Understanding E-mail Addresses

An e-mail address has a lot going for it. First and foremost, it is possibly the closest thing to having a truly permanent address—one that is transferable from country to country and that can be accessed throughout the world. This portability is a key reason that many people who travel a lot subscribe to one of the major international on-line services, such as CompuServe or AOL. No longer does traveling prevent you from reading your mail.

Second, it is so much more flexible than a traditional mailing address, which changes every time you physically change street addresses. And if you have chosen a reliable Internet Service Provider (ISP) or on-line service, then your address is theoretically active forever, or at least until you stop subscribing to the service.

The ability to read an e-mail address and break it down into its respective parts is very important, not just because you should have a clear understanding of where you are sending messages, but also because it could help solve delivery problems when a message is returned as undeliverable.

All e-mail addresses have a simple structure that is composed of the following unique components:

1. A person's name or unique ID
2. The host computer that holds this person's mailbox
3. Additional subdomains further identifying the network where the host computer is located
4. The type of institution (e.g., com, edu, mil, gov, org, or net)
5. A two-letter country code (e.g., NZ, UK, JP, or AU)

The "@" signifier, pronounced *at,* is used to separate the person's name from the actual address elements. Each subsequent subdomain is separated with a dot ("."").

Examples of addresses and their interpretations follow:

1. Nigel.Rowe@Mosby.com
2. 72530.1024@Compuserve.com
3. SWhiteman@libsci.mit.edu
4. DeanHaskell@wyatt.akld.co.nz

Functionality
The way the search engine operates in the various services on a network. This includes the way the browser works, how the interface functions, and how search strategies are handled by the search engine (e.g., Boolean operators, truncation, plurals, etc.). Just think FUNCTION; the way it operates.

The first two examples are straightforward enough, with example 1 identifying the person as working at a commercial institution (com) called Mosby and example 2 identifying the addressee as a subscriber of CompuServe. Example 3 illustrates a situation in which the computer hosting the user's mailbox (libsci) is just one computer in a larger network (mit), and the "edu" identifies it as an educational site. Example 4 locates the host computer "wyatt" on the "akld" network and identifies it as a commercial (co) computer located in New Zealand.

Institutional codes help identify the type of organization for the host computer. "Com" (or "co") is short for commercial and indicates a business location; "mil" means military; "edu" is short for educational; "gov" represents local and national government organizations; "org" is a nonprofit organization; and "net" represents a network.

The country code is almost always used as part of the addresses outside of the United States, and it is safe to assume that an address without a country code is located in the United States. Often users' locations are effectively masked if the address is tied to one of the major on-line services such as CompuServe or AOL, because the users are often free to create their own unique e-mail IDs.

For messages to be sent properly, e-mail addresses must be typed exactly as they appear, complete with any punctuation and other symbols; however, there is usually no distinction between lower and upper case characters. Although there are variations on how different mail systems connect to the Internet, and correspondingly varying address formats, the rule that the user ID or name is placed on the left of the @ sign and the address on the right is strictly observed. A notable exception is CompuServe, where addresses are composed of a member ID separated by a comma (72530,1024) within CompuServe itself, but separated by a dot if the e-mail originates from outside CompuServe (72530.1024).

⚡ **POWER TIP**

It is very easy to send a reply to messages for which you are one of several recipients and learn later that everyone saw your response when you only intended for one person to receive it. Depending on what you said, this sort of mistake can prove very embarrassing. When replying to messages, be sure that the *To* field in your reply lists only the people you want to receive the message. Delete unwanted names. If your e-mail software does not allow you to delete, then manually compose a new message, copying the addresses when necessary.

Gateway
A special-purpose dedicated computer that connects otherwise incompatible networks and routes data packets from one network to another.

E-mail Management

A few simple rules can make your e-mail experience a lot easier, especially when it comes to remembering addresses and storing copies of messages. All e-mail software has some form of address book. Learn how this works and get into the habit of storing all of your frequently used addresses, along with any additional information that will help identify the entry.

Often an address by itself will not say anything about the owner (e.g., 72530.1024@Compuserve.com). Unless this address was tagged with the person's name in the address book, it is possible you would not be able to identify it later. Most e-mail software attaches this name tag to the actual address, so the previous example shows up on messages as being from "72530.1024@CompuServe.com <NigelRowe>."

An advanced feature of some software lets you build mailing lists of selected addresses in your address book. With this feature, it is easy to send a message or an e-mail newsletter out to a large number of recipients by simply selecting the mailing list as the recipient of the message. This saves the effort of manually inserting multiple addresses into a message.

Similarly, keep copies of your important outgoing and incoming e-mail. Sometimes deleting e-mail as it is read can seem the best thing to do, but chances are you will delete something that is needed later. The best solution is to store or archive all messages for at least a week after receipt, and then choose the ones to be deleted. Your e-mail should be viewed as nothing different from ordinary postal mail. Consequently, treat junk e-mail the same as you would regular junk mail, that is, do not save it. Personal letters or business notes and memos may be saved or printed if necessary for future referral.

Some of the best e-mail programs have a facility in which different folders can be created, each storing messages under different headings. Other e-mail programs simply store all e-mail in an outgoing folder and an incoming folder. In the case of the latter, it is important that you minimize the amount of saved mail, otherwise the task of sorting new from old could be time consuming.

The simple task of copying your e-mail to labeled archive disks can enable you to keep copies of all your important messages and minimize the clutter in your mail box. Unless you receive a lot of mail, an archive floppy disk for each year is a good starting point.

Gopher
A system of interconnected menus. Each menu option could be a document or a pointer to another menu. Selecting an option takes you to that resource.

⚡ **POWER TIP**

Overall, e-mail is very reliable, but unlike ordinary mail for which the authenticity of a message can be confirmed by a signature or a postmark, e-mail has no similar mark of authenticity. For someone who knows what they are doing, it is an easy process to forge an e-mail address and send out misleading or inflammatory information. Always check before acting on any e-mail message when you cannot verify the contents by other means.

Sending Attached Files

There comes a time when a simple message is not enough, and you need to attach an accompanying file. This file can be any number of things: graphics or photos, word processing documents, spreadsheets, database files, or even a computer program. Most e-mail software handles these attachments in the same way. First, you create the message and then select the *attach document/files* option. Usually a file selection window will pop up and you select the file or files that are to be sent.

When the message is sent, the software automatically converts a copy of these files to the MIME (Multimedia Internet Mail Extensions) format. MIME ensures that everything contained in the message can be reassembled and recognized at the receiving end. This process considers the fact that e-mail messages are divided into smaller data packets for transmission. When these packets are reassembled at their destination, it is easy for uncommon characters to get mistranslated along the way.

This does not affect simple text files, in which all characters conform to ASCII (American Standard Code for Information Interchange), but highly formatted files (e.g., computer programs, complex word processing files, or desktop publishing files) can contain any number of unique characters. MIME converts these nonstandard characters into the correct ASCII format.

If your e-mail program does not perform MIME conversions automatically, then a separate converter program is needed. The attached file is first run through this program, and the resulting converted files are sent as e-mail messages. If the conversion program produces five files, then each file is sent as a separate message. At the other end, the recipient of the message will need to use similar conversion software to convert each message back into the original format. Chapter 5, "Optimizing Internet Software," explains how to use these conversion programs.

E-mail Software

cc:MAIL

This excellent software package is produced by Lotus Development Corporation, and is found mostly in business environments and local area networks (LANs). It is available in two major versions, one for the office (cc:MAIL) and a standalone (cc:MAIL Mobile) for use when traveling or accessing your mail from home. Key features include filters for presorting incoming mail according to various criteria, rules for managing new and existing mail, and a spell checker. cc:MAIL is available for Windows and the Macintosh.

Gopherspace
All of the material available on Gophers throughout the Internet.

Pegasus Mail

This is a popular Windows alternative to cc:MAIL that was developed in New Zealand and is available free of charge, for both LANs and standalone PCs. This package has many of the same features as cc:MAIL, as well as additional features especially for managing attached files and launching multimedia attachments.

Eudora

This program is available in two versions: Eudora Light and Eudora Pro. The major difference between the two is that Eudora Light is free and has fewer features than Eudora Pro. This is probably the most popular e-mail software available; many ISPs offer Eudora Light as part of their initial software package. Eudora was originally written for the Macintosh and remains the best Mac e-mail package.

Netscape

This is the only Web browser with a built-in mail program. This is extremely useful when you are surfing the Web and have a need to send e-mail. A very useful feature is the ability to attach a text version of any Web page to your message. With the latest versions of Netscape (2.0 and above), e-mail messages can be composed exactly like a Web page with graphics and hypertext links. These versions also offer an address book.

CompuServe

The CompuServe CIM software features a message filing system with full search capabilities. Copies of all outgoing messages can be filed automatically if this option has been chosen in the configuration section.

Note: all messages remain on the CompuServe system until they are transferred to the In-Basket, saved to the filing cabinet, or dealt with while connected.

Other key e-mail features of CompuServe include the following:

- With SmartRules, e-mail can be retrieved via pager or by voice mail using a toll-free number anywhere in the United States.

- AutoForward and AutoReply rules. Automatic notices can be sent to senders (all or selected) of new messages alerting them when you are on vacation or otherwise unavailable.

- An address book that can be configured to store individual addresses and mailing lists, and leave room for comments

- Message limits within CompuServe are 2MB and outside CompuServe, 50K (messages larger than 50K can be sent but this is not recommended)

- A single file can be attached to a message. All multiple files or nontext files must be manually converted using conversion software before being attached to messages.

- Spell-checking software is available as an add-on component.

- A 100-message maximum for any individual mailbox. This limit includes unread and read mail. Once this limit is reached, any new mail is returned to the sender with a message saying the mailbox was full.

- Mail deleted in error can be restored as long as you have not closed the mail box window.

With the present versions of the CompuServe CIM software, sending a message to customer service and some other in-house departments requires you to use a special e-mail window within the appropriate area. This bypasses the usual method of composing e-mail, and no copy of the message is kept. The only way to avoid this is to manually copy the message (highlight it and cut and paste into a new file) before sending.

Sending attached files is another area of concern. If the file is sent to another CompuServe address, there is no problem as long as the correct file type is identified in the *File Type* dialog box. However, to send an attached file through the Internet to an address outside CompuServe the file must be converted to MIME format and then sent as an ordinary message. This process requires software beyond the CompuServe CIM package. (See Chapter 5, "Optimizing Internet Software," for a detailed explanation of how to accomplish this.)

America Online

All versions of AOL software contain a very simple-to-use e-mail package. Version 3 enhances this with the ability to format a message using colors, text formatting (e.g., font sizes, bold, italics, underlining, and justification), and embedded hyperlinks to Web pages and other areas of AOL. Of course, messages lose this special formatting when they are sent to addresses outside AOL.

GUI
Graphical User Interface. Windows is an example of a GUI. This allows a user to communicate with computer software by using a mouse and graphic icons to control programs.

Key e-mail features of AOL include the following:

- Flash sessions enable mail to be retrieved or sent automatically at predetermined or impromptu times.

- Outgoing text messages are limited to around 30K. Longer messages need to be split up into numbered parts. Incoming messages are limited to around 320K.

- Using Windows, a single file can be attached to a message, which the AOL software converts into a format that can be reliably sent over the Internet. Multiple files must be manually converted into a single file before being attached. The size of the message and accompanying file cannot exceed 15.8MB if they are being sent to another AOL address, and 1MB for mail through the Internet. On the Macintosh, multiple files can be attached to messages.

- All read messages are copied to your personal filing cabinet if AOL has been configured in this way. This greatly simplifies the process of replying off-line.

- Mail in the personal filing cabinet is searchable by date, sender, and contents.

- An add-on spell checker program is available separately.

- An AOL mailbox holds a maximum of 550 messages. When this limit is reached, the system deletes previously read mail first, followed by unread mail. No unread mail will be deleted until this mailbox limit is reached, although mail unread after 5 weeks is automatically deleted.

Note: All mail remains on the AOL computer system until you read it or delete it from your mail box. Reading new messages automatically tags messages to be deleted unless the message is highlighted and you select the Keep as New option. Exiting from the mailbox window deletes all mail tagged to be deleted.

Hacker
The *media's* definition: A person who "breaks" into computers without authorization. The *real* definition: A skilled computer programmer who operates computers as a hobby.

⚡ POWER TIP

With both services it is always cheaper to read and reply to messages off-line. With CompuServe, save all new mail to the In-Basket (Get Mail/Save to In-Basket). On AOL, activate a *Flash Session* to retrieve new mail. This also enables replies to be composed in a more leisurely and thoughtful fashion.

Why Does My Mail Come Back to Me?

Probably the single best feature of e-mail, and definitely the most underrated, is the Internet's "return to sender" function. Normally, this happens whenever an e-mail message cannot be delivered, and a copy of the message is returned to you. Within this message will be a copy of the original message preceded by a cryptic explanation of the reasons for it being undeliverable.

This note is strange primarily because it was automatically generated somewhere en route, usually at the point at which the message could not be passed any further. Unfortunately, no one has come up with a way to make this explanation readable to anyone but computer scientists.

The four primary reasons for e-mail to be undeliverable are as follows:

1. The recipient's host address cannot be located on the Internet.
2. The recipient is not known at that address.
3. The host address is not receiving mail, although the address is valid.
4. This recipient's e-mail account has been closed or their mailbox is full.

Examine the returned message closely. Often the reason for the problem is given in the subject line; "Host not found" or "User unknown" are the most common problems. If the subject line offers no such clues, open the message and read the contents. Often the first dozen or so lines contain the relevant information.

You should also refer back to the original source of the address and compare it with the address that was typed. Often a mistake was made in typing the address; ".org" might have been typed in place of ".com" or "NRowe" was typed when the name should have been "NigelRowe." Remember, all this e-mail is being sorted and forwarded completely by computer without human intervention, so one tiny mistake will not be corrected en route by a knowledgeable, experienced human mail handler.

Occasionally messages will be returned saying "Service not available" or "Message undeliverable for 2 days." This implies that the host computer has been disconnected for various reasons, probably for maintenance, or it is being upgraded. In the first instance, just keep sending the message every few days until the service is available and the message is not returned. In the second instance, the message did get through; you are just being told that the recipient will not see it until the system is back on-line.

WORLD WIDE WEB (WWW)

The World Wide Web is frequently confused with the Internet, which it is not, but it is rapidly becoming the most dominant part of the Internet. The Web (or WWW) provides a graphical, easy-to-navigate interface for looking at documents on the Internet. The expression World Wide Web comes from the ease with which a user can spin a trail around the Internet, visiting multiple computers in different countries in quick succession, by doing nothing more than clicking on successive hypertext links embedded in documents.

Home page
The home page is the door to the information a WWW server provides. This screen of information is hyperlinked to other documents or resources. Home pages are also called *Web sites.*

It is this seamless ability to link distant resources that makes the Web so appealing. Considering that in 1993 the Web was composed of only a few hundred computers, and by mid 1996 it contained over 50 million "pages" of information spread over hundreds of thousands of computers, it is impossible not to view this transformation as anything short of revolutionary.

The software that makes it all work is a Web browser, which performs all the tasks involved with locating and retrieving documents, formatting text and graphics, and making it possible to "hyperlink" to another document anywhere in the world.

A wide variety of browsers are available. Some are very good, whereas others leave much to be desired, and some are even built into other software. Probably the key feature of Mosaic (the first browser) that ensured its popularity was its availability free of charge through the Internet. In fact, within the first few months of its release, more than a million copies were downloaded. It is worth noting that most browsers since have also been available free, or at least free for an initial evaluation period.

To "surf" the Web, you must be equipped with a suitable browser. The three main browsers in use are Netscape Navigator, Microsoft Internet Explorer, and Mosaic. Several ISPs and on-line services provide their own browsers, and sometimes these can only be used in conjunction with their particular service. As you spend time navigating the Web you will notice that many sites carry notices advising which browser is optimal for the site. The latest versions of Netscape and Internet Explorer should work with every site, but other browsers frequently display a limited view of the site or will not allow access to it.

For the purposes of this book we will confine ourselves to discussing Netscape and Internet Explorer, as they are the dominant browsers, with 80% and 7% of the market share, respectively.[1]

A typical commercial Web site now boasts extensive multimedia content, in addition to hundreds of pages of text, tables, and graphics. This can range from animation and interactive graphics, to three-dimensional (3D) simulation, video and sound clips, and even real time chat features. New developments include video and audio "streaming," which allow for realtime video and audio signals to be received and project collaboration in which participants can write and draw simultaneously onto a common whiteboard.

With the advent of JAVA, a new Internet programming language, it is now possible to create software applications that can be downloaded from the Internet and run by a browser on any computer regardless of operating system or installed software.

To partake in JAVA, 3D, or many of the other flashier Web activities, you will need more than just a browser that can handle them. You will also need a better than average computer (16+ MB of RAM), a 32-bit operating system (such as Windows 95, Unix, or Windows NT), and a high-speed Internet connection. The latest versions of Netscape and Internet Explorer have JAVA and 3D capabilities built-in.

Host
A centrally located computer that provides services to other computers.

HTML
This is a simple programming language in which WWW pages are constructed using "tags" to indicate how and where text, graphics, and hyperlinks are positioned and formatted.

HTTP
Hypertext Transport Protocol. The hypertext glue that binds the WWW together. This protocol controls how documents are transferred from a host computer to the Web browser that requested it.

Both Netscape and Internet Explorer are available for Windows 3.1, Windows 95, and the Macintosh. New versions of each are released about every 6 months, and, consequently, there is a fierce battle for increased market share. Currently, Netscape is the undisputed winner because of its head start in introducing new features and supporting multiple operating systems. However, Microsoft's Internet Explorer is quickly catching up, with future versions promising to be integrated directly into the operating system and other Microsoft software products.

Getting Started

An understanding of how the Web operates is essential to navigating it effectively. For starters, the four key actions involved in accessing a Web document are as follows:

- Starting your Web browser software
- Opening up an Internet connection
- Typing in an address
- Selecting and downloading the document

To this add the four following activities based on a retrieved Web document:

- Further action based on the content
- *Bookmarking* the site for future use
- Printing or saving documents or images
- Using the document as a guide to learning HTML (Hypertext Markup Language)

Together these eight functions describe a typical Web session, and once these simple steps are mastered, you are well on the way to surfing the Internet. In fact, this is the whole point behind this book's title. A safari is an extraordinary adventure, exploring new territory, overcoming obstacles, and encountering mysterious creatures.

An on-line "surfari" is similar—documents waiting to be discovered or sought out, meeting new people, and overcoming problems encountered along the way. In many ways, the only real difference is that on-line there are fewer risks of being eaten alive or trapped in quicksand. However, you could still become lost and disoriented or stumble across a valuable gold mine of information and lose track of time and the distance traveled.

Accessing the Web

Unless you have a direct permanent Internet connection, you will need to open a dial-up connection to your ISP, or on-line service. If so configured, it is possible to have your browser open this connection for you. Otherwise, make the connection to your ISP and then start your browser.

The initial document you see when you start a browser is called a "home page." This can be a blank page or the default setting—which is the home page of the browser's developer. It can also be set to any other document of your choosing. For instance, starting Netscape Navigator for the first time will display the Netscape Communications Corporation home page, and until you change this setting, it will be the starting point every time you use the browser.

This is the first indication of how the browser works. The Netscape home page isn't stored on your computer; the browser, connected to the Netscape home page through the Internet, downloads it to your computer. The browser then breaks off this connection to Netscape and displays the page. This document is now stored locally on your hard drive or in the computer's memory.

Hypertext
A method of formatting words with an embedded link, so when it is selected, the link is initiated. For instance, clicking on a hypertext link could cause another document to be loaded.

Now, here is the value of a direct permanent Internet connection. If you had used a *direct* connection through a LAN, then once the Netscape home page had been obtained, your actual connection to the Internet would have ceased. Using a dial-up connection via modem and an ISP forces you to maintain an open connection between your computer and the ISP for the duration of your on-line session. (Of course, this connection time is also accumulating toward your ISP access plan, which could be so many hours of "connect time" each month, as well as any charges your phone company makes for the call.)

With the direct connection, this is all avoided because you (or your business or university) would typically be paying a flat monthly fee. The direct connection also allows documents to be accessed much faster than does a modem.

Similarly, Microsoft Internet Explorer connects you to the Microsoft Network home page. Of course, these initial connections have been made automatically by the browser, without you having to type in an address. Accessing documents by supplying the browser with the address is the next step.

Addressing the Web

All Web documents have what is known as a URL, or Universal Resource Locator. This rather grand term describes where a document is located, what it is called, and the method needed to access it. As we said earlier, browsers can replace many other pieces of Internet software; however, it is still necessary to identify the method used to access the document so the browser knows what to do with it.

A URL could look like this:

http://www.mosby.com/project/whatsnew.html

The "http://" describes the protocol used for the connection. In this case, "http" is the standard for accessing Web documents and sets up the correct process for a document to be transferred back to your computer. The next part of the URL, "www.mosby.com," identifies the address of the Web server used for this request. The server is the computer that holds the document.

In actuality, the Mosby Web server is referenced by a unique number called the Internet Protocol (IP) address (204.233.129.3), but because it is easier to remember a name than a long number, a system called the Domain Name System (DNS) translates between this IP address and a unique domain name (www.mosby.com). Both are equally valid addresses, and sometimes you will see just the number given as an address.

The third part of the address is the directory containing the document: "/project." Successive directories are separated by additional forward slashes (/). The last part ("whatsnew.html") is the document filename. Often no directory will be listed. And more often than not you will see just the basic address with no directory or document name (e.g., http://www.mosby.com), in which case the default home page (Fig 3–3) will be loaded first (usually index.html or index.htm).

Besides "http," other Web protocols include "gopher," "news," and "ftp." Some browsers automatically add the http protocol to any address, so all you may need to type is the actual server address. There is no distinction between lower and upper case in the Web server of the URL. However, on some Web servers (e.g., UNIX) this distinction is made with reference to the document name. So match the case used whenever possible.

Navigating the Web

Browsers can be operated by using the pulldown menus or by clicking on buttons on the toolbar (see Fig 3–3).

Internet
The global network of inter-connected computers that allows e-mail and other documents, including computer files, to be easily distributed from computer to computer.

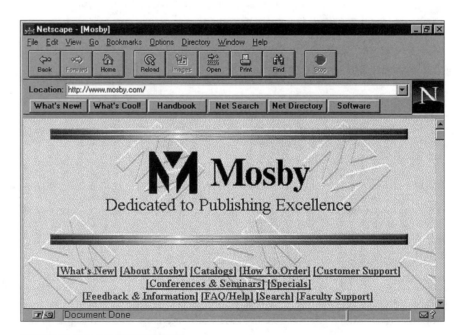

FIGURE 3–3.—*Home page of WWW.Mosby.com.*

The standard toolbar buttons are as follows:

Back or Forward

The *Back* button will reload the previously accessed page, and *Forward* returns to the most recent page. These only work with documents loaded in the current session. So if the *Back* button is "grayed" out, there is not a previous page to return to.

Home

This button loads your default home page.

Refresh (Reload)

If an error occurs while loading a page, click on this button to start again. At some Web sites you can use this feature to reload an updated page. This is especially common at sites for which the page is continuously updated (e.g., news, weather reports, or stock prices).

Open

Use this to type in a URL. If the URL has been copied from another document or an e-mail message, then this is the place to paste it. Click *OK* or press *Enter* to access the new document. With Microsoft Internet Explorer, you display previously saved documents on your computer by typing their directory and filenames. The browser will then load them like it would any other Web document. With Netscape, you load previously saved documents by choosing *File* and *Open File* from the menu bar.

Print

This prints the page currently open. Use *File* and then *Print Settings* to change the way a printed document looks.

Stop

This stops the current document from loading and is the same as pressing the ESC key under Windows. This is also the graceful way to cancel most actions that go awry.

Location/Address

This area displays the URL of the current document. You can also type or paste URLs here.

Working With Documents

Okay, the page has been transferred to your computer. What you can now do with it depends on what it contains. Most Web pages are hypertext documents—their structure allows for links to other documents. These links are embedded into the page and appear in a color different from the rest of the text, often blue. For instance, clicking on a picture may lead you to another document, or it may change the size of the picture. There are no hard and fast rules, and what happens when you activate one of the hypertext links is totally dependent on how the page has been written. Many pages are plain text with no embedded hypertext. Usually, these pages have been converted from older computer systems.

IRC
Internet Relay Chat. A form of interactive communication between computer users performed in real time using typed messages.

ISDN
Integrated Services Digital Network. A digital telephone connection that allows simultaneous highspeed transmission of voice and data.

Web pages are constructed using a programming language called Hypertext Markup Language (HTML). This language is easy to learn, and it is precisely this ease of use that has helped the Web to grow so fast. Links can reference other parts of the same document (e.g., footnotes or subject headings), link to a different document on another computer in a different country, or start up other programs. Clicking on a picture of a sheep may enable you to hear the sounds of sheep (baa!), view a video clip of sheep chewing grass, or even take a slide tour of a woolen factory.

This interconnectedness is the beauty of the Web. It is easy to start off viewing a page that expounds on sheep, and a few clicks later, find yourself on a page describing the latest photographs from the Hubble space telescope. Many Web pages reflect the interests and preoccupations of the people who built them, whereas others are the on-line equivalents of direct mail catalogues or other advertising materials. Some are as exciting and interesting as the best printed magazines, and with multimedia elements they can be as visually stimulating as television.

What Makes a Page

Pages are composed of several different elements. Text and HTML code form the main document, and pictures and multimedia items are saved as individual files. When the document is initially requested, all of these elements are transferred to your computer. If the connection is slow, or if there are a lot of graphics, downloading can take several minutes or longer. All browsers have some visual indicator in the top right corner of the screen to indicate when downloading is in progress (in Netscape this is an animation of a meteor shower; on MS Internet Explorer the Windows logo flutters against a moving sky). Additional information about the download is presented in the message bar at the bottom of the screen.

Multimedia items are usually indicated by a hyperlink. Clicking the link then downloads the file. Some sites rely heavily on these types of visual and audio stimuli, and so video and audio clips download with the rest of the page. However, because of their size and the extra time it takes to download, most sites have multimedia elements available as hyperlinks.

Depending on how your browser has been configured (and how current it is), downloaded files will run automatically as soon as they are downloaded, or a dialog box will open up that says something like "No Viewer Configured for File Type." In this case, choose the *Save to Disk* or *Save As* option and save the file to a directory on your computer.

More than likely, downloaded files will have to be uncompressed or installed on your computer before you can make further use of them. In the case of multimedia files, it is usually a matter of setting up a Viewer or Plug-In application that the browser will use to play the file. Netscape and Microsoft Internet Explorer are both configured to handle all the basic video and sound file formats without any further work. But, there are many other file types in common use that require your browser to be properly configured before they can be used.

Remembering Where You Have Been

A fundamental part of any surfing session is keeping a record of the sites visited that you would like to visit again. In Netscape, this function is called *Bookmarks,* and all you need to do is select *Bookmarks/Add Bookmark* on the menu bar to record the URL and the title of the current page in the Bookmarks folder. In Internet Explorer, this process is called *Favorites,* and choosing *Favorites/Add to Favorites* on the menu bar saves the URL. Both browsers allow separate Bookmarks or Favorites folders to be set up, so saved URLs can be better organized.

It is very easy to save dozens of Bookmarks in a single on-line session. Take the time to organize these; otherwise it becomes an almost impossible job to locate an address quickly. Also ensure that the reference name for each saved URL is accurate and descriptive. Sometimes the default name for a page is not what you will remember later.

Using Web Documents to Learn HTML

Constructing your own Web page is a relatively easy task. All the major on-line services allow subscribers space to maintain their own Web pages, so anyone can set up their own Web site inexpensively. Appendix One, "Ten Steps to Building a Web Site" describes the best means to go about this. However, a good place to learn how to build hypertext documents is to examine the pages that you visit. Using the *View/View Source* menu bar option on either browser allows you to see the HTML code that makes up a Web page.

You can even save the page to your hard drive and change or study it further (use *File* and then *File Save As* from the menu bar). If you make changes to these pages, loading the file in your browser will show how these affect the document. This is how many people have learned to write Web pages. Similarly, if while viewing a page you see an image that you would like to copy, under Windows using the mouse to right-click on the image brings up a *Save Image* option.

ISP
Internet Service Provider. An entity that provides Internet access for a fee.

Jughead
Software used to conduct keyword searches of specific Gopher sites.

⚡ POWER TIPS

It takes forever! Web servers allow lots of people to access the same page simultaneously. But whether the server can keep up with the sheer number of requests is another matter. Be patient if it takes a long time to load a page. Remember, complex pages or large files will take longer to download than simple ones.

Stop! If the downloading logo in the upper right corner of your browser is active for an unusually long time (say 5 minutes), use the Stop button to cancel your request. Try again—you might get a better connection.

LAN
Local Area Network. A group of computers in close proximity that is connected and shares common resources, such as printers and software programs.

How long should a page take to download? This depends on three things: (1) the size of the file, (2) the demand on the Web server holding the file, and (3) modem speed. Essentially, the speed of your modem is the most crucial factor. Using a 14.4K modem it takes about 1 second to download every kilobyte of information under normal circumstances. A 40K file will take about 40 seconds.

Can I speed things up? If you have a slow modem, selecting the *Turn off graphics* mode on the browser will considerably reduce the amount of time it takes to access new documents. A small "placeholder" indicates where graphics would have appeared, sometimes with a brief description of the graphic.

When is rush hour on the web? The worst times to access the Web are between 10 AM and 2 PM and from 6 PM to 10 PM. This is especially true when accessing the Web using a connection through on-line services.

I Keep Getting Error Messages!

The two most common error messages are "Host not found" and "Document not found." If the host's address has been typed correctly, or you are connecting from a hyperlink, then clicking on *Refresh (Reload)* could solve the first problem. If the problem persists, then something is wrong with the address (check your source) or the host server is unavailable.

The second error message may mean that the document has been renamed or moved, so trimming the document name from the address may get you to a point where you can relocate the original document. Sometimes you will need to truncate the directories as well. For example, if "http://www.mosby.com/whatsnew.html" doesn't work, then cutting the URL back to just "http://www.mosby.com" may do the trick. Remember, the Web is a rapidly evolving place, and as new sites are built, older sites are taken down or relocated. When all else fails, you can search the Internet for information relating to that site.

Exploring the Web

"Fun Internet Resources" (Appendix 3) lists a good number of places to start. Because the Web is an enormous information resource, doubling in size every 6 months, it is becoming increasingly difficult to locate the material you need. One of the solutions to this has been the development of search engines. These automated software tools roam the Web indexing every document and hyperlink they come across, and feeding the information back into gigantic databases such as Yahoo!, Excite, and AltaVista.

By sending a query to a search engine, it is possible to quickly search millions of documents for specific words or particular combinations of words. The search results are sent back in the form of a list of hyperlinks to the documents that matched your request. Often each link has a brief description, with further clues as to whether the page will have what you are looking for. Chapter 6 introduces the best search engines and provides strategies for more effective searches.

Limit or Limiters (also known as qualifiers) Options available in MEDLINE and other databases that allow the user to limit the entire result to be retrieved. These include limiting your result by language of journal, years of the database, type of publication, and type of study.

⚡ POWER TIP

Using a program called DOSLynx, it is possible to surf the Web under DOS. Only text pages will be visible using this method, and all complex formatting, such as tables, fonts, and color will be ignored. Graphics will be ignored or replaced with a description along the lines of "This is a picture of a sheep." DOSLynx can be run as a stand-alone program or accessed through the Internet using Telnet. Appendix 2, "Internet Providers and Obtaining Internet Software," provides more information.

USENET

Usenet newsgroups represent the de facto Internet community. This is the place where millions of ordinary people worldwide hangout, share experiences, write about their day-to-day lives, and buy and sell things. It has been said that the entire sum of human knowledge has been posted at some point in newsgroup messages, but some say they don't believe anything written in a Usenet posting. Somewhere between these two extremes is the definitive answer for what newsgroups are all about.

This is the Internet equivalent of public meetings at a town hall, a very big town hall, with thousands of rooms, each containing groups of people having distinctive ongoing conversations about any subject imaginable.

Finding a Newsgroup

There are in excess of 18,500 Usenet newsgroups. These are grouped into the following seven major hierarchies:

Comp: Computers
News: Usenet and Internet
Rec: Recreation, the arts, and hobbies
Sci: Science
Soc: Social issues
Talk: Debate on controversial issues
Misc: Everything else

There are many less common newsgroup hierarchies, a few examples of which are the following:

Alt: Alternative newsgroups
Bionet: Biology
Biz: Business, advertising
K12: Education to grade 12
JP, NZ, TW: Newsgroups for particular countries (i.e., Japan, New Zealand, or Taiwan)

These are the topmost hierarchies, and from them are lots of branches. This is a continually evolving community with hundreds of newsgroups added each year. Currently, there are around 150 newsgroups with subject areas directly related to health care issues including "alt.health.cfidsaction," "alt.med.allergy," "alt.support.cancer.prostate," and "misc.kids.pregnancy." However, well over 300 are related to various sexual matters, and there are newsgroups for authors, hobbies, pets, forms of transport, classified ads, and all popular TV shows, and newsgroups for totally frivolous subjects like "alt.barney.dinosaur.die.die.die."

It is becoming increasingly more common for private newsgroups to be established at a particular Internet location. These newsgroups can be identified by the lack of an established Usenet hierarchy as part of their names. Netscape's newsgroups are probably the most well known of these. Many of these private newsgroups are for internal use only and cannot be accessed from the Internet, but others (including Netscape) can be accessed if referenced correctly.

Participating in a Newsgroup

A message in a newsgroup is commonly called an article (or post), and although articles are similar to e-mail, they are not created using e-mail software. You must use a separate program called a newsreader to compose and read newsgroup articles. Appendix 2, "Internet Providers and Obtaining Internet Software," provides more information on obtaining newsreaders.

All a newsgroup does is bring together articles that have been posted to that particular newsgroup, arranged by the subject header. At any time there may be dozens of distinct subjects being discussed within each newsgroup.

When you access Usenet for the first time, you will need to compile a list of the newsgroups in which you are interested. Your Usenet source should have a list of all the newsgroups it carries; this is available as a searchable database or a file that can be downloaded. You then subscribe to these newsgroups in the manner prescribed by your newsreader software.

There are also other options to be set, such as the address of your news source and your e-mail address. Modern newsreader software also allows you the choice of whether you want to receive just a list of new message headers or all articles complete with full text. Sometimes the *Headers Only* is the preferred option if the newsgroup carries a lot of traffic. You can then work through the message headers off-

Login
The process of identifying yourself as an authorized user at the start of a computer session.

line, tagging only the articles that interest you. During your next session these "tagged" articles will be retrieved. This not only saves on the amount of unnecessary postings to wade through, but also could dramatically cut the amount of time you are on-line, thereby saving on connect charges and your time.

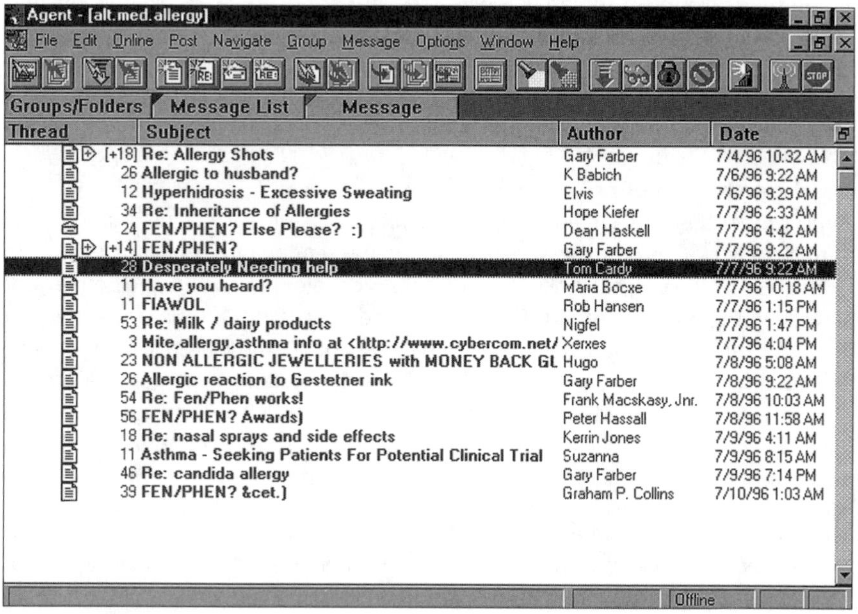

FIGURE 3–4.—*Example of Newsgroup articles.*

Mailing list
An automatic means of including everyone in the circulation of e-mail messages sent to a specific mailing list.

In Figure 3–4, you can see an example of articles posted to the newsgroup "alt.med.allergy." Each subject appears on a separate line and clearly shows the author, message length, and the date posted. Replies to articles are grouped together; for instance, the message titled "FEN/PHEN" has 14, and "Re: Allergy Shots" has 18. If an article has replies to it, then the total number of these is indicated alongside the subject header. If there are no replies, then the message length is the number alongside each message, which tells how many lines of text there are. Clicking on a message will display it or expand a list of replies.

These postings have all the same elements of an e-mail message. There are *To, From, Date,* and *Subject* fields, along with other unique fields that reference the place of the message in the "thread" of an ongoing subject. Newsreader software uses these references to display articles in the correct sequence. So for instance, if someone had posted a message with a car for sale, the next message in the thread would be a reply from someone asking the price. Subsequent articles would then expand on this, with more people getting involved.

Unfortunately, articles have a habit of drifting completely away from the original subject and someone joining the conversation later on (when all the earlier articles have expired) will see a subject saying "Car for Sale!" and will open up the articles to find everyone now talking about trekking in the Himalayas. It is easy to change the subject header so it reflects more of the current discussion, but this never seems to happen.

Mapping
The user enters a conventional "textword," term, or phrase that is "mapped" to the appropriate MeSH. (This is either by choice or done covertly by the search engine.)

If you select a subject thread you will discover people asking questions, posting replies, and just plain talking. There are also lots of people who do not take an active part in the discussions, preferring just to read the articles posted. They are called, perhaps unflatteringly, "lurkers." Many lurkers are newcomers who are still getting a feel for what the newsgroup is all about.

Posting to Newsgroups
Replies to articles can be made by posting a follow-up article to the newsgroup or by sending a private e-mail message to the original sender. Often, you may want to quote part of the original article so your reply is coherent to someone who may not have seen the original posting. This can be done by copying the relevant article and pasting it into your reply. Usually the more than symbol (>) is placed in front of each line to differentiate it from your message. Several newsreader programs insert this symbol automatically when you reply to an article. It is considered good form to quote only the most relevant passages and not the entire message. Adding a "Re:" to the subject header also indicates that it is a follow-up reply.

New threads may be created by simply posting an article with a new subject. Remember, newsgroups are public forums, and although articles may seem like ongoing conversations among only a few people, there is a surprisingly large amount of interest by those not directly contributing to the discussion.

An article usually contains plain text, but it is possible to convert pictures or other binary files into a text file that can then be imported or pasted into an article. Obviously this message will need to be converted again before it can be used, and a lot of newsreaders handle this automatically. However, you may need to save the article to a separate file and then manually run it through the conversion software. Articles composed like this will be much larger than usual and will often be split into multiple parts, each part labeled in sequence. Usually the subject header will indicate if this is the case. A lot of these types of postings contain pornographic images and will be found only in those newsgroups.

When a new article is sent to a newsgroup, Usenet distributes this around the entire Usenet system, which is hosted on computers all over the Internet. So when people access their favorite newsgroups, the material they are reading can be located on a local Usenet computer host, rather than a Usenet host in another country.

Frequently Asked Questions
Newcomers to Usenet should read the articles in the newsgroup "news.announce.newusers." There is a wealth of information about how Usenet operates and the "do's and don'ts" of composing and posting articles.

Because of the limited amount of storage space and the sheer volume of new articles (1 million+ every week), articles are usually only kept available for a short period (usually 7 days) before expiring. This unfortunately causes a lot of similar questions to be asked over and over, much to the annoyance of regular newsgroup participants.

A scheme has developed whereby most popular newsgroups have a person (or several people) who maintain the "FAQ" or Frequently Asked Questions list. This FAQ explains what the newsgroup is about, its history, and any rules and attempts to answer all the common questions that newcomers might ask. The FAQ is updated regularly and posted every month or so to the newsgroup. Often this is the best place to look before asking questions related to the newsgroup or Usenet itself. There are also Web sites that maintain a collection of all the FAQs, usually with some sort of search mechanism.

Some newsgroups are moderated, meaning that all posts are directed to a moderator instead of posted directly to the newsgroup. The moderator examines new articles for content and appropriateness. Most newsgroups, unfortunately, are not moderated, so there are many inappropriate articles, which can be short annoying "I agree" type messages, advertising, offensive language, incorrectly posted articles, and multiple copies of the same article. In small newsgroups this is not such a problem, but in the bigger newsgroups where hundreds of new articles are posted every day, this "signal to noise" ratio can be very low.

Accessing Newsgroups

Depending on how you access the Internet, it is possible that your business or institution is a Usenet host, in which case the system administrator should be able to give you all the information necessary to get connected. If this is not the case, you can access newsgroups through your ISP or on-line service or by subscribing to a Usenet news provider. Most of these places will provide you with the appropriate newsreader software or will advise you as to what you will need. CompuServe and America Online for instance, have newsreader capabilities built into their existing software.

Usually there is not an extra charge to access newsgroups, because they are regarded as a basic part of any Internet service. However, gaining access through a dedicated News provider can ensure that you receive all newsgroups available and also all articles that are posted. Many ISPs and on-line services restrict or limit the types of newsgroups they carry, and sometimes they do not reliably provide all the articles.

On the other hand, a separate News provider operates solely to ensure an uninterrupted Usenet service and will go to far greater lengths to ensure your continued satisfaction. But this means you pay an additional fee to access their service. See Chapter 5 for more information.

Newsreader Software

Newsreaders come as two distinct types: (1) those that only allow newsgroups to be read on-line and (2) those that enable articles to be downloaded for reading and composing replies offline. If you access the Internet using CompuServe or America Online,

Medical subject headings (MeSH)
The *Annotated Alphabetic List* is a massive printed thesaurus made up of hundreds of thousands of clinical, biomedical, pharmaceutical, and basic terms. These indexing terms are called MeSH and are used by the indexers to create MEDLINE.

then you need nothing extra to read newsgroups; however, there are several key features about each service that should be clarified.

CompuServe

- Newsgroups can be accessed by a computer running Windows, DOS, or Mac.
- Single articles or entire threads can be saved to a disk for reading off-line.
- Articles can be searched by subject, author, or date.

America Online

- Articles can be downloaded automatically, by using the *FlashSession* feature, to the personal filing cabinet for reading or replying off-line.
- Articles containing pictures or other nontext files can be decoded easily by the *FileGrabber* feature. When a nontext message is opened, a dialog box appears asking if you want to decode the file or save it to decode manually.
- The full text of all newsgroup articles in the personal filing cabinet can be searched.

Agent

This is the best newsreader available for computers running Windows. It is available in two versions, Free Agent, which is available at no cost, and AGENT, which contains more features and must be purchased. Separate versions for Windows 3.1 and Windows 95 are also available.

Key features include the following:

- Archive folders can be created or copied.
- Articles that have been read can be archived to folders or saved on a disk.
- Message headers can be downloaded and tagged for later retrieval.
- Off-line reading and replying are available.
- Pictures and other objects can be decoded automatically.
- There is a built-in e-mail package with an address book.
- Filters process e-mail and newsgroup articles according to rules.
- A *Kill Files* feature includes filters that allow for articles to be ignored if they contain key phrases or they come from particular individuals.
- The software can be configured for several different news sources.

MacSoup

This is a very good shareware program for the Mac. Key features include the following:

- Message headers can be downloaded and tagged for later retrieval.
- A *Kill Files* feature indicates filters that allow articles to be ignored if they contain key phrases or they come from particular individuals.
- An e-mail program is built in.
- Multiple mailboxes with separate filters are included for sorting mail.

MEDLINE

MEDLINE is a collection of bibliographic citations, now numbering in the tens of millions. MEDLINE is licensed to more than 100 vendors, who mount it on their own retrieval systems.

Reading Newsgroups With a Web Browser

Many Web sites allow access to current newsgroups and archives of old postings. Several major sites have been established that enable users to search postings using criteria such as author, key words, and date. These sites have been constructed to allow articles to be read and replies to be sent without an additional newsreader. See Chapter 5 for more information.

Netscape is unique among Web browsers because it has a very good built-in newsreader. Unfortunately it is also the slowest way to access newsgroups. All mail is read on-line. Netscape also hosts a collection of private newsgroups through its Web site (select User Groups on the contents page).

Version 2 of the Microsoft Internet Explorer is equipped with only a rudimentary on-line newsreader, although a more elaborate version is available as an add-on. Microsoft also runs a large number of private newsgroups. Look for the "Microsoft." newsgroup hierarchy.

TELNET

By using Telnet it is possible to operate a specific computer through the Internet as easily as if it were on the desk in front of you. This ability is very handy when you are traveling and need to access files located on your desktop computer way back where. By remotely accessing your system (if it is up and running), you can access programs, read your e-mail, and transfer files.

Telnet is one of the oldest Internet applications, but it is rapidly being superseded by the graphic user environments of Windows and Mac OS. Unfortunately, most long distance work is relegated to tasks that can be run through a command line interface (like DOS); these are primarily text and accessing menu options. But this makes it ideal for accessing remote databases, on-line library catalogs, playing games, and other specific textbased Internet applications.

A modern use for Telnet is internally within large companies to allow offsite workers the ability to run computer programs in the main office. Within such an internal network, it is possible for a much wider range of customized programs to be operated than could possibly be maintained on each user's personal computer.

Telnet sessions are started by running the Telnet software and supplying the name of the computer you wish to access. When the connection is made, a login and password request will be initiated, which then clears the way for you to use the remotely connected computer. Typically, most public Telnet sites allow you to log in as a guest (type "guest" at the login prompt), and supply your e-mail address as your password (or type "anonymous").

Metathesaurus
Part of the Unified Medical Language System (UMLS) project at NLM, the Metathesaurus is made up of hundreds of thousands of terms, from diagnostic classification schemes to preferred names of procedures. This massive thesaurus, of which MeSH is but a small part, is part of an effort to interpret the terms entered by users into the generally more powerful terms used in the original indexing process.

Because you are accessing a remote computer, the functionality of the computer you are sitting in front of is restricted only to those keyboard commands that the remote computer can understand. Usually this means most function keys are disabled, along with any customized keyboard commands. This can prove to be a frustrating experience until you are more familiar with it. Most Telnet commands are sent by using the page up and page down keys and multiple-key sequences (e.g., controlH or controlA) and using the arrow keys to navigate menus. The most useful command to learn is the *Help* feature, which you can usually reach by using ctrlH or by typing "help."

MIME
Multipurpose Internet Mail Extensions. A standard format for encoding files that are attached to e-mail messages so they can be sent reliably through the Internet.

CompuServe offers a Telnet service and provides listings of the most popular Telnet sites. America Online does not offer Telnet as a built-in feature, but it is possible to use additional Telnet software and take advantage of your AOL TCP/IP connection to open a Telnet session. Many smaller on-line services and ISPs offer Telnet access as the entry point or an additional way of accessing their systems.

Windows 95 features a Telnet program called, amazingly enough, Telnet. Using it is as simple as starting your Internet connection and then clicking on the Telnet icon in the Accessories folder. There are a large variety of other Telnet programs available for use. The most popular Windows program is called EWAN, which is available free. Appendix 2, "Internet Providers and Obtaining Internet Software" gives more information about obtaining Telnet software.

⚡ **POWER TIP**

It is possible to access CompuServe using Telnet. This is a very useful service when you are traveling or otherwise unable to use your everyday computer and need to read or send e-mail. Start Telnet and type "Compuserve.com" as the address. At the host prompt type "CIS" and then your normal login. CompuServe is setting up a new mail system, so if a mailbox has been transferred to the new system, mail can only be sent and not read using this method of access. Still, this is a useful workaround when using a computer not loaded with CompuServe software.

INTERNET MAILING LISTS

A mailing list is a collection of names and addresses gathered for a common purpose; for instance, you may have a mailing list showing the e-mail addresses of all your former school friends. Many e-mail programs (e.g., cc:MAIL or Eudora) allow you to address a message to a mailing list rather than creating a lengthy recipient list each time you want to send everyone the same piece of e-mail. Your personal mailing lists are maintained by you as a part of your e-mail address book.

Internet mailing lists are a different kettle of fish entirely. These are automated programs that enable messages to be sent to a large group of people with similar interests, who may not already know each other. When a message is sent to one of these mailing lists, it is automatically forwarded to everyone who subscribes to the list. Internet mailing lists serve the following three main purposes:

- The list can provide a focal point for a particular interest group.
- The list administrator can send information to everyone on the list.
- People on the list can send information to all the other list participants.

Modem
MOdulator-DEModulator. A device that converts data so information can be transmitted through telephone lines to other modems or computers.

Subscribing

Internet mailing lists must first be subscribed to, and in so doing your name is added to the list of recipients. When someone wants to send a message to the mailing list, e-mail software is used to compose a message that is then sent to the mailing list address. Most mailing list addresses begin with the name of the list software, which could be "Listserv," "Majordomo," or "Listproc." This format makes them easier to distinguish from other Internet addresses.

Once you have subscribed to a list you will start to receive all the articles that are subsequently posted to it, but probably the first message you will receive is a message welcoming you to the list and containing important information about how to "unsubscribe" from the list. Print this message and keep it handy, because you will need to refer to it when you decide to stop participating in the mailing list.

Use the following syntax examples to subscribe or unsubscribe to lists hosted by one of the three main mailing list servers:

Listproc: SUBSCRIBE [listname] Firstname Surname
           UNSUBSCRIBE [listname]

Listserv: SUBSCRIBE [listname] Firstname Surname
           SIGNOFF [listname]

Majordomo: SUBSCRIBE [listname]
           UNSUBSCRIBE [listname]

In the [listname] field, enter the name of the mailing list; these commands should appear as the first and only line in your e-mail message. This message should be sent to the mailing list e-mail address, which could look a bit like: LISTSERV@SURFARI.UMYB.EDU

The subject line can be left blank or could say "Subscribe."

Professional Information

In a sense, Internet mailing lists are more immediate versions of Usenet newsgroups, albeit with a much tighter focus and a greater percentage of participation. There are a variety of mailing lists available; many of these are widely advertised and talked about. But there are also a number that are less public. It is these lesser known mailing lists that are probably the most worthwhile to join.

There is probably more professional and career-oriented content to be found in mailing lists than in Usenet newsgroups, and this has everything to do with visibility and accessibility. Usenet is widely available, but it is impossible to know who is reading it at any given time because it is a public forum with few rules or restrictions.

Multitasking
Running more than one program at the same time on the same computer. For instance, printing a document while editing another.

With a mailing list, an interested person first must discover the mailing list address (not always an easy task) and then subscribe to the list. Because a return e-mail address is required, it is always possible to keep track of who receives the list. Some lists attempt to get all new subscribers to qualify their reasons for joining by requiring a short message introducing themselves and their interests.

Every mailing list has an administrator or list owner who handles the day-to-day maintenance and who answers newcomers' questions. If need be, the administrator can remove or add individual's names to the mailing list, but otherwise the processes of subscribing and unsubscribing and delivery of messages are automated by the mailing list software.

Sometimes mailing lists are moderated, which means that all messages posted to it are subject to review before they are forwarded to the list subscribers. This has the welcome effects of ensuring that people stay on the topic, defusing arguments, and weeding out unnecessary messages (like gratuitous advertising).

Many mailing lists, especially those with a lot of traffic, send out digests rather than individual messages. A digest collects multiple messages to be sent out at specific intervals. The advantage is that you receive one e-mail digest containing perhaps 30 messages, rather than 30 individual e-mail messages. This process can make it a lot easier to manage messages, but the downside is that replying to specific messages is no longer easy; quotes and return addresses must be cut and pasted manually.

The Usenet newsgroups "news.lists" and "news.answers" carry an updated list of all publicly accessible mailing lists every month.

⚡ **POWER TIP**

When replying to a mailing list message, you can reply to the mailing list as a whole (the default choice) or send a private message to the original sender. If you are replying privately, check to ensure your response is not also going to the mailing list address. A quick look at the "To" line should confirm this.

FILE TRANSFER PROTOCOL

FTP is the means by which files are transferred around the Internet. These files can be text, multimedia, shareware, or commercial applications. Increasingly, it is becoming the means by which new software is provided to end users, especially people using the Web to access software libraries. FTP is used mostly for downloading files, but it is also the method by which files can be uploaded to another computer.

Initiated via a variety of methods, FTP is typically started automatically by a Web browser or Telnet session, but a program known as an FTP client can be installed on your computer. The latter option provides the most flexibility in accessing files on a remote computer system and also allows for files to be easily uploaded.

An FTP session involves opening an Internet connection, starting your FTP client, and logging on to a host computer. Unlike Telnet, which allows you to control a remote computer, FTP only allows you to examine file names and download a copy of them to your computer. Your level of access to the host computer is usually limited to certain directories, with the ability to upload to only one directory.

Unless you have an access account with the host computer system, you will need to log in as an anonymous user. At the login prompt type "anonymous" (if this does not work try "guest"). If a password is requested, your e-mail address is all that is required.

You are then free to browse the accessible directories and choose the files you wish to download. Ending the session, or logging off is as simple as closing your FTP client program.

National Library of Medicine (NLM)
Located in Bethesda, Maryland. Among numerous other projects, NLM indexes 3,800+ peer-reviewed clinical journals by using the *Annotated Alphabetic List* (a thesaurus) Medical Subject Headings (MeSH). This process creates a bibliographic database called MEDLINE.

⚡ POWER TIP

Sometimes an FTP site provides descriptive or "readme" files with detailed information about other files at the site. These are usually plain text, and depending on your FTP client, you can read these without having to download them first. Reading these files before downloading other large programs can save you the time and effort of copying programs that will not run on your computer.

GOPHER

Before the Web there was Gopher, which was the first successful attempt at making distant Internet resources easily available. Unlike the Web, however, Gopher documents do not contain embedded hyperlinks, graphics, or multimedia content.

Newsgroups
(See Usenet.)

Netiquette
The conduct, decorum, and attitude applied while using the Internet.

Navigation through "Gopherspace" is made possible by navigating around Gopher menu pages. Each menu option can be a document or a pointer to another menu. And like a Web browser, Gopher software knows when to start other programs, such as FTP or Telnet, to retrieve or access particular types of documents. Access to Gopher servers at other locations is made possible by selecting the main menu option for *Other Gopher Servers* or by selecting a menu option that references a document at the other location.

Because of its popularity, there are a lot of Gopher resources that are still not accessible by any other means. So although the rapid development of the Web has eclipsed Gopher's success, there is still a large demand for those documents located on Gopher servers.

Web browsers have the ability to access Gopher resources without additional software. When using a browser, you can distinguish a Gopher site from others by its URL (gopher://) and the fact that only hierarchical menus will be displayed. Clicking on any menu item will "burrow" deeper into the Gopher site.

Gopher was first developed at the University of Minnesota, and this is still the best place to begin an exploration of Gopherspace (Gopher://gopher.tc.umn.edu). Appendix 2, "Internet Services and Software," gives more information about obtaining separate Gopher software.

VERONICA AND JUGHEAD

As Gopher became larger and more standardized, the need to search through Gopher resources quickly for information became very important. Veronica was developed to regularly index all Gopher menu resources on the Internet and make this information available to all Gopher servers. To use Veronica you will need to locate it on your local Gopher server or another set of Gopher menu pages. A successful Veronica search will yield a custom menu page of items matching your search parameters. Selecting any one of these items will take you to the relevant document or other resources.

Veronica is not good at searching specific Gopher sites, so her erstwhile companion, Jughead, was created to search using key words from menus on a specific Gopher server. Although the process is known as Jughead, you will rarely see a menu item saying "Jughead Search." Instead look for a menu item that looks like "Keyword Search of UMN Gopher Menus," which stands for, "Search all Gopher Menus on the University of Minnesota Gopher System."

ARCHIE

Locating specific files on the Internet is difficult. On-line services like CompuServe and AOL maintain large libraries of the most popular files that can be easily searched, but FTP has no built-in search functions. Archie was developed as a means of searching files that are available via FTP.

The Archie filename database is constantly being updated, but in mid 1996 there were more than 2 million files at more than 1,000 anonymous FTP sites. Archie can by accessed through the Web, Telnet, or a separate Archie client program on your computer.

Unfortunately, searches are restricted to the filename or part of the filename. So to initiate a search you must know at least some of the filename. Do not just search on filenames containing ".txt" unless you are prepared to wade through the 50 gazillion files with this prefix. Appendix 2, "Internet Providers and Obtaining Internet Software," gives more information about how to access Archie on-line or obtain Archie software.

Network
A collection of systems and services that include databases, consumer information, bulletin boards, and all the things in Systems and Services that is available for free, for a cost in a proprietary set-up, or through the Internet.

WAIS

With so much information available on the Internet, finding documents that contain specific information is often difficult. To help solve this, WAIS (pronounced "ways"), short for Wide Area Information Servers, was established to provide a regularly updated database of indexed documents.

WAIS databases are located all around the world, so a WAIS search can be specific to just one computer server or all WAIS databases. It is commonly found on many Web servers, allowing easy searching of the server's entire contents. It is more powerful than Veronica alone because it allows for the entire document to be searched and not just the document title.

Searches can be general, that is, any information on computers, or very specific using Boolean search operators (such as AND, OR, or NOT) to create a complex query (e.g., find documents containing computers and operating systems not Unix or mainframes).

Like FTP and Archie, WAIS can by accessed through the Web, Telnet, or a separate WAIS client program on your computer. Appendix 2, "Internet Providers and Obtaining Internet Software," gives more information about how to access WAIS on-line or obtain Archie software.

INTERNET RELAY CHAT (IRC)

IRC is realtime conversation accessible through Telnet or separate IRC programs. This is the on-line equivalent of CB radio, with participants hanging out in thousands of topic-specific Internet chat channels and typing messages to others similarly engaged. It is possible to be active in several channels at the same time and also to send private messages to other IRC users. Depending on the software you use, it is possible to receive notices saying who is in the channel at any given moment and the nicknames of people entering and leaving.

If planned in advance, several people from around the world can converge in one channel and conduct a real-time meeting, with goals beyond those of just chatting. Newer IRC software allows for use of live video and audio during a session, along with file transfers. IRC software is widely available for DOS, Windows 3.1, Windows 95, and the Macintosh. Appendix 2, "Internet Providers and Obtaining Internet Software," provides more detailed information.

Reference

1. Pitta J: The cutting edge: Showdown on the Web: Microsoft, Netscape battle for Net dominance. *Los Angeles Times,* July 8, 1996.

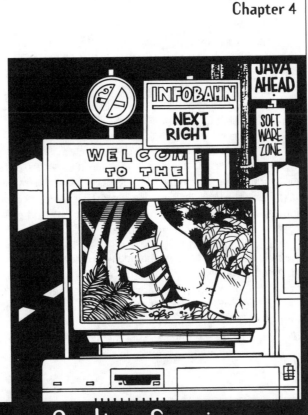

Chapter 4

Choosing an On-line Service

INTERNET SERVICE PROVIDERS AND ON-LINE SERVICES

In Chapter 2 we discussed the important distinction between an Internet Service Provider (ISP) and the commercial on-line services like CompuServe and America Online (AOL). Compuserve and AOL offer an extensive array of exclusive content that can't be found anywhere else on the Internet, and an ISP provides only the means to access the Internet.

Recently, however, this has become more confusing because all the commercial on-line services now provide full Internet access. This comes as a standard part of their existing on-line service or as a separate service whereby you receive only a basic Internet connection. In this regard, there is now no difference between ISPs and on-line services.

So how do you make the decision about your Internet access? Previously we posed a list of questions that should be used to determine whether an ISP would meet your needs. But even this might not be enough to sort the wheat from the chaff, especially because most ISPs offer a standardized range of features that vary little from one plan to the next.

Glossary Terms O–P

On-line/off-line
To be connected to another computer via a network or modem, and the reverse.

On-line services, however, have a depth of original content that enables them to be considered over and above ordinary ISPs. And because their pricing structures aren't that much more expensive than a bare-bones Internet connection through an ISP, these services are more attractive Internet providers. Therefore, this chapter will offer more information about how the on-line services differ from one another and will also help to identify some other means of gaining access to the Internet.

Within the United States, there are three major on-line services: America Online (with 6 million members), CompuServe (4.5 million members) (Table 4–1), and Prodigy (1.5 million members). A number of smaller companies follow: Microsoft Network (MSN), Delphi, and the Well. Internationally, mostly in Western Europe and Asia, there are a number of regionally based on-line services, but CompuServe is the predominant force in providing international connectivity.

The hallmark of most of these companies is the simplified process of getting connected. America Online pioneered the brilliant marketing strategy of inserting its software inside computer and trade magazines. After a few years, CompuServe and Delphi used this advertising method to put their software in the hands of prospective new users. If you have a computer and a modem, then one of their free disks is all it takes to connect. If you use Windows 95, then instant access to the MSN is available without having to do anything more than clicking on the MSN logo on the desktop.

Operating system
A collection of programs that controls a computer's operations, enabling users to run their own programs and use other devices connected to the computer (e.g., printers, mice, and scanners)

TABLE 4–1.—Key Features of AOL and CompuServe

Feature	CompuServe	AOL
DOS interface	Yes	No
International network/membership	150 countries	Partial (Europe, Japan, Asia)
ISDN dial-up	Yes	No
Basic Fee	$9.95 per month	$9.95 per month
Number of Internet hours included each month	5	5
Frequent user plan	$24.95 for 20 hours, $1.95 each additional hour	$19.95 for 20 hours, $2.95 each additional hour
International communication surcharges	$3.00 to $10.00 per hour using local access numbers (US$)	$6.00 to $42.00 per hour using local & long distance numbers (US$)
Free magazinze	Yes	No
Free home page	Yes (1 MB)	Yes (2 MB)
Threaded forum messages	Yes	No
Integrated filing. System	Yes	Messages/Usenet only
External newsreaders, e-mail programs	Yes	No, must use AOL software
TCP/IP Winsock supplied	Yes	Only with AOL version 3

CompuServe

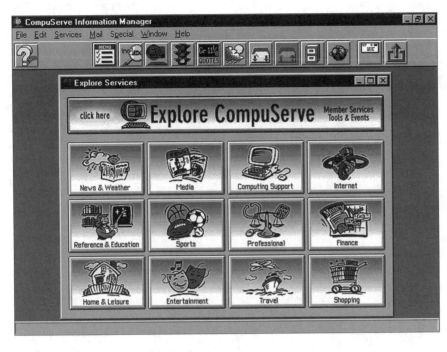

FIGURE 4–1.—*CompuServe WinCIM software interface.*

Packet
Data sent across a network are composed of data packets. An e-mail message might be sent as several packets.

CompuServe (Fig 4–1) is the longest established commercial on-line service, providing computer services to companies and individuals around the world for 3 decades. With 4.5 million members, it now is a close second behind AOL's 6 million–strong membership base. However, it attracts a much higher number of computer industry professionals and business executives than does any other on-line service.

Other than its longevity, CompuServe boasts an extensive range of information content, ranging from computer product support to the latest in health care research. Much of this is supplied in conjunction with outside information providers and, as such, is accessible by paying a premium above and beyond the ordinary CompuServe membership fees. The cost for these premium services ranges from several dollars per hour to $20 per hour, priced in minute increments. Premium services are denoted by a '$' symbol in all menus and icons.

Key Content Areas on CompuServe

Time Magazine, CNN, People Magazine, Rolling Stone, Sports Illustrated, Books in Print, exclusive access to parts of the Time/Warner Pathfinder Web site, ZD Net (contents of popular computer magazines and software libraries), Executive News Clipping service, United Connection (Air and travel bookings), and Worlds-Away—a three-dimensional chat world populated by other CompuServe members, using three-dimensional graphics to simulate real-life activities—are all available on CompuServe. Information USA is a popular area that explains how to seek out

U.S. government information and U.S. phone directories (searchable by address and name). And PaperChase and IQuest provide "front ends" to hundreds of other external databases containing millions of published journals, books, and government publications.

Information is grouped under 12 broad subject headings and is accompanied by associated forums containing messaging areas, software and file libraries, and conferences.

CompuServe's best feature is its breadth of support for computer products. This support ranges from providing forums for every type of hardware and software product, as well as the whole gamut of Internet and communications issues, to supplying libraries with the latest software patches and upgrades for most computer types.

Accessing CompuServe
Presently CompuServe is accessed by using one of several methods:

1. Dial-up shell account, using any basic communications package

2. CompuServe's own CIM graphic software (WinCIM for Windows 3.1) and MacCIM.

3. Off-line CompuServe Navigator software (Windows version, CSNav and the Mac version, MacNav). These programs automate access and reduce connect time by quickly retrieving and sending messages, files, and reports.

CompuServe plans to transfer all of its services to a Web-based format late in 1996, which will by necessity replace all current access methods with a common Web browser interface.

Access speeds range from 300 bps (bits per second) to 56 Kbps ISDN (Integrated Services Digital Network).

Internet Connections
CompuServe is accompanied by a Web browser called Spry Mosaic, which provides basic Web browsing capabilities. A full range of other Internet tools are provided as standard, including FTP, Gopher, Usenet, and Telnet. You are free to use these software tools or supplant them with others.

CompuServe comes with a built-in TCP/IP (Transport Control Protocol/Internet protocol) stack, allowing any SLIP/PPP (Serial Line Internet Protocol/ Point to Point Protocol) compliant software to be used in conjunction with it.

CompuServe members can construct their own Web sites and have these hosted through CompuServe.

International Connections
CompuServe can be accessed at local and long distance telephone rates in more than 150 countries. Use the keyword GO PHONES for access numbers in the United States and around the world. Communications surcharges apply in many countries.

Page
See *Home page.*

Parallel port
Attached to most computers to transmit data to another device (usually a printer) using parallel transmission, that is, sending data simultaneously over separate wires.

America Online

Within a few short years, AOL (Fig 4–2) has rapidly become the largest on-line service. Its content is comprehensive and ranges across the spectrum from personal interests to professional issues. There are forums and chat groups for almost any subject. Particularly strong areas are those relating to Sports and Entertainment and Children's Education.

Key Content Areas on AOL

ABC News, *New York Times, Newsweek, Wired,* MTV Online, ZD Net, *Consumer Reports,* chat rooms, News Profiles (news clipping service), Library of Congress Online, and People Connection (live chat) are available on AOL. America Online also "hosts" several areas on behalf of professional organizations; the organizations maintain their own content, and access is available only to members of the relevant organizations.

Several features allow for AOL to be personalized for different members of your household. In fact, each AOL subscription can include up to five different people, each with their own screen names, mailboxes, and filing cabinets to store retrieved materials. Each additional account can be separately configured with parental controls or personal preferences for software settings.

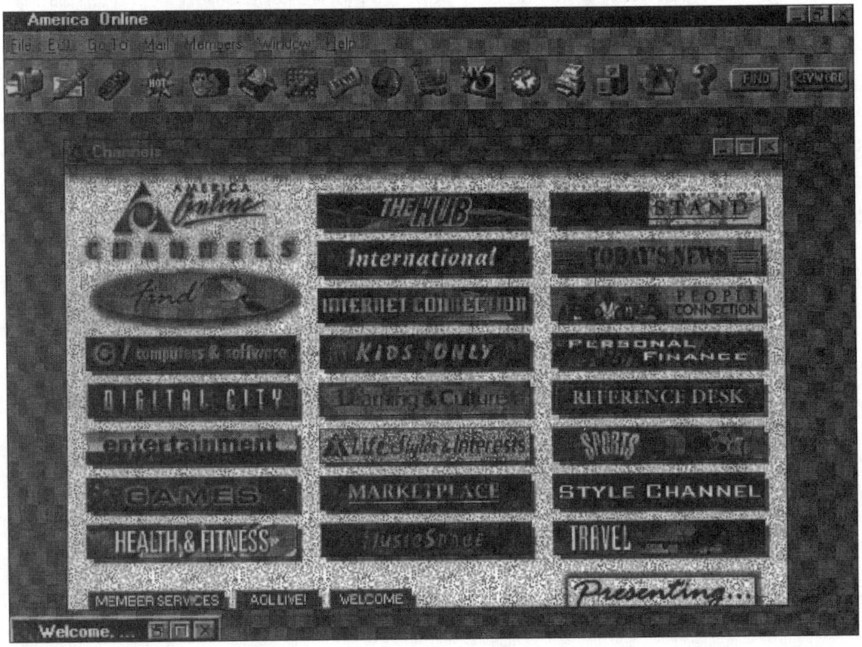

Plug-in
Software applications that attach to Web browsers and extend their capabilities (e.g., video, 3D, animation, audio).

FIGURE 4–2.—*AOL Software Interface.*

Plug and play
A standard way of setting up hardware and software automatically. When installed, the plug and play device identifies itself to the operating system so it can be configured without further work.

Accessing AOL

America Online can be accessed only by using the proprietary AOL software (Windows and Mac). Version 3 comes complete with its own TCP/IP stack, which allows for other SLIP/PPP compliant Internet software to be used in conjunction with it. Unfortunately, this does not include external e-mail or newsreader software, which will not connect to AOL.

By using the FlashSessions feature, it is possible to minimize connection time by scheduling an automated access session to collect or send e-mail and retrieve subscribed Usenet articles. These sessions can be run at any time, with or without your supervision.

Access speeds range from 2,400 bps to 28.8 Kbps, although AOL can also be reached through any TCP/IP connection allowing superfast access.

Internet Connections

A built-in Web browser is standard with the AOL package, although it leaves a lot to be desired. America Online is planning to replace this browser with a choice of Microsoft Internet Explorer or Netscape Navigator. A useful feature is how Web sites have been integrated into many AOL areas, so forums may contain links to external Web resources, as well as to internal AOL resources.

Other built-in tools include FTP, Usenet and Gopher. Telnet is available through external Telnet software, which must be obtained separately. The File Grabber feature of the Newsreader software automatically decodes pictures and binary files from Usenet newsgroups.

Members of AOL can construct their own Web sites and have these hosted through AOL.

International Connections

Global access to AOL is available through the AOL Global Network and Sprint Net. This carries a hefty surcharge outside of the continental United States and Canada, although local access numbers are available for many foreign cities. Access speeds vary, but 14.4K seems to be the optimum speed available. Use the keyword AOL-GLOBALNET for a list of international phone numbers.

⚡ **POWER TIP**

If you are traveling outside the continental United States and have another account through CompuServe or an ISP, use this connection to make a TCP/IP connection to AOL and avoid the costly communications surcharges.

WOW!

After bombarding the country with television commercials and splashy ads in *Time, People,* and the *Wall Street Journal,* in 1996, CompuServe launched its new consumer on-line information service, WOW! This is a "light" version of existing CompuServe content, essentially a collection of its best and most accessible features. These include The Weather Channel, Reuters news services, *Sports Illustrated, Consumer Reports, National Geographic, Grolier's Interactive Encyclopedia,* and chat rooms.

The emphasis for WOW! is on providing simple access to the Internet with a user friendly graphic interface that incorporates a customized version of Microsoft Internet Explorer. This allows a seamless link between proprietary WOW! content and that of the Internet. Basic e-mail and a Usenet newsreader are available as part of the WOW! package, but these can be easily replaced with other, better SLIP/PPP software.

This is still a new service, with many potholes still to be filled. However, the following key features make it an appealing prospect for someone who wants Internet access:

- A free 1-month trial membership
- Unlimited use, including unrestricted access to the Internet for $17.95 per month ($14.95 per month for existing CompuServe members)
- Up to six users can share a single account (with individual e-mail addresses)
- Parental controls to block or restrict Internet access for children

Of course, there are some drawbacks to WOW! You can only use WOW! if you're running Windows 95 and have a CD-ROM drive. A Macintosh version of WOW! is scheduled for release in late 1996.

Sprynet

CompuServe also provides a global Internet access package called Sprynet. This provides complete Internet access in more than 150 countries, with over 480 POPs (Points of Presence) to choose from. Access speeds go up to 28.8 Kbps. Pricing plans in countries other than the United States and Canada are very competitive and include unlimited access. Coverage is extensive in the United Kingdom and Europe. Unlimited pricing plans are available in the United States for $19.95 a month, including a startup software package.

Global Network Navigator (GNN)

This is AOL's barebones ISP. There is little proprietary content, although the GNN home page has a continually changing series of materials, including "the Best of the Web." Subscribers to GNN can build their own Web home pages and have access to exclusive GNN software to help them achieve this. At present, each subscriber receives 20 MB of space to store the home page, which surpasses every other ISP.

Below are other services available to GNN subscribers:

Smart Hotlist: This maintains a catalog of your favorite Web sites and automatically monitors them for changes or additions.

POP
Point of Presence. A geographical location where an Internet service provider maintains a dial-up connection for modem users. For example, an ISP based in San Francisco could have POPs around the country.

Virtual Places: You create an *avatar* (a graphic representation of yourself), which you can then use to represent yourself during on-line chats with other Virtual Places users. Avatars can display gestures and other expressions, adding to the communication experience. You can also pull together a group of on-line friends and take them on a guided tour of your favorite Web sites.

GNN provides 20 hours of Internet access per month for $14.95, with additional hours priced at $1.95. Access is provided through more than 1,000 POPs in the United States and Canada. Worldwide access is available through the AOL Global Network, with hefty communications surcharges.

OTHER ON-LINE SERVICES

Prodigy

Once upon a time, Prodigy was one of the leading on-line services; unfortunately, it never received the same amount of attention that was bestowed on CompuServe and AOL, despite being the first service to offer complete Internet access. In 1996, its owners (Sears and IBM) sold it, and its future is uncertain.

The strongest areas are its chat rooms and mailing lists, where every conceivable interest is catered to, and quite a number hold interest to people seeking health care information. Users can create their own chat rooms and can limit who has access.

A variety of pricing plans are available, but the one of most substance is 30 hours a month for $29.95, with additional hours priced at $2.95. Access speeds are available around the United States at up to 28.8 Kbps.

The Microsoft Network

Launched at the same time as Windows 95, MSN was originally intended as a serious competitor of CompuServe and AOL. Its integration in the Windows 95 desktop, meant that Internet access was only one click away for all Windows 95 users. The unexpected sudden popularity of the Web changed all this, and MSN is still struggling to find its place. By the end of 1996, the entire service will have been migrated to a fee-based Web site, with substantial parts of its content available free to everyone who visits.

Whether MSN will become anything other than just another Web site, remains to be seen. Certainly Microsoft is moving on to bigger and better things, as witnessed by the MSNBC cable TV and Internet news operation.

Microsoft Network does provide full Internet access and proprietary content, although very little relates to health care issues. Access costs are $6.95 per month, including 3 free hours and additional hours priced at $2.50. Access speeds are available right up to ISDN, although these will become faster once MSN becomes Web-based.

Proprietary
A service that has its own software protocols and is connected by modem to an individual user.

Protocol
Describes a formal method of describing data formats and the rules two computers must follow to correctly exchange that data.

Delphi

This is another on-line service that is going through a major restructuring after having been sold several times over the past 5 years. Proprietary content covers a wide range of interests, especially computer and business issues. Multi player games are also well established, along with chat rooms and special interest forums. A variety of content relates to health care.

Delphi is unique because it allows users to create and maintain their own forum areas, with complete control over who has access and over the content.

Subscribers can build their own Web home pages, and each subscriber receives 10 MB of space to store the home page. Access costs are around $20.00 a month for 20 hours, with additional hours available at $1.80 per hour.

Proxy server
Some networks are not connected directly to the Internet but are protected by a firewall. Proxy servers forward requests for information through the firewall to the requested server and return the information to the user.

The WELL

Started in 1985 by the folks who published the Whole Earth catalogs and the *Whole Earth Review,* the WELL (Whole Earth 'Lectronic Link) has an interesting and eclectic set of subscribers. Because its membership hovers in the 10,000 range (not the millions), there is a strong sense of community.

Set loosely by topic, each discussion area is called a conference and may be open, limited, or closed. Several cover health care topics, both classic and modern, with lively discussions. Files are available for downloading.

Like Delphi and Prodigy, the WELL, too, was sold in the recent past. The new management aims to run the business as a for-profit venture while trying to maintain the best of the WELL's qualities. For example, a handful of conferences look at the WELL itself, its internal and external developments, what the problems are, and how to resolve them. The management team is not only known by name, but also all members of this team read and post in the conferences themselves.

Complete Internet access is available in addition to the WELL's other services. Unlike CompuServe and AOL, the WELL has set up a package of shareware programs (including Netscape, Eudora, and Agent) for those who want Windows access. The WELL also provides basic e-mail and text-based Internet access. Several years ago, a (now former) WELL member created a free program called Sweeper to automate conference reading and posting, saving connect time and telephone charges. Local access is available in more than 250 U.S. cities. Pricing plans start around $15 a month.

CONCLUSION

The continued success of the Web has certainly forced all of the on-line services to re-evaluate their offerings in the midst of so much material being freely available. CompuServe and AOL are experiencing a dramatic slowdown in new memberships.

It's too early to say whether the interest has peaked in the type of services offered by CompuServe and AOL. After all, at an unbeatable price they still maintain a depth and breadth of information that is unavailable anywhere else.

Proxy services
All data traffic is checked by a proxy before being sent through a firewall and on to the receiving computer. The proxy, hopefully, prevents an untoward event.

The sheer vastness of the Internet makes it a tremendous task to locate specific resources of interest. At least in this regard, on-line services manage to break it down into more manageable clumps that can be found time and time again (with a degree of certainty that they will still be accessible). However the shakedown of the small players shows no sign of abating, and there are clear signs that this uncertain future is speeding up the defection of existing subscribers to transfer to the larger on-line services or ISPs.

Regardless of how this all plays out in the foreseeable future, CompuServe and AOL will be in a much stronger position to survive if they continue their present trend of moving away from proprietary access software like CIM or the AOL software package, and toward software packages such as Web browsers that do not depend on just one service. The next chapter details the methods whereby your existing CompuServe and AOL software can be adapted to better suit this new environment.

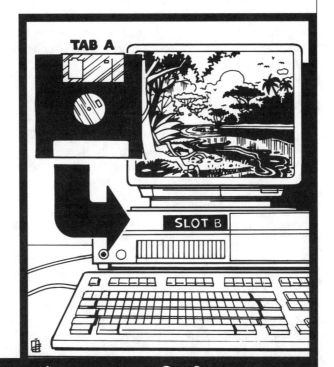

Chapter 5

Optimizing Internet Software

There comes a time when your existing software no longer cuts it. It could be that newer versions are available with better time-saving features, that you have changed operating systems, or that you just want to try a different program. One of the great things about TCP/IP (transport control protocol/Internet protocol) applications is that you are free to swap from one to the other, and even replace certain components, without compromising your ability to get on-line.

This is perfectly illustrated by the Windows and Mac CIM software that comes with CompuServe. By itself, the program takes care of your basic Internet needs (e.g., e-mail, WWW, Usenet, Telnet, Gopher, and FTP), and although these are all easy to use, they only operate with the most basic of features. For instance, when reading Usenet newsgroups, it is not possible to review articles that you have already read without first resetting the default settings. And even then, the articles may have expired and be no longer available. Using an external newsreader resolves this problem and conveniently provides additional options for accessing and searching articles.

Glossary Terms S

SCSI
Small Computer Systems Interface. A standard way of connecting devices to a computer, usually for data storage. It is a faster alternative to parallel interface.

This chapter assumes an intermediate knowledge of Internet software and computer operating systems. The focus is in identifying the techniques and strategies that will help you assemble the best collection of software tools for your Internet surfari. For ease of reference all these tips have been grouped under headings that correlate to their broad subject areas.

SDI
Selected Dissemination of Information. A popular feature on some proprietary systems, SDI is a function whereby a "folder" is created with a search strategy in it, and whenever the database (usually MEDLINE) is updated, any citations that match the strategy are "tossed" into your folder for convenient viewing.

WWW BROWSERS

Sending E-mail in Microsoft Internet Explorer (MSIE)

There is no built-in e-mail program in MSIE; however, if you have an external e-mail program and are accessing the Internet through an Internet Service Provider (ISP) or CompuServe, you can configure your external e-mail software to be launched automatically by MSIE when needed.

The following instructions will work with all versions of MSIE, Windows and Mac.

Step A

1. In any Desktop Window select "Edit/Options" on the menu bar.
2. Click once on the "Filetypes" tab.
3. Scroll down until you reach URL:MailTo protocol.
4. Click once on "Edit."
5. Under "Actions" highlight "Open."
6. Click once on "Edit."
7. Use "Browse" to select your external e-mail application.
8. Click once on "OK."
9. Click once on "Close."

Step B

Configure your e-mail software so messages can be sent and received from your Internet provider. If it is not already configured, you will need to read the instruction manual that was supplied and have this set up before proceeding.

Step C

When using MSIE, type "mailto:" in the "Open Internet Address" box (use File/Open). This launches your e-mail software. Sending mail from this point proceeds in the usual manner. Close your e-mail software when you are finished.

With a CompuServe connection, you can only send e-mail messages using an external mail program; you cannot receive them. To do this, you still need to use your WinCIM or MacCIM software.

Setting Your MSIE Start Page to a Blank Page

When first installed, MSIE sets up the URL "http://www.msn.com" as your default home page. Until this is changed, each time you start MSIE this is the first page you will see. You can specify any URL as a start home page, including files on your own computer, but starting MSIE with a blank page is not so straightforward.

1. Create a new file using Notepad (TeachText on the Mac).
2. Leave the file empty and call it "Homepage.htm" and save.
3. Close this file and start MSIE.
4. Click "File/Open," find "Homepage.htm" and open it.
5. Click "View/Options" on the menu bar.
6. Click the Start And Search Pages tab, and then click "Use Current."

Whenever you start MSIE in the future, it will begin with this blank page.

Configuring Netscape for Multiple Users

Netscape stores all its default settings, including your e-mail address and configuration preferences in a file called Netscape.ini. When two people want to use the same version of Netscape they are forced to use this same set of user preferences and the same default bookmark file. Obviously this doesn't allow any flexibility in recognizing two different users with varying e-mail addresses or ISP connections, as well as separate bookmark lists.

The solution is to create a different Netscape.ini file for each user. By creating a new directory or folder for each user with its own version of the netscape.ini file, you can then make a modification to the command line instruction that starts Netscape, pointing to the relevant user's file.

This solution will also allow you to run different versions of Netscape on your computer, configured for either different ISP's or other changes.

Windows 3.1

1. You first need to create a new directory to store all your configuration files. Copy to this directory your existing netscape.ini file.

2. Create a new program icon. (In Program Manager select File, New/Program. Select New Program Item and then click on OK.)

3. In the Program Item Properties window, type a description for this program (e.g., Nigel's Netscape).

4. Use Browse to locate the program file (e.g., Netscape.exe). The path and file name of the program will then appear in the Command Line dialog box.

5. Position the cursor at the end of this line and add a space and the following: -i c:\netscape\netscape.ini (substitute c:\netscape with the directory you created in step 1.)

6. Click on OK. The new program icon will appear in Program Manager.

Search capabilities
The way in which the search engine treats the search strategy that has been entered in the blank box(es). Capabilities include Boolean operators, the use of parentheses, the ability to refine or limit the search, and the mapping to MeSH.

7. Double click this icon to start Netscape and then work through all the configuration options that are applicable for this user.

8. Repeat steps 1 through 7 for each additional user or version of Netscape.

Windows 95

Search engine
The programming or software applications behind the functionality, in other words, the machine that drives the search capabilities inherent in the network.

1. You first need to create a new folder to store all your configuration files. Copy to this folder a copy of your existing netscape.ini file.

2. Create a new desktop shortcut for your Netscape program file

3. Select the shortcut and right-click on it while the icon is highlighted.

4. Select Properties.

5. Click on the Shortcut tab.

6. Click once in the Target dialog box and position the cursor at the end of the line.

7. Enter a space and then type: -i c:\netscape\netscape.ini (substitute c:\netscape with the folder created in step 1).

8. Click on OK.

9. Double click this icon to start Netscape and then work through all the configuration options that are applicable for this user.

10. Repeat steps 1 through 9 for each additional user or version of Netscape.

Macintosh

You will have to configure MacPPP for each different user with their appropriate ISP details, user name and password before making the connection. If you are using an existing ISP account but just want separate preferences, this will not be an issue.

The way to set up your separate configurations is to do the following:

1. Install and run Netscape at least once.

2. Create a folder for each user.

3. Put a copy (not an alias) of Netscape in each folder.

4. Put a copy (not an alias) of /MAC HD/System Folder/Preferences/ Netscape F into each user's folder. When you first run Netscape, a Netscape F folder is created in the preferences folder. This is the default folder and a copy of this folder needs to be placed in each user's folder.

5. Create a Netscape folder and put an alias to point to the individual user's preferences file. Double clicking on the appropriate Alias will start that user's copy of Netscape and use the Netscape F folder in that user's folder.

CompuServe

Using an Alternate Browser

With the current versions of CompuServe Information Manager (CIM 2.0 and above), Spry Mosaic is offered as the built-in browser. Clicking on the *Internet Browser* button launches Spry Mosaic. Unfortunately, Spry Mosaic has many shortcomings, not least of which is its inability to recognize many of the new HTML features, especially those popularized by Netscape and Microsoft Internet Explorer (MSIE). Not all is lost, because it is simple to replace Spry Mosaic with the browser of your choice. The following guidelines assume Netscape is the replacement browser.

Windows 3.1 (WinCIM)

1. Obtain and install the 16-bit version of Netscape in the directory C:\NETSCAPE.

2. Open the file C:\CSERVE\CIS.INI using Notepad or a similar text based word processor.

3. Make these changes to the following section:

   [External Applications]

   http=C:\NETSCAPE\netscape.exe /SDDE
   ftp=C:\NETSCAPE\netscape.exe /SDDE
   news=C:\NETSCAPE\netscape.exe /SDDE
   gopher=C:\NETSCAPE\netscape.exe /SDDE

4. Save the file and exit Notepad.

5. Copy the file winsock.DLL from the C:\CSERVE\CID directory to the C:\NETSCAPE directory.

6. Netscape should now be the default browser under WinCIM.

To replace Spry Mosaic with MSIE, complete all the steps as outlined above, replacing Netscape with the location of your MSIE file. As this book was going to press, CompuServe announced new licensing agreements with Netscape and Microsoft that are intended to make Netscape or Internet Explorer the standard browsers with CIM. Further information is available on CompuServe (GO WCIMGENERAL).

Windows 95 (WinCIM)

Note: To use a 32-bit version of Netscape you must be accessing CompuServe via a Windows 95 dial-up connection and not using the 16-bit dialer that comes with the WinCIM software. Otherwise, use the steps as outlined above. Version 3 of WinCIM will be available as a 32-bit application. Further information is available on CompuServe (GO WCIMTECH).

Search history
A record of the various search strategies performed and their results. This can be shown somewhere on the system. In proprietary systems there is also the ability to save your search histories, and sometimes the bibliographies retrieved. This can also lead to saved Searches, in which the user can save the strategy and/or the results of a search somewhere on-line (and eventually on the Internet), to be run again, without having to re-enter the terms.

Macintosh (MacCIM)

Make the changes as previously outlined to the file "CompuServe Config" located in the CompuServe Settings folder. Further information is available on CompuServe (GO MCIMSOFT).

Search strategy or query
The term(s) entered in the blank box(es) to "tell" the database what subject is being sought.

Using an External Newsreader With CompuServe

CompuServe provides two means of reading Usenet newsgroups, a textbased DOS newsreader and a point-and-click Windows or Mac option. Both are functional, allowing you to select articles based on the sender, subject, or date (GO USENET). However, saving copies of articles and following ongoing message threads takes a lot of effort. CompuServe (unlike AOL) has made access to its Usenet system very open. You can use most external newsreader programs once they have been configured to access the CompuServe newsgroup host.

This process involves installing an appropriate newsreader program and specifying the details necessary to login to the CompuServe system and retrieve the articles you are interested in. AGENT (or Free Agent), the best newsreader available, requires little in the way of setting up and integrating into your existing package. Not only does this allow you to read downloaded messages off-line, but you can also compose replies via e-mail or newsgroup and easily archive or search older messages.

The following scenario assumes you are using Windows 3.1 or Windows 95 and have chosen AGENT (or Free Agent) as your newsreader software:

Step A

1. Install AGENT on your computer.

2. Start AGENT and select "Options/General Preferences" from the menu bar.

3. Click on the "User" tab and complete the details about yourself, especially your e-mail address and full name.

4. In the News Server Authorization section, check the "Server requires authorization login" and type your user name. This is your CompuServe ID, complete with comma.

5. You are free to check "Remember password between sessions," or you can be prompted for your password each time you log on. Be careful that you type your password correctly.

6. Click on the "System" tab.

7. Enter one of the following host server names into the "News Server" entry box:

   news.compuserve.com
   dub-news-svc-1.compuserve.com
   dub-news-svc-2.compuserve.com
   dub-news-svc-3.compuserve.com
   dub-news-svc-4.compuserve.com
   dub-news-svc-5.compuserve.com
   dub-news-svc-6.compuserve.com

   Note: When you identify a specific server, you may have a harder time getting connected. Your connection may close unexpectedly or be timed out. Just have a little patience and retry as soon as you are given an error message. You could also reset the "News Server" to a different value. Be aware that the "news.compuserve.com" server is a combination of all the other servers, so it is not the most reliable server to use.

Server
Computers on a network are all connected to a host machine called a server, which then coordinates all computer activities. A WWW server is the computer that actually stores Web files and regulates access of users.

8. Enter "Mail.compuserve.com" in the "E-mail Server" entry box.

9. Click on the "Dial-up" tab and complete the information relating to the dialup session you want to connect with. Most of the time you will start AGENT as part of an already open CompuServe session, so you will be able to skip this part.

10. Click on "OK."

Step B

1. Select "Online/Refresh Groups List" from the menu bar.

2. This will start up the process by which a list of all available newsgroups is downloaded from CompuServe to AGENT.

3. This could take some time to complete, but once it has finished, you are free to browse through this list and select the groups you wish to subscribe to.

4. Select "Online/Get New Headers in Subscribed Groups" from the menu bar.

5. This will download the current article headers for each of your newsgroups. You can then select the articles you want to retrieve.

Once these steps are completed and AGENT is performing to your satisfaction, you can close AGENT or continue to use it further. Closing AGENT will leave your CompuServe session active, but closing the CompuServe connection will also shut down AGENT.

This only briefly touches upon what AGENT is capable of, but experiment with its features and you will find that it is a powerful addition to the CompuServe service.

Downloading Files in CompuServe

Sometimes when you download a file in CIM, only part of a file is received or the on-line connection breaks off part way through the transfer. You can restart this download session and download only the remainder of the file. For large files this can save a lot of time.

If an error like this occurs, restart your CIM software and login again.

1. Relocate the original file.

2. Download it again.

3. A message will pop up saying the file exists and giving you the options of deleting this file or resuming the download.

4. Answer "Yes" to Resume Download.

Set building
A record of the search history that is compiled as results are retrieved. Each search strategy and its result becomes a set. Then the sets can be combined in various ways by the user.

America Online

Using an Alternative Browser

Note: Windows Version 3 of AOL comes complete with its own winsock.DLL file located in the AOL\Winsock directory. Before using an alternate browser with version 3, rename any copies of winsock.DLL that reside in the C:\WINDOWS directory to winsock.OLD.

Windows 3.1 and AOL Version 2.5

1. Rename any other versions of winsock.DLL in your C:\WINDOWS directory to winsock.OLD. This will ensure only the AOL Winsock is used.

2. Obtain and install the 16-bit version of Netscape in the directory C:\NETSCAPE.

3. Download the AOL winsock.DLL file (keyword NETSCAPE).

4. Move this file to the C:\NETSCAPE directory.

5. Restart Windows and login to AOL.

6. Start Netscape by switching over to Program Manager and double-clicking on its icon.

7. You can now use Netscape to surf the Web!

8. You can use Ctrl/Tab to toggle back and forth between AOL and Netscape.

Windows 95 and AOL Version 2.5

Follow the aforementioned steps, but in place of step 5: Minimize your AOL window and select Netscape from where it has been installed.

Note: You cannot use a 32-bit version of Netscape with AOL.

Macintosh and AOL Versions 2.6 and Below

You must be running version 2.5 or above of the Mac AOL software and have System 7 or higher with MacTCP or System 6.0.5 with Communications Toolbox installed. To determine which release of AOL you are running, select "About America Online" from the Apple menu. If you do not have the latest release, go to Keyword Upgrade and order it on-line.

1. Obtain and install Netscape for the Mac.

2. Start up AOL and login in as normal.

3. Start Netscape.

4. You can now toggle back and forth between AOL and Netscape.

MSIE: Follow the aforementioned steps substituting MSIE for Netscape wherever necessary. You cannot use a 32-bit version of MSIE with AOL.

If you experience problems running Netscape Navigator or any other Web browser, you can undo the installation and return to your original configuration by removing the new winsock.DLL and replacing it with the previous versions you renamed.

E-mail Messages Within the AOL Browser

You can send e-mail messages from within the AOL browser without having to switch back to AOL and starting the e-mail program. With the AOL browser open, type "mailto:" with the e-mail address of the recipient immediately following the colon (no spaces). This will launch the "Compose Mail" window, and you can then fill in the remaining information. After the message is sent, you will be returned to the Web browser.

Displaying Article Headers in Usenet Newsgroups

For Usenet articles, the default setting displays only the Subject, Date, and From information. However, there is a wealth of other information available in the message header.

1. With AOL running, use keyword Newsgroups to reach the Usenet area.

2. Select "Set Preferences."

3. Select the appropriate headers option (show headers at top or bottom).

Changing the Order of Usenet Articles

1. Bring up the same "Set Preferences" menu.

2. Change the current article order selection.

Shareware
A means of freely distributing software for evaluation by end users, with the intent that, if it is used regularly, the user will forward a fee to the author of the program. Shareware works on the honor system because there is no means of knowing who uses the program. Some shareware is set to work for only a few weeks (or months).

Adding Signatures to Usenet Articles

From the "Set Preferences" screen you can also create a unique signature. This signature will be added to the bottom of every Usenet article you create. Signatures usually contain information about you, such as your address and affiliations, but often feature a favorite quotation or reference Web site URLs.

Downloading Files in America Online

Whenever you download a file in AOL, you are given the option of downloading now or later. Choosing the later option provides the opportunity of queuing several files, which could then all be downloaded in a single session while you do something else. There is even a checkbox that when checked will disconnect AOL at the end of a successful file transfer, so you do not need to keep checking your computer if it's left unattended.

Sometimes a problem occurs when downloading a file, and only part of a file is received or the on-line connection breaks off part way through the transfer. AOL provides for this download session to be restarted with downloading of just the remainder of the file and not the entire file. For large files this can be a godsend.

If an error like this occurs, restart AOL and login again.

1. Select "File/Download Manager" from the menu bar.

2. Click once on "Show Files Downloaded."

3. Double click on the appropriate file name.

4. Click once on "Download Now."

5. A message will pop up asking if you want to resume the file download; answer "Yes."

USENET NEWSGROUPS

Can I Get a More Reliable Usenet News Feed?

Yes you can! CompuServe and AOL have undoubtedly made it easy to access newsgroups, but they do not provide a very reliable link to the hundreds of thousands of new messages posted daily. In fact, sometimes entire message threads are not accessible through these systems.

The alternatives are to pay for a direct news feed from some other source or sign up with an ISP that provides a full news feed.

Several companies now offer this type of service; Zippo and AirNews are the most prominent. Zippo offers several different plans, starting off with a basic $12/year package of around 4,500 newsgroups. Super Zippo, which is $69.95 per year, gives

Shell account
The simplest means of accessing the Internet. Instead of connecting your computer directly to the Internet, you dial into an Internet host and operate software on the host machine.

access to 18,000+ newsgroups, plus an e-mail address, space to host a home page, and access to a substantial FTP archive of Internet software. AirNews costs $9.95 per month and only provides access to newsgroups (18,500+).

Zippo also maintains a free public "Direct Read News" service that is available to anyone with a Web browser with access to 4,500 selected newsgroups.

Further information is available at the following Web sites:

AirNews
http://www.airnews.net

ZIPPO
http://www.zippo.com

SLIP/PPP
Serial Line Internet Protocol/Point to Point Protocol. These protocols allow your computer to be connected directly to the Internet using TCP/IP. The newest protocol is PPP.

Can I Read Old Usenet Articles?
Several sites on the Web archive old Usenet articles. Most of these archives are related to newsgroups about computers, software, and the Internet. However, a major site, called DejaNews, exists solely to provide an easy means to search through tens of millions of ordinary Usenet articles.

Presently, most Usenet articles for 1995 and 1996 are available, and there are plans to extend the archive back even further. Articles are searched through a Web browser, and this can be a simple search by subject or a complex search specifying key words, author name, date, and specific newsgroups. For each successful search, a hypertext list is created that displays the results. You can then select the entries that look the most promising, and the original article will be presented.

Once an article is displayed on the screen, you can treat it like any other Usenet article, that is, you can post a reply or read the article that preceded it or those posted in response to it. You can also select the original sender's name for a "profile" of the other newsgroups the original sender has posted articles in and the number of articles posted. This can be very useful in determining the sender's credibility on-line, especially on controversial subjects.

This is a free service, subsidized by advertising. DejaNews is available at

http://www.dejanews.com

Digital Computers provides the AltaVista Search Engine on the Web. AltaVista provides an index of the past few weeks' worth of Usenet articles. It is accessible at

http://altavista.digital.com/

Change the "Search" setting to Usenet.

SETTING UP MULTIPLE WINSOCK CONNECTIONS

SPAM
Sending multiple copies of the same message to Usenet newsgroups. (Not recommended, unless you want to be flamed in return!)

Sometimes it is desirable to have several different methods to access the Internet installed on the same Windows computer. This could be because you wish to use the modem to access an on-line service directly, but you still want to use a direct network connection to use Netscape. Or you may wish to use the services of two Internet providers (e.g., AOL and CompuServe.) Each method requires a different winsock.DLL file to be running.

Because only one winsock.DLL file can be present in the Windows directory at any given moment, it is necessary to delete the existing file and replace it with the new file each time the other service is accessed. Because all the files are called the same (winsock.DLL), this can become a confusing issue. The only easy way to tell them apart and to know which one is currently loaded is to examine the size and date of the file by using File Manager or Windows Explorer.

The best solution is to create a short batch file under DOS, which automatically swaps the appropriate files and also checks to see which version is presently loaded. Now it is just a simple matter of running this batch file whenever the TCP/IP stack must be changed.

The Bookmarks disk accompanying this book contains an example of this batch file (WINSW.BAT).

The file performs the following four functions:

1. Checks existing winsock.DLL file and identifies which version is loaded.
2. Offers a choice of versions to load.
3. Makes the change.
4. Reports which version is loaded.

This process eliminates any confusion and ensures the correct winsock.DLL program is available. On PCs this swap can be made from within Windows, and it is not required that Windows be restarted for the change to take effect, although any open Internet programs will need to be closed and restarted under the new TCP/IP stack.

⚡ **POWER TIP**

To switch between winsock.DLLs:

Create a batch file called WINSW.BAT (use Notepad or any word processor and save as an ASCII file in the C:\ directory.

Type the following commands exactly as they appear here:

```
echo off
REM Routine to swap Winsock files from Windows 95 to CompuServe
REM and vice versa
CLS


ECHO
IF EXIST C:\SOCK.TXT GOTO MESS2
IF NOT EXIST C:\SOCK.TXT GOTO MESS

:MESS
ECHO CURRENT Winsock is CompuServe
GOTO CONTINUE

:MESS2
ECHO CURRENT Winsock is WIN95
GOTO CONTINUE

:CONTINUE
ECHO
ECHO
ECHO (A) Setup CIS Winsock
ECHO
ECHO (B) Setup WIN95 Winsock
ECHO
ECHO (C) Exit (setting remains the same)
ECHO
choice /c:abc Enter Choice
IF ERRORLEVEL 3 GOTO END
IF ERRORLEVEL 2 GOTO WIN95
IF ERRORLEVEL 1 GOTO CIS

:WIN95
CD C:\WINDOWS\WINBACK\
COPY winsock.DLL C:\WINDOWS
CLS
ECHO
ECHO
echo Current setting is for WIN95 access
COPY C:\WINDOWS\SOCK.TXT C:\
ATTRIB C:\SOCK.TXT +R
PAUSE
GOTO END
```

Subheadings
Subheadings (in MEDLINE) represent 80+ clinical features, like diagnosis, etiology, adverse effects, and the like, that can be attached to a term to specify its emphasis. They are usually noted as two-letter acronyms, like DI for diagnosis, when found on the search or in the citations. Sometimes subheadings are included in a limiting function, because they often limit the number of citations retrieved.

```
:CIS
C:
CD C:CSERVE\CID
COPY winsock.DLL C:\WINDOWS

CLS

ECHO
ECHO
echo Current setting is for CIS access
ATTRIB C:\SOCK.TXT -R
DEL C:\SOCK.TXT
PAUSE
GOTO END

:END
EXIT
```

Systems or Services
The databases, book content, journals, news services, and the like that make up the network.

When this batch file is run, it first checks for the presence of a file called c:\SOCK.TXT. If found, it knows the winsock.DLL file loaded is the 32-bit version. If this file is not found, then the CompuServe winsock.DLL is the one present. If this needs to be changed, the appropriate Winsock is copied to the Windows directory. Note that all these files are copied from the directories where they are originally stored.

If you had not already worked it out, this particular sequence changes the TCP/IP stack from being a 32-bit connection to one that is used via CompuServe. But this can easily be adapted to swap between a CompuServe Winsock and an AOL Winsock. In fact, it is this swapping of Winsocks that caused no end of fuss when Windows 95 was first released. On installing Windows 95, the install program replaces any existing winsock.DLL file with the Microsoft version, which effectively stops other TCP/IP reliant software from operating when it cannot find the appropriate Winsock. Windows 95 never deleted any communications software, but it did cause a few problems for the unsuspecting. But now you know how to avoid this happening to you.

On Macs, configuring multiple versions of MacTCP is definitely more problematic, because more is involved than just swapping files. You should definitely consult with the technical support personnel at your ISP, or read the manual that came with your Internet software.

DEALING WITH COMPRESSED FILES

The main reasons for compressing files are to reduce the size of a file or combine multiple files into one file. The end result is less time is required to download files. In the DOS/Windows world, the most common program used for compressing files is PKZIP. A "zipped" file has the extension .ZIP, but it can also have the extension .EXE, which indicates that the file is selfexpanding. A .ZIP file by itself requires a copy of an "unzip" program to uncompress it. The most common program used for this purpose is PKUNZIP. Older compression methods are still in use, and files compressed by using these methods can be distinguished by the extensions of .ZOO, .ARJ, and .ARC.

On the Mac, compressed files are "stuffed" by using a program called STUFFIT (.SIT; .SEA, which is selfexpanding) or they are converted into a format called BINHEX (.HQX). STUFFIT is used for compressing and uncompressing files and can also handle files converted using BINHEX.

To decompress Mac STUFFIT and BINHEX files on a PC you will need a copy of the PC versions of these programs or a multipurpose PC file conversion utility. PC ZIP files can also be converted on the Mac with the appropriate conversion utilities.

File Encoding
In Chapter 3 we discussed how e-mail software converted nontext files into a MIME format that allowed sending these files as e-mail messages. Many of the most popular e-mail programs handle MIME conversion automatically, whereas others require manual conversion of the files and then pasting the file into a new message or attaching it to the e-mail message.

MPACK and MUNPACK are the most popular PC-based programs for performing MIME conversions. MPACK is used to encode files and MUNPACK is used to decode e-mail messages that contain MIME files. A message that contains a MIME-encoded file usually includes a note at the beginning of the message indicating the file is MIME encoded.

To decode a message like this, first save it to a text file, making sure to include everything in the message. Then launch your conversion utility, in the case of Windows, use MUNPACK with the command:

Munpack filename

where "filename" is the text file containing the message. The attached file will be saved to its original file name. Any accompanying notes are also saved to a file.

On the Mac, BinHex is the encoding option most used for nontext file attachments.

Usenet File Encoding
Within Usenet newsgroups, a different conversion method is used to convert binary files and graphics into a format that can be accessed in newsgroup articles. UUEN-

CODE (Unix to Unix Encode) is the method used for Windows and Mac. Many Usenet newsreaders (including America Online) can automatically decode Uuencoded articles, otherwise a separate UUDECODE program is required. Uuencoded files sometimes end with the file suffix such as .uue, or .uu1, or .uu2. WinCode is the most popular Windows program for encoding and decoding files. UULite is the best Mac program for this purpose.

TRANSFERRING FILES BETWEEN A PC AND A MAC

Swapping files between a PC and a Mac is not easy. First, the floppy disks are formatted differently. Macs can read and write to a PC disk without additional software, but PCs need conversion software. ASCII on a Mac means something different from ASCII on a PC-ASCII files on a PC contain a linefeed code denoting when a new line starts, whereas Mac ASCII files have a carriage return code. This has the unfortunate effect of removing all line breaks when a Mac ASCII file is opened on a PC.

Mac files are also constructed differently, comprising what are termed *data* and *resource forks*. All Mac communications software, by default, recognizes this unique structure and converts files into a single binary file using the MacBinary file format before uploading. When the file is downloaded onto a Mac system, the files revert to their original structure. PC files, on the other hand, are self-contained.

Most graphic file types will run on each system without further conversion. However, TIFF graphics on the Mac must be saved in a PC TIFF format.

Chapter 1 discussed using emulation software for running PC programs on a Mac. The other solution is obtaining a Mac-to-PC file conversion utility that should, in one stroke, remove all of the problems involved in transferring files from one system to the other. MacOpener is the most versatile of these programs available on the PC, allowing Mac disks to be read and formatted, in addition to translating and converting file formats.

Sometimes the easiest method of transferring a file from a Mac to a PC is to e-mail the file to yourself or a colleague from a Mac, and then access your mail using a PC.

Appendix 2, "Internet Providers and Obtaining Internet Software," provides more information on acquiring compression and encoding software.

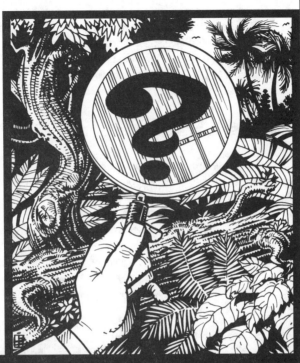

Chapter 6

Searching

"I Know It's Got to Be Here Somewhere"

A LITTLE INTRODUCTION

The excitement of knowing that you are capable of accessing an immeasurable repository of information is soon replaced by the nightmare of how to find a specific site or document. With 15 billion words, 30 million pages (and counting), no particular order, no comprehensive index, and no bound volumes, the Internet's World Wide Web (WWW or Web) represents the most expansive "library" ever assembled. Your halcyon days of carefree surfing are done, and you simply want to find a patient education document that discusses Crohn's disease. (Site and document are often used interchangeably. For our purposes, the site is generally the organization that provides the information. The information is the document.)

The egalitarian Web offers incredible stores of data to anyone with a modem and an Internet hook-up. Although initially the content volume was indexed with simple tools, the Internet has lately experienced an extraordinary growth of pages and documents. The Internet developers and designers are now formulating tools that are

Glossary Terms T–U

T1/T3 LINE
High-speed digital telephone connections.

TCP/IP
Transport Control Protocol/Internet Protocol. These two standards dictate how data travel from point A to point B on the Internet.

quickly becoming as sophisticated as the search capabilities of the pre-existing on-line commercial databases. Such features are familiar to users of services, such as Grateful Med and PaperChase, in which controlled vocabularies and advanced search capabilities help to retrieve specific articles. Paradoxically, as the Web grows, the reality of universally effortless searching becomes less possible. To stay one step ahead of the crowd and to use the Web productively, you must learn some tricks of the librarian trade, as well as the utility of the individual search tools.

USING THE SEARCH ENGINES

Trying to impose order on chaos, the Internet has *search engines,* electronic cataloging and registering tools that break the information on the Web into manageable bits and return an on-line list of sites, documents, pictures, and sound or film clips. Generally, these are commercial ventures that generate revenue in various ways, but are almost always free to the user. You enter a query or search strategy, wait for the pages or documents to be listed, click on the desired listing, and ideally, the document appears on the screen. This massive job of culling information from Web pages (graphic), and Usenet newsgroups (a large network of text-based newsgroups, similar to bulletin boards) is now handled by more than 250 search engines (see Eleven Search Engines).

Search engines find their existent and potential data by sending out software agents (the "librarians") called *spiders,* also known as robots or scooters, that follow the labyrinth of the Web, searching and building indexes that can be scanned in seconds. Not all search engines are created equal. Only a few cover the Web exhaustively, by the Universal Resource Locaters (URLs) they tag and the thoroughness of their indexing of the pages and documents. Retrieval depends on how the search engine gathers its information and how well the search engine accommodates your inquiries. Using one search engine does not guarantee that *all* the information existent on amniocentesis and pregnancy will be returned. Conversely, a search engine, depending on its search capabilities, might return thousands of irrelevant documents.

Search engines operate in two prevailing areas. The first domain, typically (although not consistently) embodies the entire Web and all its content. These search engines offer a keyword search function or a combination subject list (which facilitates browsing) and keyword function. These global search engines include Digital's mammoth AltaVista (http://www.altavista.com) and the McKinley Group's innovative Magellan, (http://www.mckinley.com).

Within the search engine, there is a search query field in which you enter the keyword(s) of interest, for example, *leukemia,* and the search engine returns a list of sites or documents about that subject. Or you can choose a subject category, as in Yahoo! (http://www.yahoo.com) where the "Health and Medicine" section is broken down into hundreds of categories, each one leading to numerous health related pages.

One of those sites (with keyword searches or subject browsing) might be the University of Pennsylvania's Oncolink (http://www.oncolink.upenn.edu/). Oncolink's site-specific search engine represents the less apparent, second general area of search engines, those of individual institutions or groups. These search engines limit themselves to the content particular to the institution's or group's Web site that is so large it needs its own search engine and interface to find information within the site. Generally, the discussion of search strategies that follows refers to both domains of searching, although the global search engines tend to be more sophisticated in their search capabilities because of the size (huge!) of their realm.

Telnet
The means to access other computers from a remote location and control them as if they were sitting in front of you.

Following the metaphor of the WWW as a traditional library, a browser, such as the ubiquitous Netscape, acts as the front door, and the search engine is the vast, automated card catalog. (This library metaphor must be used cautiously, for the Internet does not have collection development policies, traditional cataloging, or even restricted hours, as does a conventional library!) Search engines come in all shapes and sizes, from concept types, such as the visionary Excite (http://www.excite.com) to the inverted word type, such as Inktomi (http://www.inktomi.com) which only has to store an index and not the actual documents.

SEARCH STRATEGIES

Whether you use a broad-based search engine or a smaller, site-specific search engine, the issue remains the same. How do you find what you need? Following are tips to becoming a competent searcher on the Web, but first, a discussion about search queries. The two biggest problems encountered with retrieving adequate information are the following:

1. Getting nothing relevant when asking a question
2. Getting overwhelmed with too much information

Generally, a question goes unanswered, not because there is no answer, but because the inquiry was not phrased properly. Although search engines try to address this deficit by noting every word in a document, the chance of retrieving lots (tons) of extraneous material is far too high for the busy health care professional.

CONSTRUCTION OF A SEARCH

A query or search strategy consists of one or more keywords (or phrases, company names, or personal names) believed to be part of the title or body of a Web page. Most search engines have a single open box or *field*. Multifield boxes that accommodate more than one term and other search capabilities are being developed for some search engines. Generally, to the side or below the field(s) is a short explanation of how to enter the strategy or how to do sophisticated searching.

KNOW YOUR SEARCH ENGINE!

Considerations

The problem for the user comes with the variety of search engines and their search capabilities. Although their goal is the same—to retrieve information for the user—their methods are often somewhat different. Let's look at some of the advanced search features that affect what you enter in the field and what is returned to you. The on-screen instructions, or the help files, will let you know whether the search engine accommodates the following options:

- Boolean Logic
- Stemming and truncation
- Automatic truncation and exact word matches
- Concept searching
- Phrases or case sensitivity
- Word proximity or proximity
- Field searching
- Nesting or search set manipulation operators

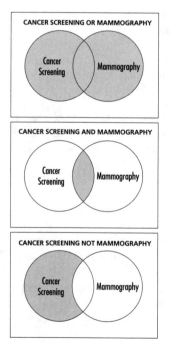

OR Operator
Any one of the terms are present (more than one term may be present).

Such a query would return documents on cancer screening (any sort, prostate, colon, etc.) or any documents on mammography. Expect a large retreival rate with "OR."

AND Operator
All terms are present.

Such a query would return documents on cancer screening that discusses mamography (no prostate, colon, etc., would be included). Expect a large retreival rate with "AND."

NOT Operator
The first term is present, but not the second.

Such a query would return documents on cancer screening types (prostate, colon, etc.) except for those on mamography. Expect a more specific retrieval with "NOT."

FIGURE 6–1.—*Search engine.*

Most search engines employ some form of **Boolean logic** expanding or limiting the expected results by placing the proximity operators AND, OR, NOT, between individual terms (Fig 6–1).

The AND retrieves the documents that include all the terms. For example, for a *single* document that discusses *both* measles and mumps, you would enter: measles AND mumps. Retrieval rates are generally lower (or certainly more specific) with the AND operator.

The OR retrieves *any* of the terms in *any* document. So, measles OR mumps would include *all* the documents that included *either* measles or mumps, but not necessarily *both*. Retrieval rates are generally much higher using the OR operator. Entering (measles or rubella) and mumps would give you yet another retrieval, for you are seeking a broader set of measles articles, but they must include mumps.

The NOT eliminates a related subject from the general document pool. So, if you wanted documents on communicable diseases in children, and you already had enough information on mumps, but not nearly enough on measles, you would enter: measles NOT mumps. *Caution:* You may lose some valid documents here; if there is a single article that discusses measles *and* mumps, you will lose it by ridding the list of the mumps articles.

Some engines perform the Boolean by default, or implicitly, whereas others offer the user the ability to customize the operators. The implicit Boolean environment is generally annoying to the seasoned user because OR is the default operator. Imagine, if you enter "health maintenance organizations," you get all the entries on health, all the entries on maintenance, and all the entries on organization, a significant percentage of which are irrelevant to the original inquiry. In such a case, you should consider using a search engine such as Open Text, (http://www.opentext.com), in which you can customize health maintenance organization as a phrase or in which you can indicate the more appropriate operator, AND, between the terms, facilitating a more targeted retrieval. Sometimes, the implicit operator is AND, and you might want to create a larger pool with the OR operator.

Various search engines control what is called stemming and truncation. *Stemming* is an automatic operation in the search engine that reduces the keywords (not phrases) to their root word, such as fibrosarcoma to fibro, and the search continues using that root word. Your results would then include fibroma, fibrosis, and fibrositis, which, although useful, might be irrelevant to your original search. *Truncation,* as performed by the search engine, is a default setting in which the search automatically looks for variant word endings. If you enter prostat, you will get prostatic, prostate, prostatitis, etc. The difference between the two is that you control the level of truncation, putting in the root, while stemming assumes what you want the root to remain.

Some search engines have *automatic truncation,* so if you enter cardio, because you want something on cardiomyopathy, the engine may well return cardiovascular, car-

Terms or Keywords
The words that are usually seen alongside the blank boxes on a network's interface. "Enter term(s) here." Terms or Keywords refer to any sort of word, phrase, or, in the case of MEDLINE, MeSH that is being entered in the search box. Terms, textwords, keywords, or MeSH relating to a particular subject, can also be referred to as the "search" or "search strategy."

diographic, cardiology, and other words beginning with cardio ad infinitum—far more than you ever anticipated. Other search engines perform *exact word matches.* In other words, they match exactly what you have typed. If you typed prostat, that is what will be returned, which in many cases, will be nothing. In either of these cases, there is usually an option for the user to switch off the default and instruct the search engine about whether you want truncation, or exact matches.

To add yet another dimension of distinctiveness, some search engines, such as Excite, perform *concept searches.* You want documents on the economic implications of managed care programs. You enter: economic AND implications AND managed care organizations (MCOs). You get back documents on that subject, but you also retrieve documents on related topics such as the effect of MCOs on health care and the role of an HMO or an MCO that could include information or aspects you had not considered. Such hand-holding ability is done by the search engine that is programmed to retrieve statistically similar documents, even if they lack one or more of the key words you entered. This may be more than you need, but it could retrieve documents you would have otherwise missed.

Phrases and Case Sensitivity

As demonstrated with the health maintenance organization example used earlier, the ability to enter phrases is a useful one. Also, some search engines are *case sensitive,* meaning that if you want Munchausen's Syndrome, typing "munchausen's syndrome" will not find what you want. The capital letters must be typed in. In other search engines, the case is irrelevant. This is an especially important concern when entering terms such as proper names, procedures, or countries.

Some search engines have *word proximity,* in which you can note where you want to find the word within the document. The *proximity operators,* such as those offered by Infoseek (http://guide.infoseek.com), are words or characters that insert between two key words to specify how close the words should be for the document to be returned. For example, if you were searching about nursing ethics, the use of a proximity operator that specifies "next to each other" would give you the phrase, nursing ethics. The proximity operator of "near each other, in any order," would retrieve more documents; perhaps a document with a discussion of nursing, a few lines on the hospital environment, then the term "ethics" would be returned. The two words, nursing and ethics, are not together, but the document is relevant to your search.

Field Searching

Simply want to look at your search topic in the title, author's name, abstract, or keyword list? Many search engines now offer field searching, an effective way of limiting a large retrieval.

Nesting or Search Set Manipulation

This is the fancy stuff. A simple search on infectious diseases, which would retrieve thousands of sites or documents with some search engines, could be managed by using parentheses. For example, (tuberculosis or Hantavirus) and (pediatric or children) and United States, would give you the documents that covered tuberculosis or Hantavirus, only in children, not adults, only in the United States, not worldwide, a much more succinct search than retrieving documents on all the infectious diseases in the world.

Some engines compensate for this lack of specificity by letting you repeatedly add terms to the original query, but this does not allow for how you wanted the retrieval to be emphasized. As search engines "mature," this is one feature that will be accommodated, in the search field or through multiple fields.

Text-based
A document that contains only textual characters (no graphics).

THE SEARCH

You have found one or more search engines you like and figured out the basics of keywords, Boolean logic, and stemming. You want to see what the Web has to offer regarding calcium channel blockers and myocardial infarction. Remember, there are two types of search engines, the broad-based engines, such as Yahoo!, and the site-specific engines, such as that of the Atlanta Reproductive Health Centre (http://www.ivf.com). Generally, you must run the search through the first level, unless you have "bookmarked" a site previously, and can simply return to it for another search.

You begin with Yahoo's search engine. You do a search on myocardial infarction and retrieve nothing. AltaVista gives you 6000. Open Text yields 370. What to do? (See Fig 6–2 for an example of performing the same search with different search engines.)

TWO PROBLEMS

Any discussion of searching on the Web is confused by the fact that no two of the biggest search engines cover exactly the same territory (e.g., URLs, pages, or documents) in exactly the same way (e.g., different interfaces or Boolean logic). As a rule, because of the size of the Web, the lack of any systematic "collection development," and the liberal definition of what constitutes a document, the retrieval yields (except in a catalog-based system such as Yahoo!) are fairly large. So, although it is unusual to get too few hits (as happens in conventional on-line databases), some considerations follow.

How Can I Increase My Hits?
If there are too few hits, it could be that the terms were not entered properly or were spelled incorrectly. Do check search engine instructions if you are not certain how to enter the term (remember the discussion about implicit Boolean logic and default truncation). More likely, the term you used, such as myocardial infarction, was too specific.

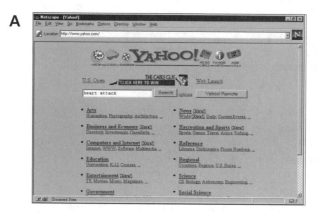

FIGURE 6–2.—*Search engines.*

D
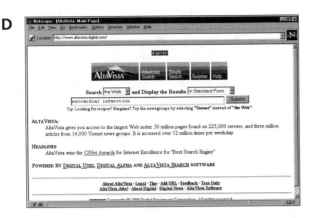

E
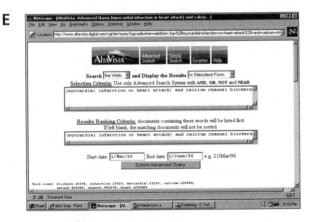

Depending on which search engine you've used, take note of these small, but important points.

Hyphens.—Did entering calcium-binding test the mettle of the machine? Try calcium AND binding, or try (calcium-binding) as a *phrase.*

Proper Names.—Do you need to enter A. Lincoln, or Abraham Lincoln or Abraham and Lincoln, or Lincoln, Abe?

Apostrophes.—Tourette's syndrome. Will it accept the "'s"? Or should you simply try Tourette?

Don't forget, *phrases, case sensitivity,* and *stemming and truncation* can affect your search strategy too.

Learn the Art of Synonyms and Acronyms.—Remember, this is the WWW, not a conventional MEDLINE medium. A lot of the material is written for, and used by, the public and a variety of health care professionals. The language is eclectic, if not eccentric. A subject like myocardial infarction, is also known as coronary arrest, heart attack, heart arrest, heart failure, and MI. Try those terms, (with an implicit or controlled OR between the terms for a larger yield).

Acronyms are pervasive and important, especially in medical terminology. Entering acquired immunodeficiency syndrome probably will not get as many returns as entering AIDS; entering DRGs will be more successful than entering, diagnostic related groups.

How to Find Useful Synonyms and Acronyms. —The following are tips for finding help:

1. Look at the Web sites themselves, they can give hints.
2. Ask colleagues.
3. Look in printed reference tools, dictionaries, or thesauri.
4. Pay attention to the media, television, and popular magazines.
5. Ask patients; diseases are given nicknames and known by slang terms, too.
6. Ask a librarian.
7. Join a Usenet group; ask for ideas on search terms or strategies.

Ironically, by entering a broad search strategy, you may get too many documents.

How Can I Limit My Hits?

Browse your list. Ascertain, by the short descriptions of the sites, the terms most often used. In our example, probably heart attack. Depending on the search engine, you can *nest* related subjects (see Nesting or Search Set Manipulation), so the system will return (heart attack and myocardial infarction) and (calcium channel blockers) in one document.

Adding more terms or phrases with an AND operator, rather than an OR as you would to increase results, is also a way to trim your result. Sometimes the search engine itself allows for some limitation factors. For example, you can limit the amount of documents retrieved, the years covered, and the geographical area. And don't forget that *field searching, word proximity, stemming and truncation,* and *nesting* can all be used to fine-tune a search strategy.

Perhaps you retrieved inappropriate documents. The word you entered could be a *homonym.* Remember fourth grade grammar? Homonyms are words that are spelled the same but have a meaning different from the one you have in mind. For example, if you are a hospital administrator looking for documents about discharges, you do not want to retrieve clinical articles about runny noses or sites that help auto mechanics diagnose battery problems. Until search engines can ascertain the context of a word in a document that they are working on, the only way to alleviate this problem is through strategy and search capabilities. You can enter the terms with parentheses and a proximity operator, (patient AND discharge) NOT batteries, or scroll through the inappropriate sites.

More important, when too large a result is retrieved, recall the "Lincoln's Hat Rule." A patron asks the librarian for books on the Civil War. "Too big." How about the last two years of the war? "Too vague." I really want to know about the Gettysburg Address. "What about it?" Well, I want to see a picture of what sort of hat Lincoln wore when delivering the Gettysburg Address. So, if all you want is information about myocardial infarction and calcium channel blockers, by all means, enter just that.

ELEVEN SEARCH ENGINES

As with any reference tool, you will find that individual search engines will become favorites, whereas you will rarely use others. Let's take a look at some of the most conspicuous or innovative search engines on the Web (Table 6–1), those that provide a comprehensive database of Internet sites and offer the advanced search features that we have touched on previously.

Caveat

In the interest of lessening confusion and because this environment evolves as we "write," this table is neither exhaustive nor completely instructive. Indeed, some of these features may have changed during the writing of this book. It is meant to steer you to eleven popular search engines and get you started. Remember, search engines also have on-line instructions about their search strategy protocols. Although it is sometimes hard to locate or difficult to understand, on-line information can be helpful to those who persevere. This is an adventure! There is information at the end of this tunnel! If you want to delve further into individual search engines, refer to the literature listed at the end of this chapter.

To address the disparities between search engines and the material they retrieve, designers are trying to create the dream Web search engine—one that would send the search strategy to the Web's biggest search engines, such as Infoseek, clNet, or Galaxy, collate the returns, eliminate redundancies, and send back the relevant results. MetaCrawler (http://metacrawler.cs.washington.edu:8080/index.html) takes a good stab at it, although it takes some time to return the results, retrieval is sometimes inconsistent, and there are *more* than the top eleven search engines. It is a wonderful time-saver when you need documents quickly. The c!Net (http://www.search.com), a "search engine clearinghouse," provides direct access to more than 250 search engines that are organized by subject. It also lets users customize their own page of up to 20 search tools.

Tree or Hierarchical Tree
Each MeSH is part of both a broader or narrower area. For instance, Lyme Disease is part of the larger "tree" of Bacterial and Fungal Diseases, then down one limb of Bacterial Infections, it is part of Spirochaetales Infections and has branches leading off of it as well. In some systems various parts of the tree can be picked to increase or narrow your search. In some systems, the term can be exploded within its tree to include all the MeSH that fall in that category.

TABLE 6–1.—ELEVEN SEARCH ENGINES

Search Engine	Basics	The Downside	Highlights
AltaVista http://www.altavista.digital.com	Indexes every word of every available Web page, 30 million pages! Includes Usenet Default search setting: Simple Queries OR Relevancy ranking: Yes Truncation: Not automatic Field search: Yes	Response time can be slow A relative newcomer, but making a big splash No duplicate detection It is *so* big! You really need to work at trimming down a search	Search commands and features similar to traditional on-line commercial database services Boolean operators, AND, OR, NOT, NEAR in advanced search Search examples easy to find Phrase searching with double quotes
DejaNews http://www.dejanews.com/	Usenet articles Default search setting AND can be changed to OR Relevancy ranking (scoring) Returns *hyperlinked* to author and article headings Wildcard, * to alter truncation		Power Search offers query filters by newsgroup; "Thread" Search into related news Archives of articles, too Helpful Help function, especially the FAQ (frequently asked questions)
Excite http://www.excite.com	Concept-based navigation tool, relates subjects to one another Services indexed: WWW pages, Usenet Classified, and Reviews Size: 1.5 million Web pages Default search setting: "Fuzzy AND," both AND and OR are used, with higher weight given to results with both terms Relevancy ranking: Yes Truncation: Words are stemmed to roots, e.g., magical is stemmed to magic	Concept and keyword searching can give large numbers of irrelevant hits Some confusion over keyword/concept searching, and +/- or Boolean operators Does not tell you total number of returns	Because of the special software, results are fast Usenet discussion groups, search refining, concept searching! Boolean operators AND +/- to add or eliminate words Advanced search tips are helpful Phrase searching
HotBot http://www.hotbot.com (In public beta testing, June 1996)	Capable of indexing and searching every word on the Web Services indexed: identified 50 million documents, 35.8 million in the beta version Usenet coming Default search setting: AND (OR is available) Relevancy ranking: In a way, words used in title ranked higher than words used only in text Truncation: Currently, no; exact word match. Enter cardio, get cardio. If you want cardiomyopathy, put that in.	Still in public beta testing, sometimes bugs are evident, but seldom Some users do not like the green background, others do No proximity operators yet, but they are coming	Superior design on the interface and search engine; you can add search fields as you need them Search words, phrases, persons, and URLs Exports popular Boolean operators via the pop-up interface More direct access coming Modifiers (e.g., must, must not) available Location (e.g., country), date, and other limiters available Well thought out and executed; this is the one to watch The Help function uses a screen with identifying script, quite clever Good FAQ also
shot			
Infoseek http://guide.infoseek.com	Searches retrieve most relevant matches Includes related topics to explore, and news from popular sources. Services indexed: WWW pages, e-mail addresses, Usenet Size: 400,000 documents Default search setting: OR Relevancy ranking: Yes Truncation: Key words default to stem	Not as many categories as competing services Sophisticated searching difficult because of the search syntax, but worth working at Usenet postings, magazine articles and some other services have a fee No Boolean operators; (+/-) used for including or excluding keywords Must capitalize proper names Charges apply to some services	Precise, few false hits Allows for customizing and searching just a portion of the Web or the entire Web Proximity operators, link two terms with a hyphen to retrieve only those docu- in which those words occur near each other Phrase searching optional (put the phrase in quotation marks)
ments			
Inktomi (ink-to-me) http://inktomi.berkeley.edu/query.html	Indexes entire document (full text); at the word level, not subject level Only noncommercial search service Services indexed: Web documents Size: 2.8 million pages Default search setting: OR Relevancy ranking: Yes Truncation: None Common endings such as "ed" and "ing" are eliminated, and a root word is used for the search	Quirky search syntax, does not recognize Boolean operators or punctuation No description of sites No proximity operators No phrase search	Uses exclusion and inclusion (+/-) for refining searches Relevancy ranking on the description It is fast Good for sophisticated searches

Search Engine	Basics	The Downside	Highlights
Lycos http://www.lycos.com	Fast and comprehensive Includes, videos, sounds, and graphics Services indexed: WWW pages, FTP (file transfer protocol), Gopher Size: 3.6 million pages Default search setting: OR Relevancy ranking: Yes Truncation: Automatic	Too many hits? Process to refine search is relatively unwieldy Phrase search: None Proximity operators: None AND operator does not always operate properly	Huge database, more hits than most Browse by subject Various finding capabilities, from specific people to entire sites on a subject Boolean operators: AND, OR Truncation: Automatic; type in cat, get catheter, catholic, et cetera. Just want cat? Type the word with a period at the end You can customize what the output looks like You can match prefixes and disable the truncation default
Magellan http://www.mckinley.com	Size: 1 million pages Numerous services, including searches by category and across the entire Web Default search setting: OR Relevancy ranking: Yes Truncation: Yes	A search box and a lengthy list of categories make for a confusing interface Slow response No Boolean operators; use +/- for including or excluding keywords	Choose rated and reviewed sites, or entire Net Neat starred rating system; might help some users decide between multiple sites Magellan's Search Box to enhance one's own Web site
Open Text http://www.opentext.com	Services indexed: WWW pages Size: 1 million documents Default search setting: AND Truncation: Automatic Phrase search: Yes Relevancy ranking: Yes Plurals and word variants allowed	Sometimes low precision on the retrieval list	Extraordinary advanced search capabilities Boolean operators, AND, OR, BUT-NOT Proximity operators, NEAR, FOLLOWED BY. Search refining; can combine search strategies! On each retrieved entry, you can visit the page, see a list of the lines on the page containing matches to your search query, or search for similar pages Offers three types of searching: simple, weighted, and power, with increasingly sophisticated options
WebCrawler http://webcrawler.com	"Random-links" feature to find unusual and new sites List of 25 most-visited sites on the Web Services indexed: WWW pages, FTP, and Gopher Size: 250,000 documents Default search setting: AND Relevancy ranking: Yes Phrase search: Yes	The default return of only 25 hits per page might be annoying if you are covering a broad range of topics	Fast, because it is not searching the entire Web Boolean operators, AND, OR Nice place to start Helpful search tips Offers title, then summary, so there is not so much to scan
Yahoo! http://www.yahoo.com	Browse and search subject categories 200,000 Web sites in 20,000 categories Default search setting: AND or OR, you choose Limit search to specific category No phrase or field search	Categories and content are chosen by Yahoo! staff, so what you find may not be as complete or selective as some of the other services Only title, URL, and comments are indexed Small, but delivers	Updated daily Categories make browsing easy; organized in general sections from health to science Hyperlinks to other search engines for additional searching Augmented by Open Text's indexing and search engine Good!

URL

Universal Resource Locator. This describes the location of an Internet address and the communications protocol used to access it. This can be a simple site address (i.e., http://www.Mosby.com) or a specific document (i.e., http://www.Mosby.com/index.html).

Individual search engines, such as Magellan, Excite, and Point (http://www.point-com.com) have taken the approach of rating or reviewing sites or offering meatier descriptions of sites, so the user has a bit more on-line help to decide between multitudinous entries. Also very intriguing are the MNI System's Achoo (http://www.achoo.com) dedicated to becoming the most comprehensive directory of health care information sites (see Chapter 9) and NLightN (http://www.nlightn.com). NLightN's "universal index" searches databases such as

MEDLINE and PsycINFO, as well as newswires and reference materials—all at once! Quarterdeck's new Windows utility, called WebCompass, is a common gateway interface (CGI), that does the footwork of sending your strategy to various *resources,* such as Yahoo! or Lycos, collects the responses, eliminates duplicate sites, and presents them in a single list. WebCompass has many special features, including an *agent* that retrieves and indexes documents that were selected in a previous search, and automatically performs searches for you—like an electronic clipping service.

ONCE THE RESULT IS AVAILABLE

You are looking at a list of 75 retrieved documents; some of them have immediately recognizable authoring entities, such as the American Nurses Association, the National Cancer Institute, or the American Holistic Medical Association. But many are unfamiliar. Most search engines rank by a scored *relevance ranking,* computed on how frequently your search term(s) appear in the retrieved document. The higher the number, the higher relevancy; the more relevant articles (regardless of when they were created) appear first in the list. Arguably, they may not be the most relevant documents to your search, but generally they are on target. (Interestingly, in some search engines, such as AltaVista, while the terms you enter are being "ORed" and thousands are returned, the most relevant documents float to the top of the list.) Users accustomed to chronologically based databases, such as MEDLINE, in which the most current document is listed first, will need to browse the list retrieved to determine currency.

How do you choose which site to click on and view? It can be hit or miss, but generally one or more descriptive sentences inform you about who sponsors the site and what information is there. Once you are in the site, the same criteria that were used to develop *Mosby's Medical Surfari* can be implemented to measure whether the site is useful to you. The criteria are as follows:

- Authority: the credibility or longevity of the university, specialty society, or professional group that established the site.

- Contents: Is the material useful, unique, accurate, and compelling? View the site as you would a book; scrutinize the content for its beneficial aspects.

- Organization: Is the information easy to get to? If it takes more than a few clicks to get to something useful or interesting, then it is buried too deep. Is the information broken down into logical portions? Does it have an initial table of contents that helps establish where the other material lies?

- Currency: Does the site have clear and obvious pointers to new content? Is new material particularly well highlighted?

- The "Look": Appealing graphics? Attractive background color? Innovative icons? Although these are not crucial to the content transference, these features can separate one site from another.

- Internal Links: More and more sites are including other Web sites in their content. Sometimes finding just one site can open up a world of related sites, saving time and effort. These links can be saved as you go along, with your *bookmarks* where you have created folders for various subjects.

- Search Engine: Within the site, is it easy to use?

GETTING SOPHISTICATED

Really pressed for time? Need fine-tuned documents? Want to try new things? Some hints follow.

1. Start small: Yahoo! indexes relatively few documents, and the realm searches are small. It is a good place to start and has a serviceable "Health and Medicine" section. It will not overwhelm you on your first visit. And it is democratic—if it does not have what you asked for, it offers, among others, Infoseek and Open Text to let you go further.

2. Go directly to a specialty or university site, such as the Arizona Health Science Library's terrific "Nutrition and Health" site (http://hinet.medlib.arizona. edu/educ/nutrition/html.)

   With its own search engine and voluminous content, you can initiate a search on nutrition and aging the that will be more focused than if you used Lycos's search engine and retrieved thousands of documents.

3. Try the networks. These large content entities, such as MedScape, HealthGate, BioMedNet, and the National Library of Medicine, offer access to MEDLINE and a myriad of other clinical and patient information services. Those will be discussed in Chapter 8 as part of general health information. Their search engines are a study in and of themselves. Generally, because their goal is to make clinical information easily accessible to the health care practitioner, their content will meet your needs more succinctly than browsing multitudinous sites through a general search engine.

4. Discover Usenet. Usenet, short for user's network, is one of the vestiges of the text-based Internet. People "assemble" to discuss hundreds of topics related to specific themes. Usenet is best searched with DejaNews, a search engine that can help you find the many Usenet newsgroups and specific articles within those groups. Whether you use alt.support cancer or sci.med, there are sure to be some discussion groups just for you.

5. Backing out of an on-line address. You are in a pediatrics site, you hotlink to a site on childhood leukemia that links you to the middle of a large university site on pediatric mental health. The URL, or address, is some 60 characters long, and you wonder how you can get to the beginning of the Web site (short of clicking to go

Usenet
USErs NETwork. With more than 18,000 subject areas (newsgroups) and millions of users worldwide, Usenet is the biggest Internet resource. New messages are posted to an initial site and then distributed around global computer networks. Because of the high-traffic volume, most messages are deleted after a set period, usually a week.

to the home page). "Back out" of the address by erasing all the characters and leaving, for instance, the http://www.health.com, which will give you the home page of the site.

6. Using the "Go to:" field as a search engine. In Netscape, the Go to: field, in which you enter a familiar URL, can also be used, in a haphazard but frequently useful manner, as a search engine. Try various combinations of acronyms, such as www.aoa.com or www.emt.edu and you may hit a large site, even before you start a search engine on the trail.
7. Just try it. The beautiful irony of the Web and of searching is, although it is becoming more complex, the search engines are generally designed to return *something*. Trial and error is not necessarily a bad way to find what you want. Save the perusal of the help files for one of those rainy days. Ask colleagues what their favorite engines are. Enjoy this heady environment.

THE DREAM SEARCH ENGINE

Search engines have come a long way during the last year and will continue to evolve and proliferate. Features such as interfaces that *force* the user to enter phrases or Boolean operators, search functionality (how a search engine operates) that more closely emulates that available in commercial on-line databases, and more annotation of sites and documents, will allow users to handle the riches available on the Web without feeling as though they have opened Pandora's Box. Now, if only they could figure out how to have a tiny, holographic, cyber-librarian, who was available for search inquiries.

Bibliography

1. Courtois MP: Cool tools for Web searching: An update. *Online* 20(May/Jun): 29–36, 1996.

2. Egan J: Ready, set, search. *US News & World Report* 120(Apr 290):64, 68, 1996.

3. Pfaffenberger B: *WEB Search Strategies.* New York, MIS:Press, 1996.

4. Steinberg SG: Seek and ye shall find (maybe). *Wired* 4:108–114, 172–182, 1996.

5. Zorn P, Emanoil M, Marshall L, et al: Searching: Tricks of the trade. *Online* 20(May/Jun):17–28, 1996.

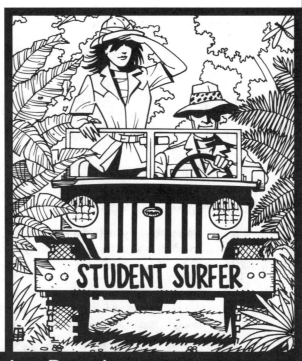

Chapter 7

Rules of the Road

NETIQUETTE, SECURITY, AND VIRUSES

At times, the Internet can be intimidating, especially to new users. This dilemma is compounded not only by having to learn how to get around, but also by having to learn how not to alienate other Net citizens by asking questions that have previously been asked. For individuals new to the Net, it would be helpful to spend as much time as necessary seeking out frequently asked questions (FAQs) lists. These can be found posted on Web sites, newsgroups, and in CompuServe and America Online (AOL) forums. In fact, by using a Web browser and one of the many available search engines, most questions can be answered fairly quickly.

Netiquette

Netiquette developed as a means of ensuring that Internet users didn't lose sight of the fact that on the other end of the software and TCP/IP (Transport Control Protocol/Internet Protocol) are real people, with the same rights, feelings, and expectations as you. That said, netiquette is more or less self-imposed. There are no Internet police who will break down your door if you violate one of the rules. However, there

Glossary Terms V–W

VERONICA
Very Easy Rodent-Oriented Netwide Index to Computer Archives. Veronica was developed to index all keywords on Gopher menus across the Internet.

are some people who will let you know when you have strayed beyond the norm. In some circumstances, your ISP (Internet Service Provider) or on-line service might impose some restrictions if things get out of hand.

The rules of netiquette are simple and easy to follow. For the most part, they relate to e-mail and Usenet messages, but they can also be applied to other Internet activities.

Don't say anything you wouldn't want to see posted in a public forum or read out-loud in a court room. You may think private e-mail will be seen only by the recipient, but it can be easily forwarded to others. Most companies routinely backup all the files on their computers, so multiple copies of your message may exist and be accessible to others.

DO NOT TYPE MESSAGES IN ALL CAPITAL LETTERS! This is the on-line equivalent of shouting. It is also very difficult to read.

It is not a good idea to overly criticize another person's grammatical or spelling errors. Remember, people from other countries and cultures do things differently, and your helpful comments may not be seen as such.

If you must criticize someone, then seriously consider doing so through e-mail and not posting the message in Usenet or in a public forum. You may find that the object of your criticism is only too willing to engage you publicly in a verbal free-for-all. Or worse, you may become embroiled in a "flame war" as others are pulled into the fight.

Occasionally you may find yourself the victim of an unprovoked or unnecessary on-line response. Be warned that some users wouldn't think twice about eviscerating you in public. Unless you really want to respond (and most of the time the intent is to lure you into a protracted encounter), ignore messages from such users or, in cases in which these users are abusive, send private e-mail to the sysop (system operator) of the forum or to the postmaster at that user's ISP (address mail to Postmaster@isp.com [substitute "isp" with the appropriate ISP name]).

Junk e-mail should be deleted or returned to the sender. Usually a reply that asks to be removed from the mailing list is all it takes, but sometimes junk e-mail is constructed by using a forged return address or no address, which makes taking any kind of action difficult. Again, forwarding a copy of the message to the postmaster at your ISP or the sender's ISP could solve the problem. AOL and CompuServe, in particular, go to great lengths to stop this kind of unsolicited mail.

If you post a question to Usenet and it is answered publicly or privately, it is a good idea to summarize the answers in a posting for the benefit of others. The nature of Usenet ensures that some people may see only some of the answers but not the original question (or vice versa.)

The Golden Rule of Usenet is to consider "What Will This Message Contribute?" If you agree with something that's been said, don't immediately send a

Virus
A computer program that automatically copies itself, infecting computers and computer disks, usually without the user's knowledge. Unless detected and removed, some viruses can damage computer programs and files. Many available software programs will detect and remove computer viruses.

reply saying, "I agree." Reply only if you have something extra to add. Likewise, if someone posts a message offering a catalog or a photo of their pet sheep, don't reply to the whole Usenet newsgroup saying, "Send to me as well." Instead, send this type of message by private e-mail. Usenet is flooded with "me too" messages, and it just adds to the volume of stuff for users to wade through.

These simple rules go a long way toward ensuring that bandwidth isn't wasted and making the Internet a little more user friendly.

SECURITY ON THE INTERNET

As more people become active on the Internet, the thorny question of security becomes ever more prominent. Some believe that the very nature of the Internet, a freewheeling frontier town with few rules, is the way it should be. But with more and more commercial business being conducted through the Internet, this state of affairs isn't conducive to the day-to-day handling of transactions and authenticating individual identities.

In fact, the freewheeling nature of the Internet has made assuming the cyberspace identity of another person or even remaining completely anonymous very easy. Obviously this poses a problem for anyone who must verify the identity of another person on-line.

On the other hand, Internet software routinely supplies more personal information about its user than was previously the case. This information can be used to build a detailed profile of your on-line habits, socioeconomic status, job, interests and hobbies, opinions and prejudices, political affiliations, and other private information, including where you live.

Does this shock you? It should. Any intermediate to advanced Internet user could probably build a comprehensive dossier on the lifestyle of another Internet user in just a few hours. A determined computer hacker, with more advanced skills and software tools, could find out as much about you on-line as could any seasoned private detective.

The biggest problem here is not what others can discover about you, but what information you post on the Internet. Usenet is probably the most telling example, because easily accessible tools can reference everything you have ever posted in any newsgroup. Read individually they probably don't say much, but, examined as a whole, they speak volumes about your interests, your opinions, the hours you are most likely to be on-line, and more. Would you want a prospective employer to read everything you've ever posted?

If you don't post many Usenet articles, then you're probably safe, but it does pay to sit back and examine the things you are sending into cyberspace. Now don't get confused. What we're talking about here are the Internet activities that are directed toward a wide audience (e.g., Usenet or mailing lists) and Web surfing. The e-mail

WAIS
Wide Area Information Server. A software system used to search indexed databases on remote computer systems.

sent to individuals is fairly harmless, and most likely what you say will be a reflection of how well you know the receiver.

We want to elaborate on the following four main areas of concern. In no particular order of importance they are listed below:

1. Personal information disclosed while on the Internet
2. Cache files and history or access logs stored, detailing the places you visit
3. Verification of on-line identities
4. Credit card information

Web browser
Software used to access WWW pages. Mosaic was the first browser, but was supplanted by the more powerful Netscape Navigator.

Personal Information

When you visit a Web site, your browser gives out information about your system. This includes the type of browser and operating system you are using, your IP address, the URL of the site you are linking from, the time of your visit, and the name of the file you access. This information is stored in an access log at the Web site and is used to generate statistics about traffic to the site. Typically, many sites use this information to determine the origins of their callers' links. For example, if you had reached the site by clicking on an advertisement at another site, this information would be invaluable in determining which advertisements were the most effective.

However, if you worked for a company like Blue Cross and were seeking competitive information from another health care insurer, perhaps Aetna, then anyone at Aetna could see from their access log that someone from Blue Cross had been seeking information about a particular product or service. From both perspectives this knowledge could be valuable competitive information.

Cookies

Netscape and MSIE (Microsoft Internet Explorer) both allow the use of a file called a "cookie." When you visit certain Web sites, bits of information relating to your visit are stored in a cookie file on your computer. Then when you next visit the same site, the cookie is retrieved and the information it contains could determine what happens next. For instance, a customized page could be shown, configured to your interests (using the cookie information). This page would be different for each visitor, depending on the contents in each one's cookie file.

If your version of Netscape Navigator (2.0 and above) is running Javascript (Netscape's built-in scripting language), then your e-mail address also could be transmitted. To give users more control about what types of information is collected, versions 3 and higher of Netscape Navigator and MSIE both provide for user monitoring of the information that is transmitted in cookie files.

And if you wanted to, you could delete the cookie files from your computer. They are clearly labeled in the directories or folders containing your Web brrowser program files. Examining the cookie file on your system using a word processor is about the only way you can tell which sites collect information in this manner.

Cache Files and History or Access Logs

Web browsers have a feature that facilitates how they provide information to the screen. This feature saves a copy of all accessed documents and graphics on your computer so only the parts of the document that have changed in the intervening time are downloaded when a site is visited again. This can dramatically decrease the time needed to construct a page. These files are referred to as cache files.

Now, although this sounds convenient on the surface, it also means that anyone can sit down at your computer and review the files in your cache, which will show the Web sites you have been visiting. Of course, if you have been scanning the "new job wanted" Web pages while at work, and your boss happens to discover these files in your cache, well… you get the picture.

Webmaster
The person in charge of a Web site.

Cache files tend to recycle themselves after a few weeks of moderate activity, replacing older cache files with newer ones. But it is possible to manually delete all the files in your cache by using the following steps:

Netscape Navigator
Click on Options/Network Preferences/Cache
Click on "Clear Disk Cache Now" and reply "OK" to the prompt
Click on "OK" to exit.

MSIE
Click on View/Options/Advanced
Select Temporary Internet Files/Settings
Click on "Empty Folder" and reply "Yes" to the prompt
Click on "OK" to exit.

AOL Web Browser
Select Members/Preferences/WWW
Click on "Advanced"
Click on "Purge Cache" and reply "Yes" to the prompt
Click on "OK" to exit.

CompuServe Spry Mosaic
Select Tools/Options/Advanced
Click on "Empty Disk Cache" and reply "Yes" to the prompt
Click on "OK" to exit.

It's a good habit to clear your cache files periodically as well as to clear out older files that are just gathering dust for the foregoing reasons. All of these browsers also allow you to adjust the size of your cache. Five megabytes seems to be the optimum size by consensus, and this is the default setting for several browsers.

History Files
Netscape and MSIE both maintain a history file that contains basic information about every Web site you have visited. Typing the following into Netscape as URLs (in the

Open Location text field) will produce the results listed in parentheses:

about:global (lists all the places you have visited and when)
about:cache (lists all files in disk cache)
about:image-cache (lists all image files in cache)

If you delete this history file (c:\netscape\netscape.hst), it will start rebuilding itself the next time you use Netscape.

No equivalent listing is available in MSIE, but the contents of the history folder can be viewed by clicking on "Go/Open History Folder." The contents can be deleted as required.

Access Logs

When you access the Web through a LAN (Local Area Network) connection, information about the sites you visit is also collected locally on your LAN server. Usually this information is used to help determine whether the system is working optimally. But increasingly, employers and institutions are using the information to keep an eye on the activities of their employees and users. Usually the only information retained in these access logs is the URL of the site visited, the date and time of the visit, and the IP address of the computer used to access the information.

No neon sign flashes in the computer room saying, "Nigel just visited the casino games site." And unless someone examines the logs carefully (or runs them through an automated search routine), there is only a small chance of someone discovering where you've been. But for the most part, this monitoring is restricted to whatever information can be gleaned from these access logs.

Verification of On-line Identities

One of the more difficult tasks on-line is ascertaining the identity of others. People can mask their identities by many means. In the CompuServe and AOL systems (and most other commercial on-line services), you can adopt a variety of nicknames. There is no obligation for these nicknames to bear any resemblance to your real name. Indeed, AOL even allows you to change your nickname as often as you like and, therefore, to have an e-mail address that constantly changes (e.g., Michelle42@aol.com).

By using the AOL example, it would be easy to assume that Michelle is a woman; indeed Michelle's postings may support this assumption. But short of actually meeting this person, there is no easy way to verify the true identity of the user. In recent years several cases have been documented of people building extensive on-line relationships and discovering much later that hotMary@aol.com is really 15-year-old Bob42@aol.com.

As discussed in Chapter 3, forging an e-mail address so it seems that a message is coming from someone other than the real sender is possible. It could be a big mistake

World Wide Web
WWW. The graphic part of the Internet, which is comprised of multimedia and hyperlinked documents that allow easy access to other Internet resources.

to take any disturbing e-mail or Usenet article at face value. Always try to substantiate the information from another source before acting on it.

Anonymous Remailers

This said, there are several legitimate reasons to conceal a true identity, for instance, someone requesting information about an embarrassing medical ailment. The anonymous remailer allows users to conceal their identities. These remailers are automated systems that allow you to send untraceable e-mail.

When you use an anonymous remailer, you send your e-mail to the remailer, which is another computer on the Internet. The remailer replaces your identifying information with an "anonymized" address. It then sends the e-mail to its final destination. The absence of a recognizable return address tells the recipient that it has gone through an anonymous remailer; usually a short notice inside the message also informs the recipient of this fact.

Probably the most prominent anonymous remailing service is based in Finland, and it can be reached by sending an e-mail message to help@anon.penet.fi. Some anonymous remailers require you to have an account with them, which means they know your identity. This is primarily a safeguard against use of the service to commit crimes or harass others.

Credit Card Numbers

When you start using the Internet to make on-line purchases, it is quite likely that you will be asked to fill in an order form with your credit card details. Many sites can now handle these types of transactions securely. That is, when you hit the send button and the order form is transmitted back to the site, it is processed in such a way that no one else can use the information it contains. Typically, this information is encrypted.

However, many sites are not set up in this way. You can usually tell the difference because a secure site will make certain that you know that it is secure, whereas the site that isn't may just have a warning about the possible hazards of supplying this information.

The key idea to remember is that supplying credit card information on the Internet through e-mail or a form on a Web site is inherently no more unsafe than giving it to someone over the telephone or in a crowded check-out line in a store. Every time you disclose your credit card details, it is possible for someone to overhear or to observe the transaction. In fact, many retail stores routinely discard duplicate credit card slips with the trash.

Over the last few years, the media have become frenzied over the unsecured nature of the Internet, and have caused many people to view it as an unsafe place to conduct business. The bottom line is, don't give your credit card information out to anyone on-line with whom you don't feel comfortable. Similarly, don't post it in a public place, such as Usenet.

VIRUSES

Viruses are small computer programs that attach themselves to other programs and floppy disks. When these "infected" programs and disks are used, the virus could act maliciously. Sometimes a harmless message appears on the screen saying you are infected, but it is just as likely that the virus could start deleting files on your computer or altering their contents. Because most viruses operate invisibly in the background, you could be unaware of the presence of a virus for quite some time.

Software is available that scans your computer and disks for signs of viral infection. If incorporated into your system, every time you start your computer or download a new file the scanner could see that you remain virus free.

Most files you download (especially those from major software vendors or on-line services like CompuServe or AOL) have already been checked. But files downloaded from elsewhere or borrowed from a friend should always be scanned before use.

⚡ **POWER TIP**
The best way to handle the potential for a virus is to create a directory or folder on your computer in which all new files and programs are stored. After scanning these files for viruses, you can use them as usual. The presence of any files in this directory or folder reminds you that they haven't been checked yet.

In recent years, there has been much discussion about viruses contained in e-mail messages. Quite simply, it is impossible to infect a computer with a virus simply by reading your e-mail. This is because a virus is a computer program, and as such it must be run to start operating. Your e-mail is only read, not run. However, a virus can arrive by e-mail if it is in an accompanying file, and this file is then run.

Note: Never activate an accompanying e-mail file or encoded Usenet article without first scanning it for viruses.

One of the most common methods for your computer to be infected with a virus is leaving an infected floppy disk in the disk drive. When you next turn your computer on, it will attempt to boot, or start, from this disk. This process transfers any virus from the disk to your computer, so get into the habit of removing all disks from disk drives before turning a computer off.

Part 2

Internet Medical Resources

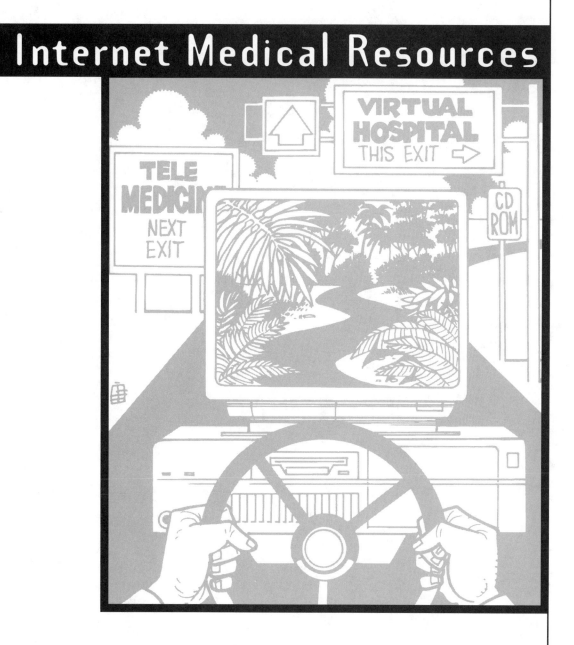

Chapter 8

Medical Networks

Where Once Only Librarians Dared to Tread

For quite some time, the only avenue for health care personnel, librarians, and other professionals to find on-line medical information was to use a proprietary dial-up system such as MEDLINE from the National Library of Medicine (NLM). Providers then encouraged on-line searching of MEDLINE and other databases with delivery systems such as PaperChase, Grateful Med, BRS, and DIALOG. Silver-Platter and Ovid offered similar off-line services on CD-ROMs (compact disks–read-only memory). Networks evolved, including the LAN (local area network)-based services such as Ovid, and proprietary services such as Physicians' Online (POL) that provide not only MEDLINE, but also drug databases, AIDSTRIALS, and the like.

Now networks are finding a home on the Internet. Some have made the transition successfully; others have achieved connection through the Internet, but their functionality (the way they operate) remains essentially like proprietary systems. There are also impressive Web sites with substantial content and marvelous links to additional sources, but they do not provide an on-line bibliographic service like MEDLINE.

We will be reviewing the main features and commenting on the serviceability of five networks. As health care content on the Internet evolves, the denotation of what constitutes a network will become more definitive. Here are the criteria for inclusion in this rather short list.

1.   The service must offer MEDLINE. Although additional content on the forward-thinking Internet networks includes consumer books, other databases, drug information, and news services, MEDLINE remains the flagship of the health care information fleet. MEDLINE, with its millions of citations to clinical literature, is the standard by which bibliographic content should be judged. It continues to be the place to start and often the place to finish when looking for peer-reviewed literature. This criterion excluded many sites, such as BioMedNet. They will be covered in the General Medicine portion of "Health-Related Information."

2.   The service must not be supported primarily through commercial sponsorship or "piggybacking" its MEDLINE provider from another site. Commercially sponsored sites tend to be more an amalgamation of other sites than of original content. This is not necessarily bad because it allows for an enormous user base and for exposure to many other sites. Still, for this section it eliminates sites such as J. Tward's Multimedia Medical Reference Library. Piggybacking, or borrowing another site's search engine, suggests liberal borrowing that is a commendable way to make MEDLINE available to

the multitudes but also indicates that functionality that is not on par with services that have developed their own search engines. This eliminated sites such as Cyberspace Telemedical Office, which will be reviewed in the "Health-Related Information."

3. The service must be an Internet application. In other words, even if it uses Internet protocol, and you can access the Internet from the service, or vice versa, the nonexistence of browser functionality eliminates the network from consideration. The third criterion removed two potential sources, POL and PaperChase. Although POL has made large strides in building a medical community on-line and bringing MEDLINE (free) into the home and office, without browser enhancements or Internet functionality (for example, you cannot use the browser's "back" button, and there are no hyperlinks within POL itself), it is not represented here. PaperChase is a beneficial source of on-line medical information. Its search capabilities, such as set building and mapping to Medical Subject Headings (MeSH), and the like should be emulated on the Internet. Unlike Grateful Med and SilverPlatter though, the two services have not made the complete transition to the Internet, and consequently, they are not included here.

No two of these networks are exactly alike. Some, such as Ovid, have extraordinary search capabilities similar to those available in proprietary services. The use of Boolean logic, limiters, MeSH, and document delivery is handled in various ways by individual networks. As you will see content is substantial, yet variable between the networks. What all the networks do possess is MEDLINE and other databases, and an inventiveness, interface design, or arrangement and inclusion of content unprecedented in the on-line medical world. So watch while they grow in capability and usership, and enjoy the adventure. You will find everything from a chapter on acupuncture to research on tamoxifen. You can even find a Civil War photograph of Lincoln (There's that hat again! See Chapter 9.) (http://wwwoli.nlm.nih.gov/databases/olihmd/olihmd.html).

THE NETWORKS

HealthGate
http://www.healthgate.com
HealthGate Data Corporation
380 Pleasant St.
Suite 230
Malden, MA 02148
Customer service: (800) 434-4283; e-mail: support@healthgate.com

Sponsor and Main Audience.—HealthGate Data Corporation; consumers, health care professionals, information specialists

Access and Cost.—Registration, password, and ID are needed for free MEDLINE with basic and advanced search capabilities. Password and ID and $14.95 per month are needed for a subscription to the "MedGate Access Plan" (MGAP), which includes MEDLINE, a news wire service, and more than eight other clinical databases. A *non-subscription,* transaction access plan (TAP) of the previously mentioned services and other databases (see "Content" section for this network) is available for 25 cents per citation, which *includes* an abstract (this can add up, be careful). "Consumer Health Information" has individual book chapters priced at $2.00, and the "Well-Connected Consumer Health Reports" charges $5.00 for documents about specific diseases. There can be charges paid to NewsPage (http://www.newspage.com), the information provider on the news wire service. Some databases, such as EMBASE, charge a small fee for the full citations to be displayed. *Advice:* Although the $14.95 price is a good deal, if you only use MEDLINE, use it free; it even includes abstracts!

The "Look" and Site Organization.—It is quite plain and pedestrian for all that is offered. HealthGate uses scripted hyperlinks; icons are not used. The organization is fairly straightforward. Choose free MEDLINE, MGAP, or TAP, give your password and ID, and the choices of databases and interface are available. Other services, such as Consumer Health Information and MDX Health Digest are available from the home page.

Content and Currency.—The last 2 years of MEDLINE are offered free from the National Library of Medicine (NLM); MGAP offers 1966 through the present; you enter the range of years you want to search. Clinical journals (more than 3,800) in English and other languages are indexed. MEDLINE is uploaded weekly; other services are somewhere in that ballpark. The Newswire Service is uploaded daily. Other databases offered by MGAP, the TAP, or both are the following:

- Ageline
- AIDSLINE
- AIDSDRUGS
- AIDSTRIALS
- BIOETHICSLINE
- CANCERLIT
- Diagnostic Procedures Handbook
- EMBASE
- HEALTH
- Medical Software Reviews
- Consumer Health Information
- MDX Health Digest
- MMWR (*Morbidity and Mortality Weekly Report*)
- Newswire Service

Interface and Search Engine.—There are two levels of interface, on free MEDLINE and MGAP/TAP. The *Basic* search function has one blank box for entering your term(s). If you enter lung transplantation emphysema, the AND operators (see Chapter 6 for a discussion about using the operators) are assumed, so the search returns citations on lung transplantation as treatment for emphysema. Boolean operators are not successful. The advanced search function, *advanced search page* (ASP) has multiple blank boxes in which you can specify "words in any field" or limit retrieval to words in the title, abstract, or as an author's name. Boolean operators (13 of them, including AND, OR, NOT, and ADJ) are available. There is no obvious MeSH mapping, but there is a *ReADER* technology that "translates" your terms automatically into the search query needed in the database you are searching. This is admirable, but not as controlled or powerful as Internet Grateful Med (see section of this network later in this chapter). There are no subheadings or other ways to fine-tune a strategy (unless you add terms to the original strategy).

Note: MeSH is important in this and subsequent descriptions because it is a "controlled language." The ability of the search engine to map natural language or your terms to the proper MeSH term will invariably give you a larger or more specific retrieval than will a non-MeSH or natural language vocabulary. Some engines map "behind the scenes"; the more sophisticated engines allow you to decide which MeSH terms to use.

Refining or Limits.—In the *basic* function of MEDLINE and the other NLM databases, you have one language option, English (otherwise *all* languages are included). You can choose whether to include abstracts and can search the last 2 years or a specified range of articles. In the ASP, the aforementioned limits, along with age groups, some journal subsets, and all NLM article types (such as review articles) are available. Here is a clever option—if there are fewer than 1,000 citations (available in increments of 5 to 200), you can sort them chronologically or by author. Automatic plural searching is available. There is no *search history,* or record of what you have previously searched (unless you use the "back" button).

Outside Site Links.—No links are available to other health-related Internet sites.

Retrieval List, Ranking, and Document Delivery.—Citations include information such as title, title/author/source, or full citation with abstract, MeSH terms, and publication type. Clicking on the title gets the full bibliographic record. You must mark the original citation to retrieve records later. Generally, documents are chronologically listed, depending on when the original article was indexed. There is no relevancy ranking (see Chapter 6 for a discussion of relevancy ranking). Documents are individually numbered. There is no document delivery. You can get articles and chapters from some of the other HealthGate consumer-oriented services.

Help.—The only on-line help is related to the descriptions of the Boolean operators, and that needs some examples. There are no icons to steer users directly to this single bit of help. Help!

Extras and Upcoming Features.—The news wire service is a good resource. It lists 50 different medical disciplines that are hyperlinked to the NewsPage service of Individual, Inc. These are then linked to the wire stories. New drugs and procedures form the bulk of the News. The MDX Personal Health Library has four books, on medical tests, pediatrics, drugs, and symptoms, that have their own simple search engines and provide good information for $2.00 per article. PsycINFO and CINAHL (Cumulative Index to Nursing and Allied Health Literature) are coming soon, as are three new titles in the MDX Personal Health Library. Continuing medical education (CME) and full-text journal articles are on the horizon.

Comments.—The "Well-Connected Patient Library," which includes comprehensive information on a number of diseases, is available for $5.00 per topic. The selection of other clinical databases, such as EMBASE, is to be commended. The network offers "What's New In HealthGate" that keeps users abreast of changes. Two recent additions, an on-line subscription to the perennial favorite, *The New Our Bodies, Ourselves,* and a service called Healthy Woman (vibrant layout and design too!) that offers excerpts from important health publications for women, show that HealthGate has its finger firmly on the pulse of what is needed in health information. It sports substantive consumer-based information, basic clinical databases for the professional, and MEDLINE. Some further search capability in MEDLINE, including search histories, Selected Dissemenination of Informatioan (SDI), document delivery, and the like should be considered for the future. HealthGate is a beneficial, affordable, well-designed network.

HealthWorld Online
http://www.healthy.net
HealthWorld Online
10751 Lakewood Blvd.
Downey, CA 90241
Customer service: (310) 862-6116; e-mail: hwinfo@healthy.net

Sponsor and Main Audience.—Health Broadcasting Network, Inc.; MEDLINE is sponsored by BodyWise; other services are coordinated 'by founders Dave Robertson and Jim Strohecker; On-line Advisory Board of Health Care Professionals; consumers and health care professionals.

Access and Cost.—Over 20,000 pages of free-access health information. There are small charges for professional-level content and for audio tapes. The on-line journals are $2 per article. Consumer-level disease information in the Health Clinic is free. Chapters from reference texts, journal articles, and audios can be accessed for fees ranging from $2 to $5. There are no charges for MEDLINE, printing, downloading, etc. Users set up a Cybercash or "ccash" account for secure transactions for the aforementioned services. On-line purchases in the Marketplace are made by credit card via Netscape Commerce Server.

The "Look" and Site Organization.—This is the cat's pajamas, visually speaking—colorful, catchy logo and compelling graphics; it looks the most like an Internet site, rather than a proprietary database that found a new environment, such as IGM (see IGM section in this chapter). This is not just a network, it is a *Village.* The Village Icon, which produces a "map," can be used to locate individual services. A "Tour" leads to the content. The links around the Village are straightforward. You can always return to the Quick'Ndex on the top tool bar to find out where you are. Each part of the Village, for example the Health Clinic, has hyperlinks to specific content.

Content and Currency.—HealthWorld offers access to the following:

- MEDLINE, CATLINE, and AVLINE. MEDLINE (1966–present) is broken into service-able portions. There are more than 3,800 clinical journals, in English and other languages, that are indexed. MEDLINE is generally updated weekly.

  HealthWorld Online's ten major sites provide a voluminous amount of consumer-based information that seems to be current and dynamic. This consists of a large volume of alternative and complementary medicine documents, including articles, chapters from books, recipes for healthy menus, calendars for workshops on alter-native therapies, and on and on.

- Library of Health and Medicine (includes MEDLINE, reference texts, and alternative medicine journals)

- Health Clinic, which contains information and resources on conventional and alternative therapies, laboratory tests, referrals to health professionals, and specific diseases.

- Wellness Center

- Nutrition Center

- Health University

- Public Health Center

- Association Network

- Media Center

- Home Health and Self-Care

- Health Marketplace (bookstores and health food stores with more than 5,000 products, protected credit card purchases)

Interface and Search Engine.—The interface is single open box in the Library of Health and Medicine and in MEDLINE. There are a number of search engines. The HealthWorld search uses Excite's (www.excite.com) search engine. You enter terms, and with Excite's "fuzzy and," that puts all the words together, the more words you enter, the more specific will be the response. Excite also offers a "Query by Example," in which you can click on a retrieved citation and obtain other citations that are conceptually related. The search engine for MEDLINE uses NLightN (www.nlightn.com), a distinctive search engine that uses Boolean operators (the default is AND, but OR and NOT are allowed, too). NLightN searches not only MEDLINE, but also searches other databases, abstract services, and news services and returns documents from them. (HealthWorld is exempt from criterion 3. Excite and NLightN are not borrowed from other health care *sites;* they are generic Internet-wide search engines, although you will see that they are not as powerful as a more MEDLINE-derived search engine, like that of Physician's Home Page.)

Refining or Limits.—There are none really. In the Excite engine, you enter additional terms for the HealthWorld Literature. In MEDLINE, the filters are from NLightN, which is a bit of a deficiency. There are no limiters in the MEDLINE interface for years, publication types, human vs. animal, or similar limiters. This shortcoming is being addressed. There is no refinement of the search strategy available, i.e., there are no subheadings, and there is no MeSH mapping, behind the scenes or overt. The MEDLINE citations do list MeSH, so you could subsequently enter the indexed MeSH term. NLightN is far ranging in the documents it retrieves, but for the sophisticated user, the lack of a MEDLINE-derived search engine is apparent.

Outside Site Links.—Although lacking in search and limitation capability, HealthWorld very cleverly uses generic search engines. There are links to Excite from HealthWorld. You can link to the NLightN search engine too, which indexes not only MEDLINE, but also the Internet, news services, and the like. In the Public Health Center and Association Network, there are links to consumer groups and professional health associations.

Retrieval List, Ranking, and Document Delivery.—The retrieval lists on the consumer-related Internet-type documents are hyperlinked to the document wherever it resides on the Web. Excite's retrieval lists in the HealthWorld Area are ranked by *Confidence.* Excite confidently believes (based on how the terms are entered) that these are the appropriate matches to your query. There are no numbers on the documents, and the total number retrieved is not indicated. In the MEDLINE area, NLightN produces an initially confusing hodgepodge of results. You should persevere; the ranking is based on when the NLightN sequence system discovered the document, and it is mainly chronological. The citations also include other databases besides MEDLINE. NLightN has something no one else currently has: a *review log* that keeps a record of the searches you have done and can hyperlink you back to that strategy. This is the measure of things to come! There is no document delivery.

Help.—This network exists to help, almost to a fault. In the HealthWorld section, as well as in MEDLINE, the search query instructions are just below the search fields themselves. Helpful, but a bit busy once you are familiar with it, and you must scroll quite a bit to get to bottom of the page. There is a really fine "Quick'Ndex," a categorized table of contents that has hyperlinks to the various parts of the Village. There is a section called "Guide for Professionals" that gives useful search tips.

Extras and Upcoming Features.—The extras abound. This is browsing at its best. There are legal and legislative forums, calendars of upcoming events, and a marketplace where you can buy the latest book on alternative medicine or get a shipment of goldenseal. (A "shopping basket" is provided.) The Village is a clever concept meant to build a sense of community about alternative (as well as conventional) approaches to health care. "Ask Doc Tom" (Tom Ferguson, M.D.) is a particularly thoughtful service. Dr. Ferguson carefully answers questions and helps you locate further information. A multitude of services are coming soon. Speaker's Network, Health Newswire, and Forums in Public Health are all on the horizon. Each part of the Village has a news or update function as well. NLightN will soon unveil ways to customize the retrieval list, by chronology, author's name, or source of article, which will be a welcome feature.

Comment.—HealthWorld Online is a philosophical and practical environment for self-managed care, as well as a visionary Web site. The providers believe that information makes for informed consumers and practitioners, and they want you to have all the information possible—with a heavy accent on alternative practice. Health professionals and consumers will enjoy the on-line CME in the Health University, the Nutritional Influences on Illness Database, the Government Health Information, and on and on. Although the MEDLINE functionality needs substantial work, this innovative network has enormous potential.

Internet Grateful Med
http://www.nlm.nih.gov/
National Library of Medicine
8600 Rockville Pike
Bethesda, MD 20894
Customer service: (800) 638-8480; press 4 for staff members familiar with IGM;
e-mail: gmhelp@gmedserv.nlm.nih.gov

Sponsor and Main Audience.—NLM; health care professionals and information specialists

Access and Cost.—Previously available only through conventional mail service, you can now obtain your password and ID with an on-line request form and a credit card by using Netscape 2.0 browser, otherwise you must still fill out a paper form and wait for 7 to 10 days to receive your password and ID. There are no subscription or minimum fees. The NLM charges per search, but only for the time that the search is actually running, not while you are formulating your search strategy. The connect time is 4 cents per minute, and the citation charge is 1 cent per citation you view, print, or download. The character charge is 5 cents per 1,000 characters you view, print, or download. Other charges include 6 cents per search statement and 4 cents for each 100 work units. Generally the total cost is $1.25 to $6.00 per search. Hourly rates are available if the connection time is lengthy. Student rates and fixed and flat rates are available. Access for users outside the United States who do not have direct access is coming soon.

The "Look" and Site Organization.—IGM has a clean, functional look. It includes handy icons such as "Fetch for Display," "Download for Disk," "Order Documents,"

"Other Years," "Next Records," and "Details of Search." It has a "New and Noteworthy" link to inform users of any network changes. The organization is straightforward. You choose from the initial HyperDoc screen, and off you go.

Content and Currency.—Content is primarily MEDLINE (1966–present), broken into serviceable portions. More than 3,800 clinical journals in English and other languages are indexed. It is updated weekly. Your NLM account can also include Toxnet/PDQ, and in the future, the AIDS database. It now includes Health Services/Technology Assessment Text (HSTAT) for some of the clinical practice guidelines from the Agency for Health Care Policy and Research, and there is a hyperlink to the extraordinary images from the History of Medicine Division of NLM.

Interface and Search Engine.—The interface consists of three unchanging open boxes. You are allowed to enter words as authors, as subjects, or in titles.

You can enter text words or MeSH. This is the originator of all that is medical information on-line and possesses a very powerful search engine. It includes Boolean operators; AND is the default, and OR is available. You can find "Related Terms," (MeSH terms related to the term you entered.) You can then choose a related term that is hyperlinked to more information and to the MeSH Tree Context. Such a term can then be used as the major topic in the search to make it more specific. You can "Analyze Search," which shows the search history; i.e., which terms were used and what they retrieved individually and together. After choosing related headings, other terms, or qualifiers, or subheadings (such as surgery, therapy, or etiology) can be applied as limiters, which is a very potent search capability. You can nest (see Chapter 6 for a discussion of nesting) terms together with parentheses, for example (a and b) or (c and d) and e. For those wondering if the functionality of Grateful Med transferred to the Internet, the answer is "Yes," with a few exceptions that are discussed later in this section.

Refining or Limits.—You can limit by one of four languages, one of four publication types, and "Study Groups," "Age Groups," and "Beginning and Ending Year". (There are not as many choices as with Grateful Med.) Refining is also done with the MeSH and subheadings mentioned earlier. After you enter a term, you will not realize how multilayered and powerful IGM is unless you try the "Find Related" icon. It leads to the *Metathesarus,* that leads to "Concept" and more terms, which leads to subheadings. Give it a whirl!

Outside Site Links.—None, except to other NLM services.

Retrieval List, Ranking, and Document Delivery.—The original short citations include title, author, source, and NLM ID. Clicking on the title gets the full bibliographic record, including an abstract and MeSH terms. You must mark the original citation to "fetch" records later. Other than a total number, and a 1 out of 10 numeration, documents are not individually numbered. This is a small but annoying element when you are trying to access if you have already seen the citation in an earlier search.

Generally, the citations are chronologically listed (depending on when the original article was indexed.) There is no relevancy ranking. You can download all or part of the retrieval set at once. You can order documents (articles) through Loansome Doc or e-mail a set of retrieved citations to yourself or someone else.

Help.—There is an "I" icon that is always available to describe how the other functional icons work. There is also a "New User's Survival Guide," that is *exemplary,* covering everything from a simple first search to using the Metathesaurus to downloading. You can e-mail the developers.

Extras and Upcoming Features.—Even if you don't find a related term for a phrase you entered, such as "abuse control," IGM will map it to the proper MeSH term "child abuse" (and give you any "abuse control" hits). There are 5,000 such "Associated Expressions" in IGM, the results of which will appear first on your retrieval lists. There is an interactive tutorial coming soon. Yes!

Comments.—Although there is no NOT function on the interface, you can, for example, enter "/not hepatitis A" in the search field to eliminate a particular term from your result. A more apparent NOT function would be appreciated, as would numbered citations. The content (other than the obvious millions of article citations) is not far-ranging. For example, there are no book chapters, no CME courses, and no consumer health information. We would like to see some "set-building" capability, an SDI component, and the ability to customize the citation format. This does not detract from the idea that when it comes to NLM-produced databases, no one sets the standard higher. This workhorse of affordable, comprehensive bibliographic medical information has translated quite well to the Internet environment. The developers should be proud.

Ovid

http://www.ovid.com
Ovid Technologies, Inc.
333 Seventh Ave.
New York, NY 10001
Customer service: (800) 950-2371; e-mail: support@ovid.com

Sponsor and Main Audience.—Ovid Technologies, Inc.; institutions, health care professionals, and information specialists

Access and Cost.—Ovid, primarily a client-server, LAN-network type database provider, has hit the Internet with a BANG! The "Ovid Web Gateway" permits users to access Ovid and its Z39.50 databases using a Web browser. The Z39.50 is a powerful communications system that allows Ovid to bring databases into our lives. There is already a "pay-as-you-go" and fixed-fee structure in an ASCII format, but the Internet is new to Ovid. A free trial (the demo contains three databases and MEDLINE for 1993) of the Gateway is being offered, but soon there will be pay-as-you-go fees. Although the intricacies of billing are still to be resolved, the fixed-fee for institutions for the Gateway will probably be a minimum monthly subscription against which connect time and citation retrieval are charged against. For the general public, the pay-as-you-go fee will be (depending on the database; these numbers are for MEDLINE) about $12.00 per hour plus 20 cents per full citation and abstract (no additional charges for viewing the titles) plus telecommunications charges.

The "Look" and Site Organization.—Ovid's muted colors, distinctive icons, and clean design create an atmosphere that is at once appealing and functional. The icons at the bottom of the home page provide straightforward links to the various services. MEDLINE and other databases are part of the "NEW" section, so the databases are immediately apparent. Because of its other services, such as the Ovid Client/Server, Ovid Full Text, and Ovid Online, the Home Page also links to information about the other products and services. The other databases in the Gateway Demo—Current Contents, ERIC, and part of their full-text core biomedical collections—are also easy to locate. Within the MEDLINE demo the graphics on the icons are fairly indicative of the actions they allow.

Content and Currency.—Content! Well, it is not the same as HealthWorld Online's emphasis on alternative therapies and consumer information, or Physician's Home Page with drug interaction information, but after the initial trial period, there will eventually be more than 80 databases available. MEDLINE is updated weekly. Updates of other databases are dependent on the provider. From Bioethics Line to the PDQ Cancer Information File and from EMBASE to the Wilson Indexes will be available (for various hourly fees) from Ovid. Assuming functionality mirrors that of MEDLINE and the cost is not prohibitive, there will be an extraordinary bibliographic treasure trove on the Internet.

Interface and Search Engine.—As they say in the Dodge truck ads, "This Changes Everything." As an information provider outside the Internet, Ovid had some of the most refined functionality of any system, anywhere. This functionality has transferred admirably to the Internet. First, the basic interface consists of two blank boxes, one for keyword(s) and one for author. In the advanced version, there is a single blank box for keywords (why did they remove the author box?) and the search capabilities are more sophisticated. The system automatically assumes an operator in the search field, but you can enter Boolean logic or parentheses. Here is the beauty. Ovid is distinctive on the Internet (although some proprietary systems, such as PaperChase have it) because it "maintains state," that is, it keeps track of search terms and results and allows users to manipulate previous search results as needed. This is immediately evident in the display screen, which gives not only the result, say 33 citations, but also the search strategy and a "set" number. For example, Set 1 = lung transplantation and emphysema, Result 12. A second search becomes Set 2, and so on. You can then *combine* (AND, OR, or NOT) various set numbers to get a fine-tuned result (or a broader result). In addition to being able to search on journal, title, or body of the work, the advanced version also allows for MeSH mapping (it is, in fact, automatic, unless you shut it off), and once the MeSH tree is shown (the hierarchy of the term and its related terms), you can add subheadings to the term. In a database such as

ERIC, the terms will map to that producer's distinctive thesaurus. Naturally, the Boolean operators and similar affiliating type functions are not as crucial in the up-front boxes, because the system and the display screen allow for combining. What more could you want?

Refining and Limits.—How about this? In the *basic* mode, you limit at the outset by marking radio buttons. The options are *just* the English language (otherwise you get all languages); *full text* (of the citations that are available, you want only those that are available with the complete article); just *human* (or you get animals too); and just *reviews,* or just *abstracts* (or you get all types of articles and citations with or without abstracts). You can change the range of years searched too. And in the *advanced* mode, you have those limiters in addition to the language you would really prefer (there has never been a lot in Swahili or Urdu), particular age groups, the type of publication (e.g., clinical trial, review, or letter to the editor), type of animal, and other limiters as well. Also, as mentioned, the subheadings act as MESH limiters, and the functions themselves, with the ability to combine, make for fine tuning a search result.

Outside Site Links.—None. Well, other than all of those Z39.50 databases soon to come. No hyperlinks to other Web sites.

Retrieval List, Ranking, and Document Delivery.—The retrieved citations are numbered, and the *complete record* hyperlinks to the full citation and abstract, if one has been supplied. The author's name is hyperlinked to all other publications by that author, and the journal title is hyperlinked to the table of contents of the individual issue of the journal so you can see the other articles published with this one. But wait! If the full text of a retrieved citation is available, say an entire article on Grave's disease from the *Journal of the American Medical Association,* from the full text you can return to the list of titles you came from and see the table of contents of the entire issue. You can e-mail the article to a colleague or save the article. No relevancy ranking is available. Citations are listed chronologically, depending on when they were indexed by NLM. Speaking of citations, Ovid has a Citation Manager at the end of the citations that allows you to display, e-mail, or save your citations. And you can customize how they look—citation only, with abstract, or with abstract and MeSH terms. Other than the three substantial core biomedical collections of full-text journals (which will be such a pleasure to have available), there is no document delivery.

Help.—Help is available on the ASP and alongside the database names for more information on that database. The *help* function on the ASP is straightforward; it gives examples, and it does the job. Also, as you begin the demo, and find yourself in the advanced features with MeSH mapping and subheading, on-screen hints make the job less stressful.

Extras and Upcoming Features.—On the Ovid Web Gateway itself, what do you add to full text of the most seminal journals? More journals! What do you add to the search capability? SDI, where you make some sort of "folder" on a subject and every time there is a database update, the new citations would be placed in your folder. It's coming! Based on what is already here, you can assume these people are always thinking. Let's see what they come up with next.

Comments.—All right, this is one desirable network. It is wide ranging, it is confident, and it might well set the standard for how searches function on the Internet. Still, it is remarkably hard to figure out what Ovid does truly offer and to whom. With its servers and on-line systems and worldwide hookups and fixed fee, and pay as you go, and the Z39.50 and 80 databases and…well, it's almost too much. A bit of time should be spent on the instructional text to succinctly detail how various users can access Ovid to use MEDLINE and other clinical databases. Then clarify the gnarled pricing structure. Will the casual user or nonacademic health care professional or freelance librarian be able to afford this? For a company with such a crystal clear search capability, the transference of basic information about the services is muddied and wordy (and a bit of whimsy would be nice; this company is *so* serious). Although we can go to other networks for consumer information and drug information and news, Ovid's "Fall Line-Up" could offer document delivery (other than the full-text journal articles already offered), or perhaps the staff will figure out how we can save our search strategies and search results somewhere on the browser. Numerous clinical librarians have sent thoughts heavenward hoping that the information overseers would see fit to offer Ovid on the Internet. The day is here, and it should be visited by the masses.

Physicians' Home Page (PHP)
http://php2.silverplatter.com
Silver Platter Education
246 Walnut St., Suite 302
Newton, MA 02160-1639
Customer service: (800) 521-0574; e-mail: php@silverplatter.com

Sponsor and Main Audience.—Silver Platter Education, Inc.; "…exclusively designed for physicians."

Access and Cost.—You must register on-line to receive a user name and password. The first month is free. There is a $19.95 monthly fee for unlimited access and a $30.00 one-time sign-up fee. For physicians that have SilverPlatter on a CD-ROM, the fee is $9.95 per month. The fee for medical residents is $9.95 per month. Document delivery has charges too. Members outside the United States must pay a US National Library of Medicine International Users fee as well. There is a *free* preview of all the services on the network at all times.

The "Look" and Site Organization.—This very capable network is fairly undistinguished. It is as gray and black and white as it can be. MEDLINE (and other services) is rather hidden within the introductory text. You can also click on the "Take a Look Around" hyperlink at the top of the introduction to find it.

Content and Currency.—MEDLINE's more than 3,800 clinical journals, in English and other languages, are indexed and updated weekly. The other services seem to be reliably current. AIDSLINE and CANCERLIT are included. The MD Opinions (100 questions in the field of medicine posed for consensus and member input; includes an editorial panel), MD Digests (original articles from medical journals, presented with clinical summaries), MD Drugs (the drug interactions database), MD CME (information about accredited electronic CME programs), and MD Elsewhere (investment, travel, and lifestyle resources available over the Net) are appealing features. Core Journals on the Web (search subsets of MEDLINE focused on the *British Medical Journal,* the *Journal of the American Medical Association,* the *New England Journal of Medicine, The Lancet,* and *The Annals of Internal Medicine*) is a new, interesting approach to keeping physicians informed.

Interface and Search Engine.—The interface is designed to lead the searcher into placing a string of appropriate terms. In MEDLINE, there is a single open box, a Boolean operator option (AND, OR, NOT, WITH, or NEAR), and then another box to add other terms. The search engine is exceptional. It is a WebSPIRS-PHP, specially designed Silver Platter Information search software. The truncation on words can be customized. You can use parentheses to set off terms. You can search the author field or a combination of fields. It has a *suggest* button that gives related terms that might be useful and a thesaurus on the interface that includes related concepts. Like the printed MeSH thesaurus, this is where you find MeSH terms and subheadings.

Refining or Limits.—There is an *index.* This is sensational, although sort of hidden and misnamed. Why *index?* These are known as limiters most everywhere else. They allow for customizing the search for such factors as years, publication type, and language. The limits are then added to the search strategy. The MeSH terms and subheadings can be used for refining as well.

Outside Site Links.—The MD Internet Library offers direct and organized access to medically relevant documents and resources throughout the Internet. It is selective, categorized, and most welcome.

Retrieval List, Ranking, and Document Delivery.—The retrieved documents are numbered. The entire citation plus the abstract is shown, and before you get too far into the search, you can customize the display (e.g., just title and author) and run citations "again." This is quite civilized. The retrieval list is somewhat chronological, by when the document was indexed by NLM. The document delivery is remarkable: (1) If the citation includes a journal from a publisher that has a Web site that includes the full text of its journals, you can hyperlink from the provided Univeral Resource Locator (URL) and see if the article is there. (2) Documents are available by fax. You can order almost 60% of the articles on MEDLINE. Prices vary (depending on factors such as the original provider and copyright) from $3.50 to $20.00 per fax. The ordering information is right in the citation!

Help.—Help is available within the search interface and straightforward. There are good examples in "Getting Fancy With Your Searches."

Extras and Upcoming Features.—*Embedded annotations* are incorporated within the body of articles to find hyperlinks to related information on the subject, e.g., an article about leukemia may contain an embedded annotation that takes the user directly to more research available on leukemia. There is a fine section called "Medical Research" that offers hyperlinks to sites about research projects and research groups. As with the other networks reviewed, PHP is constantly working to improve content and functionality, especially on the databases. In development now is set building throughout your search, to facilitate manipulation of your various search results! Also, the suggest terms, thesaurus, and index functions will be displayed as icons, which, on initial review, seems to be an elegant way to offer these enhancements. Stay posted for further developments.

Comments.—PHP is one impressive service. The interfaces, search engine, and functionality are indicative of how a network ought to be executed. It could use a bit of sprucing up, and it could increase its content and user base greatly if it recognized that medicine is not limited to physicians. However, its specialization has made services such as the MD Opinions and MD CME particularly commendable. The price may be a bit prohibitive, but the product may ultimately be worth the cost. Upcoming enhancements in the MEDLINE service will make PHP quite the contender in the Internet network environment.

CONCLUSION

If there was a network wish list, these five networks together would fairly well take care of most of the details. Although librarians dream of set building, SDI, saved strategies, mapping controlled vocabulary, and other fancy stuff, it could well be that health care professionals do not need all the bells and whistles that librarians covet, in which case HealthGate and other networks with basic MEDLINE search capabilities will serve their users sufficiently. It could be that a simple search of regular words is better than getting stuck up in the MeSH hierarchical tree. Then again, the very aspects that make librarians such successful searchers will be available to you. Imagine the possibilities!

The increase in substantive consumer information, the building of professional communities, the amalgamation of alternative therapies and "regular" medicine, and the increasingly sophisticated search engines are all to be applauded. We imagine that the following are still to come: diagnostic databases, an emphasis on the politics and economics of health care, content from textbooks, annotated reviews of other health care sites, help with grantsmanship…The world is their oyster, and the networks are producing, then presenting the pearls. String them together, and your understanding of health care issues and concerns will benefit as never before.

AS WE GO TO PRESS

Other networks: Community of Science (http://cos.gdb.org), Knowledge Finder (http://www.kfinder.com), Infotrieve (http://www.infotrieve.com), and Plymouth Area Communities Medical Access (http://www.pacman.org) are evident on the Internet. They all have MEDLINE and they all have other services valuable to health care professionals. Because of space, time, and other constraints, they are not included in this current review.

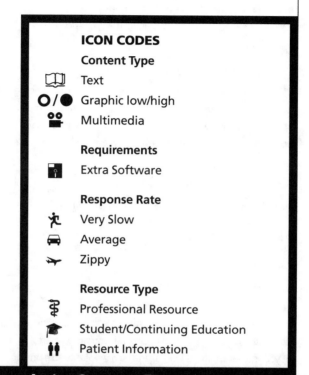

Chapter 9

ICON CODES

Content Type

Text

O/● Graphic low/high

Multimedia

Requirements

Extra Software

Response Rate

Very Slow

Average

Zippy

Resource Type

Professional Resource

Student/Continuing Education

Patient Information

General Health Care Resources

ALLIED HEALTH AND NURSING

ALLIED HEALTH

Emergency Medical Services

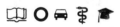

Emerginet

Provided by the National Collegiate EMS Foundation

LINKS Address: *http://www.emerginet.com/*
Cost: No charge.

This site is an excellent resource for a wide variety of emergency personnel including emergency medical services (EMS), fire, law enforcement, hazardous materials, and search and rescue. On-line articles are available from *The Global Pulse,* as are links to extensive resources, news updates, and announcements. The provider is planning the addition of continuing medical education (CME) and employment opportunities in the near future. This site has recently moved from the HVAC's Home Page, so if you like the current articles, look for back issues at http://www.ncemsf.org/ pulse/

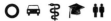

Federal Emergency Management Agency
Provided by Federal Emergency Management Agency (FEMA)

LINKS, SEARCH

Address: *http://www.fema.gov/homepage.html*
Cost: No charge.

FEMA has brought natural disaster to the Internet! This site covers the entire range of natural disasters and includes news, disaster archives, a library (photo and text), on-line publications, and extensive links to fire, search and rescue, emergency management, other federal agencies, and weather sites. Extensive information is available on-line for disaster prevention and response.

Journal of Emergency Medical Services (JEMS)
Provided by JEMS Communications

LINKS

Address: *http://wwwdot.com/jems/mainmenu.html*
Cost: No charge.

If you like on-line shopping, this is the place to be! You can check out all of the latest products gear related to EMS, fire, and search and rescue in the *Exhibit Hall* or go to the on-line *Bookstore* to order the latest publications. You will also find job listings and classified ads at this site, as well as information on several journals of interest to those in the field; but don't get your hopes up, those journal articles are not available on-line just yet. You will have to subscribe.

Medconnect (Emergency Medicine)
Provided by Medical Network, Inc.

JOURNALS, CME

Address: *http://www.medconnect.com/finalhtm/pedjc/emclbhm.htm*
Cost: No charge.

What a great site! *Emergency Medicine News at Your Desktop* is loaded with up-to-the-minute information and is a *must* for anyone wanting to keep up with the latest developments in emergency medicine. This site contains summaries from recent journal articles pertaining to the practice of emergency medicine, with *Editor's Comments* and an interactive discussion forum. By registering, you will be sent these summaries as they are available and you can join the on-line journal club. The site is well organized, quick loading, and easy to navigate, but it is bogged down by a few too many "click here to continue" pages.

National Association of EMTs

Address: *http://www.naemt.org/public/naemt.htm*
Cost: No charge.

A rather tiny site that offers information on the National Association of EMTs and their current activities.

Physical Therapy and Rehabilitation

American Physical Therapy Association

Provided by American Physical Therapy Association (APTA)

LINKS, SEARCH

Address: *http://www.apta.org*

Cost: No charge.

Several resources at this site can be searched by keyword or concept: research updates; the APTA product catalog; tables of contents for *PT* (a news magazine); and abstracts of *Physical Therapy* (a peer-reviewed clinical journal). The abstracts and tables of contents are available for most issues since January 1995. This site also provides a meeting calendar, information about the physical therapy profession in general, and more than 35 links to associations, educational programs, and related resources. One of the most interesting is Hosford's Muscle Tables, which organize information about all the muscles of the human body.

PT at Northeastern University

Provided by Northeastern University, Physical Therapy Department

LINKS

Address: *http://www.ptd.neu.edu/index.html*

Cost: No charge.

Physical therapy students at Northeastern University have on-line support for five of their classes and labs: the syllabi, discussion questions, slides, practice examinations, and lecture notes are available at this site. Web surfers not affiliated with Northeastern are welcome to view the materials. Most of the other information at this site concerns the university department itself, including employment opportunities. People planning to visit or study in Boston will enjoy the links to entertainment, cultural, and transportation resources.

Physiotherapy Global-Links Home Page

Provided by University of South Australia, Department of Physiotherapy

LINKS

Address: *http://www.netspot.unisa.edu.au/pt/or-index.html*

Cost: No charge.

This excellent collection of links gives users access to physical therapy (PT) resources with an international focus. Some links are to electronic resources (e.g., PT Web sites, Web courses, e-mail lists, newsgroups, FTP [file transfer protocol], images, databases, and Internet tutorials), while others are to publications, schools, research groups, courses, conferences, and employment notices (mostly for positions in the UK and Australia). Users will enjoy experimenting with two powerful search engines that have been incorporated into this site: AltaVista and Reference.com, which searches more than 16,000 newsgroups and more than 1,000 e-mail lists.

Dr. Pribut's Running Injuries Page
Provided by Stephen M. Pribut, D.P.M.

LINKS

Address: *http://www.clark.net/pub/pribut/spsport.html*
Cost: No charge.

This site, also titled Dr. Pribut's Sports Page, provides excellent information for patients and professionals, although the two types are not clearly distinguished. Examples of topics for patients are stretching and other preventive measures, training in hot or cold weather, sports shoes, and selecting a sports physician. Topics for professionals include biomechanics, sports physiology, and sports injuries.

Some paragraphs are too long for on-screen reading. Dozens of links take the user to other Web sites (e.g., other sports, medicine, and podiatry), information about e-mail lists and Usenet groups, and other fine collections of medical links.

Research Clearing House
Provided by The New Zealand Centre for Research and Information

LINKS

Address: *http://www.massey.ac.nz/~rchweb/*
Cost: No charge.

The Research Clearing House is compiling a database that will include research paper abstracts and the names of researchers, research organizations, and research sponsors in the field of disability and rehabilitation. This information will be available on the Web and by e-mail, phone, and fax request. In the meantime, this site maintains information about specific disabilities and conditions (e.g., autism and bipolar disorder) and about general topics such as assistive technologies and special education. Much is appropriate for both patients and professionals. In addition, there are links to gopher resources, Listservs, monographs and other publications, and Web sites for disability and rehabilitation organizations and support groups.

The National Rehabilitation Information Center Home Page
Provided by National Institute on Disability and Rehabilitation Research (NIDRR, United States)

LINKS

Address: *http://www.cais.net/naric/home.html*
Cost: No charge.

Original information at this site includes the complete text of NIDRR resource guides for patients (e.g., regarding spinal cord injury, head injury, stroke, home modification, and the Americans With Disabilities Act [ADA]), directories of NIDRR programs and other U.S. information sources, a compendium of products, a meeting calendar, *Rehab Briefs* (monographs), and abstracts of publications received. The site links to NIDRR project information, conference information, and information about helping people with disabilities to use the Internet.

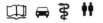 **HSTAT: Health Services/Technology Assessment Text**
Provided by National Library of Medicine (United States)

SPANISH

Address: *http://text.nlm.nih.gov/*
Cost: No charge.

The Agency for Health Care Policy and Research (AHCPR) makes clinical practice guidelines available on-line, along with quick reference guidelines and consumer guidelines. Some of the consumer guidelines are available in English and Spanish. Topics of particular interest to rehabilitation professionals include poststroke rehabilitation, cardiac rehabilitation, and urinary incontinence in adults. Each publication is searchable by keyword(s). From the welcome screen, click *AHCPR Supported Guidelines,* then click the *Submit* key.

 Ability Home Page
Provided by Ability

LINKS

Address: *http://www.ability.org.uk/home.html*
Cost: No charge.

The principal mission of this site is to make the Internet accessible and fun for people with disabilities. There are several hundred links, some of general interest, some disease- or condition-specific, including some for children. However, to see the options in each category, the user must click on each letter of the alphabet, A to Z, which can be tedious. The provider plans to expand this site to thousands of links with an on-site search engine.

 Prosthetics Research Study WWW Home Page
Provided by Prosthetics Research Study

LINKS

Address: *http://weber.u.washington.edu/~prs/*
Cost: No charge.

Prosthetics Research Study (PRS), which is funded by the U.S. Department of Veterans Affairs, conducts research on amputee rehabilitation, limb preservation, surgery, and prosthetics. The strength of this site is its *Library,* which includes a textbook, summaries of PRS projects, and a bibliography of journal articles and conference proceedings. A journal, *Virtual Journal of the Society for Computer-Aided Design in Prosthetics and Orthotics,* is said to be available, but only one article was available at the time of our visit in July 1996. There are links to prosthetics and orthotics research and education centers, biomechanics resources, and commercial products.

Occupational Therapy

O.T. Online
Provided by Kristin Levine

LINKS **Address:** *http://www.dartmouth.edu/people/lmlevine/kristin/OTONLINE.html*
Cost: No charge.

Job search on-line resources, including *PRN MedSearch* and *TheraSearch,* are main attractions of this site. Another is *OT-ONLINE,* an electronic newsletter available here with back issues to November 1995. There are excellent links to other occupational therapy (OT)–related resources, including e-mail lists, a newsgroup, commercial sites, OT Internet links, and another especially good Web site, OT Internet World (http://mother.com/~ktherapy/ot/).

The provider encourages OTs who have personal Web pages to link to this site. Committed to educating OTs about the Internet, the provider has built links to Web page creation tools, Internet tutorials, and information about Internet software (e.g., browsers and editors).

Occupational Therapy Talk Back
Provided by Tami Whitson, O.T.R./L.

Address: *http://home.earthlink.net/~whitson/ot/talkback.html*
Cost: No charge.

This site functions like a newsgroup; questions and answers are posted by e-mail. But here, when a thread has run its course (that is, when participants stop sending comments about a given topic), the e-mail is archived so it can be read by other therapists in the future. The provider runs a sister site, Physical Therapy Talk Back (substitute *pt* for *ot* in the URL given above).

Respiratory Therapy

Respiratory on the Web
Provided by Steve Grenard

LINKS **Address:** *http://www.xmission.com/%7egastown/herpmed/respi.htm*
Cost: No charge.

This is the place to start in respiratory care. Little original information is available, but the site provides links to more than 150 resources: respiratory care (RC) societies; related medical societies; job postings; hospital RC units; on-line publications; educational programs; patient education; software and equipment; pharmaceutical companies; and resources in anesthesiology, cardiology, and critical care. Unfortunately, there is no hierarchy of resources; the user must scroll through a long list.

Respiratory Care Home Page

Provided by Kristin Robinson, R.R.T.

LINKS

Address: *http://www.theshop.net/KKuhlman/resp.htm*

Cost: No charge.

This site, which is under construction, is about equally divided between resources for RC professionals and those for patients. Files for patients cover practical topics such as using an autoinhaler, using a nebulizer, and cleaning a portable humidifier. There are also answers to frequently asked questions such as "What is an RC practitioner?" and "What is asthma?" Resources for professionals include copies of articles and lectures, plus links to RC organizations, general medical organizations, and educational and employment resources.

RC-WEB

Provided by University of Missouri, Respiratory Therapy Program

LINKS

Address: *http://www.hsc.missouri.edu/shrp/rtwww/rcweb/docs/rcweb.html*

Cost: No charge.

A fascinating feature of this site is the *Lung Sounds Page,* which helps users recognize and distinguish abnormal lung sounds. The American Association for Respiratory Care (AARC) Clinical Practice Guidelines are also available, along with an alphabetically arranged list of 70 links to other respiratory care and general medical resources. This site is a subset of Lifesphere (http://www.hsc.missouri.edu), a medical Web site at the University of Missouri that has a search engine plus extensive links to Internet resources for patients and professionals.

Speech, Language, and Hearing

National Information Center on Deafness (U.S.)

Provided by Gallaudet University

Address: *http://www.gallaudet.edu:80/~nicd/*

Cost: No charge.

This site is under construction. So far it has information about more than 60 U.S. organizations for hearing-impaired persons, as well as about conferences, exhibits, publications, and state commissions.

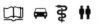

Deaf Gopher
Provided by Michigan State University

LINKS   **Address:** *http://web.cal.msu.edu/deaf/deafintro.html*
Cost: No charge.

This site is primarily for patients. It provides good guidance to educational resources, including an e-mail list, and unlike most sites, it suggests which links are best. Most of the remaining files are specific to Michigan State University or Michigan, but a *General Information* file has tips about topics such as TDD (telecommunication device for the deaf) modems and legal rights.

Net Connections for Communication Disorders and Sciences
Provided by Judith Maginnis Kuster, Mankato State University, Minn

LINKS   **Address:** *http://www.jmu.edu/libliaison/andersjl/commdis/cd-intro.html*
Cost: No charge.

An extensive collection of links in communication sciences can be found at this site. There are two ways to approach it: by type of Internet resource or by table of contents. The resource list is grouped into e-mail lists, Usenet newsgroups, on-line publications, gopher sites, FTP, Telnet, Web sites, and Wide Area Information Server (WAIS), and there is a brief explanation of each resource type. The table of contents is divided by subject matter and subdivided by resource type.

Medical Technology

Microbial Underground
Provided by Mark Pallen, Queen Mary Westfield College, UK

LINKS   **Address 1:** *http://www.qmw.ac.uk/~rhbm001/index.html*
Address 2: *http://www.lsumc.edu/campus/micr/mirror/public_html/index.html* (U.S. mirror site)
Cost: No charge.

Here you'll find a first-rate collection of links to medical, microbiological, and molecular biological resources. The provider began the project surreptitiously after his now-former superiors refused to sanction it (hence "underground" in the title). The strength of the collection is that it emphasizes electronic resources: databases of cultures and strains, on-line resources for sequence analysis, on-line publications, Listservs, newsgroups, bulletin board services, and Web courses. An on-line introductory course in medical bacteriology, written by the provider, is under construction.

Med TechNet

Provided by Western New York Microcomputer, Inc.

LINKS, CME

Address: *http://www.medtechnet.com/*

Cost: See text.

This commercially sponsored site provides continuing education for clinical laboratory scientists. PACE credits are available. There is no charge to get information about the program and view a sample course, but regular "attendance" at courses costs $59/year as of July 1996. A free 7-day account is available, and there are discounts for groups and students. The only system requirement is a monitor that displays 256 simultaneous colors. The provider also recommends Adobe PDF viewing software, which is downloadable at no charge from this site. There are links to medical laboratories, microbiology resources, and more. This site can also be accessed by Telnet (telnet://bbs.medtechnet.com) or direct dialup (set communication parameters to 8N1, then dial 1-716-688-1552).

American Society for Microbiology

Provided by American Society for Microbiology

LINKS, SEARCH

Address: *http://www.asmusa.org*

Cost: No charge.

Job search on-line resources, over a dozen of them, are a main attraction here. This site also links to information about microbiology newsgroups, a glossary of microbiology terms, on-line journals, Internet search engines, and government agencies. The original information at the site concerns the association itself: its governance, programs, products and services, and membership. All original information, including the membership list, is searchable by keyword or concept.

Radiologic Technology

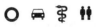

Radiation Oncology

Provided by The University of Pennsylvania, Oncolink

LINKS

Address: *http://www.oncolink.upenn.edu/specialty/rad_onc/*

Cost: No charge, except as noted.

This is an extremely well-done site that is useful to professionals and patients. Much of the information for professionals makes excellent use of computer technology, such as slides and films that are available without special software. Some of the many other resources for professionals include a technologists' area and links to BreastNet (breast cancer resources) and Uronet (prostate cancer resources).

On the *Welcome* screen, topics for patients are mixed among those for professionals, which would make them easy to miss. The substance of the information for patients is excellent: a photo-illustrated introduction to radiation therapy (geared to children but not inappropriate for adults), information about bone marrow transplantation, and practical advice about self-care, such as tiredness, mouth problems, skin care, and diarrhea.

NURSING

Nursing Net
Provided by Mark and Mary Carraway

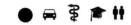

LINKS, SEARCH, JOURNALS

Address: *http://www.communique.net/~nursgnt/*
Cost: No charge.

Look here first! If you can't find what you want at this site, maybe it isn't on the Web yet. The site looks sharp. It takes awhile for the graphics to come through (load), but it is worth the wait. The menu is extensive, so you're going to be spending some time here. We recommend you do. This site is large enough that it may take you through three or four menus to find what you want; but, if you are patient, you will usually find what you are looking for. The site contains a link to Leginurse, where nurses can find out about various laws relating to nursing and how to get in touch with legislators to tell them what is on their minds. There are sites for all areas of nursing, such as emergency and intensive care, medical-surgical, and operating room. Access to several journals is available, including the *American Journal of Nursing*. There are nationwide job search engines. If all of this isn't enough, there are several Web search engines in case you still have not found what you are looking for.

Nursing Network Forum
Provided by Mid-Atlantic Network Associates, Inc.

LINKS, SEARCH, JOURNALS

Address: *http://www.access.digex.net/~nurse/nursnet3.htm*
Cost: No charge.

This site, which is maintained by United Nurses International, contains links to just about anywhere you would want to go. First, you can join various e-mail lists to keep up to date on what is happening in the world of nursing. From lists of current health care conferences to locations of medical equipment and software sites, it's all here. There are databases, search tools, on-line continuing education, and clinical information resources. Essentially all on-line nursing journals, medical agencies, and health-related organization sites are linked to this location. For a quick jump to whatever health care–related site you need, this site cannot be beat.

LINKS

Nursing and Allied Health Internet Directory
Provided by Slack, Inc. (commercial)

Address: *http://www.slackinc.com/allied/allnet.htm*
Cost: No charge.

This site provides a plethora of WWW resources for the nurse on a variety of topics, such as gerontology, occupational health, computers in nursing, emergency and trauma nursing, and hospice and home care, and it includes links to resources such as the breast cancer information clearinghouse. Several of the sites (e.g., pediatric) also have subgroupings of information and resources for parents, as well as professionals. Links are easy to access.

LINKS

Nursing Related Web Servers
Provided by University of Washington, School of Nursing

Address: *http://www.son.washington.edu/www-servers.html*
Cost: No charge.

A useful reference for the novice "surfer" who wants to see what is available in nursing. Access to some sites (e.g., pain management) is very slow, and the list of sites is restricted to nursing. Evaluation of individual sites listed is deferred to the user.

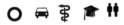

LINKS, SEARCH, JOURNALS

WholeNurse
Provided by Matt Wright

Address: *http://www.wholenurse.com/*
Cost: No charge.

The name, WholeNurse, says it all; in fact, "WholeMedicine" might be more accurate. Once you've found this site, you have found the whole world of nursing and more. Place a message in the guest book to offer feedback. Create discussion groups via the "leave or respond to a message" style message board or the on-line communication in a chat room. Resources are included for patient education about disease processes and medications. Link to the University of Pennsylvania for assistance with your résumé or go looking for a job via the Internet. An onboard search engine can help you find anything you need to know by author, title, or subject. Boundless numbers of links are available, including the *Journal of the American Medical Association* and other disciplines of professional medicine. The site is colorful and quick. Items are easy to find and access. If you want to dive into advanced medical knowledge or just blow off a little job-created steam, this is your site.

Nursing and Health Care Resources on the Net
Provided by Rod Ward

LINKS

Address: *http://www.bath.ac.uk/~exxrw/nurse.html*
Cost: No charge.

This site includes two separate sections. The first identifies resources available in the United Kingdom and information on links for a variety of specialties, including critical care. This is an excellent resource for UK nurses who want access to information and colleagues "closer to home." The second section provides information on worldwide links such as Nursenet.

Nursing and the NCLEX
Provided by Kaplan Educational Centers

LINKS, SEARCH

Address: *http://www.kaplan.com/nclex/*
Cost: No charge.

This is an excellent site for everyone. It offers excellent opportunities for nursing students approaching graduation to prepare for the NCLEX. There are resources for assistance in obtaining employment and entrance into graduate school. The site provides links to continuing education and multiple Web libraries and search engines. If this isn't enough, there are links to even more educational sites, news and information sites, and e-mail addresses for government at all levels, *including the White House.* If you are looking for references, medical or general, this is the place.

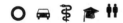

Idea Nurse
Provided by Peter Ramme, RN, CEN, CCRN

LINKS, SEARCH, JOURNALS

Address: *http://www.silcom.com/~peter/nurse.html*
Cost: No charge.

Mr. Ramme combines his talents and experience in the fields of nursing and computers to make a really neat Web site that combines a personal touch, which is sometimes absent in the larger Web sites. There are more than enough resources to keep you interested. The provider has collected articles and links to sites that he has found interesting within the field of nursing and posted them for easy access. A few words of explanation about most of the sites are presented to give you an idea of what you will see before you click on it. The provider offers a chat area and a guest book for nurses to communicate with each other. If this isn't enough, perhaps the search engines, links to job searches, collection of e-mail lists, or links to various nursing journals will be. Look at this site; it's worth your time.

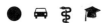

Inter Nurse

Provided by Internurse, Kirkby, Liverpool

LINKS, JOURNALS

Address: *http://www.wp.com/InterNurse/*
Cost: No charge.

Want a place to hang out? Try this site. It offers an at-home feeling with an e-mail "pal" setup and discussion options. This site gives you the chance to post reviews of literature and items of interest. On-line job posting, search, and "ask for help" areas are available. There are also links to nursing organizations, software and support groups. Here you can find a page dedicated to nurse midwives and more Florence Nightingale references than you'll know what to do with.

Nurses' Call

Provided by Lee Mahan and Sponsorship

LINKS

Address: *http://www.nurse.net/~nrs_call/*
Cost: No charge.

This is a great site, although not much is listed about the main provider. There are lots of choices of categories located on constantly available screen buttons *(Announce, Employment, Conferences, Education, Research, Mailing Lists, Who's Who, Volunteers, Directory, Guestbook, Nurses' Web, Sponsorship,* and *Feedback),* with serious in-depth information in each. Some awkward categorization, such as tucking the database entry of *DejaNews* in the *Research* button, can be overcome easily. Try the *Guestbook;* it features a message center for students, academics, and clinicians, as well as access to nursing headhunters and lists the date and time of message entry.

Nursing HealthWeb

Provided by collaborative effort of University of Michigan at Ann Arbor School of Nursing, Taubman Medical Library, and CIC Health Sciences Internet Working Groups

LINKS

Address: *http://www.lib.umich.edu/tml/nursing.html*
Cost: No charge.

The providers of this site are all authorities on computers *and* nursing. The table of contents is arranged vertically, with a brief description, and horizontally for quick traipsing. Information in a number of categories is compelling for both students and clinicians. Journals are listed with annotations about the reliability of the journal site and its contents and comments on whether annual indices are present. The world map graphic to click the geographic area for nursing education information is helpful. Under the *Communications* area, there are specialty area Listservs with tips on the subscribing (and unsubscribing!) process. The background is "ho-hum," but the contents sparkle.

MacNursing Home Page
Provided by Sylvan Rogers, R.N.

LINKS

Address: *http://community.net/~sylvan/MacNursing.html*
Cost: No charge.

This interesting site, provided by an R.N. with 20 years experience as an AAS nurse and computer expertise gained through using the computer in different nursing areas, offers a look at what nurses can do and are doing, with varied expertise. It is nicely organized with a brief table of contents that quickly—less than 2 clicks—takes you to the area you are interested in. Included are shareware products with detailed directions for downloading and using the material. A database design text, a helpful, useful feature for the novice, is included and consists of a how-to walk through on developing clinically focused nursing databases.

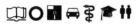

The WEBster—The Fine Art of Nursing
Provided by Kathi Webster

LINKS, SEARCH, JOURNALS

Address: *http://ally.ios.com/~webster/nurse.html*
Cost: No charge.

This site has a nice layout and an encyclopedic list of resources—with just one keystroke you can immediately access these from the home base! You name it, you can get to everything from the pulse of academia *(The Chronicle of Higher Education)* to medical bloopers and anecdotes to nursing informatics. With *Nurse Tribe* you can consult with others in your field, although you will need a software package called "Pow Wow." The WEBster is an award winner, and you are informed of that early on—so what is wrong with giving yourself a well-deserved pat on the back? A nice tutorial is available for those a little unfamiliar with the Internet. We highly recommend this jewel. Drop in and stay awhile.

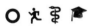

Virtual Nursing Center
Provided by Jim Martindale

LINKS, SEARCH, JOURNALS

Address: *http://www-sci.lib.uci.edu/HSG/Nursing.html*
Cost: No charge.

Everything is here, literally! It's a little overwhelming, but if you want to know the latest in the area of cardiology and primary care, you've come to the right place. The databases are nicely divided into user-friendly and rationally itemized categories. This is a fascinating collection of information that will intrigue those who are interested. The ability to browse on-line nursing journals was great, and the poison database contained fascinating information. It is a little slow and you may find yourself returning to home base a little too often, but overall, the site provides a wealth of great information. Enjoy!

LINKS, JOURNALS, CME

American Association of Critical Care Nurses
Provided by American Association of Critical Care Nurses (AACN)

Address: *http://www.aacn.org*
Cost: Membership fee for certain publications

If you work in critical care, you should find your way to this site. Maintained by the AACN, it provides information related to obtaining and maintaining the certified critical care nurse (CCRN) credential. Links to grants, continuing education, and journals are all available. Primary access is free; the membership fee is for additional information provided by the AACN. Stop by and look around.

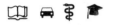

LINKS, JOURNALS, CME

Association of Operating Room Nurses
Provided by Association of Operating Room Nurses

Address: http://www.aorn.org
Cost: No charge.

This fine offering by the operating room nurses covers a wide range of needs from education to products to general information. For example, you can download a meeting proposal if you are interested in participating in an international meeting of operating room nurses.

Although it is not encyclopedic, the offerings are easy to access and will help you search for a particular continuing education offering, review a published article, or find out more about the interface of business and nursing. The ability to give feedback to the host directly on what was offered was great. Just how responsive they are to user comments is unknown.

ALTERNATIVE AND COMPLEMENTARY THERAPIES

INTRODUCTION

Alternative and complementary therapies, however they are defined and regardless of their acceptance in the allopathic or "regular" medical community, have always been an integral part of health care practice. These therapies appeal to increasing numbers of practitioners and to patients who spend significant amounts of money (much of it out of pocket) on products and treatments. As with any aspect of health care, attaining information is fundamental for the patient in choosing or complying with a specific philosophy or treatment. For an alternative *or* allopathic practitioner, information is important for investigating the philosophical or clinical components of individual therapies or for understanding the choices that patients make. The growth of user groups, sites, and documents about alternative and complementary therapies on the Internet has been explosive. The Internet could facilitate building the information bridge between alternative and regular practice that many practitioners and authors have advocated over the last few years. Networks like HealthWorld Online (http://www.healthy.net) base their philosophical foundation on embracing alternative health care, and directories like MedWeb (http://www.medweb.com) include alternative medicine in their delineation of medical categories. This suggests an amalgamation that addresses the need to find appropriate and helpful information regardless of one's clinical preferences.

Although our critique of these sites is consistent with the other sections in this guide, the subject elicits a concern that should be addressed. That is, whether the therapies, products, or practitioners are efficacious. We are not specifically judging the individual therapies, but are reviewing the inclusion of useful, substantive content on the site itself. These criteria include areas such as the authorship, existing search engine, currency, and presentation. By their nature, such criteria *generally* eliminated exclusively commercially ventures and diatribes for or against alternative practice. Because there are hundreds of sites, and because of space constraints, most sites listed in this section are directories, overviews, and catalogs. Although there are multitudinous sites on topics such as acupuncture, body work, homeopathy, herbs, Ayurevedic, chelation, and cancer therapies, we have included reviews of only a representative few. Look to the directories (especially those that are annotated) to steer you toward individual sites on particular therapies or belief systems.

The commercial sites (those that offer products, practitioners, and directories), as opposed to the catalog or university-based sites (with just hyperlinks), tend to have an array of unpublished documents, conference listings, and bits of information on therapies and conditions, but they are generally not replete with substantial content. (See HealthWorld in the Network section for a site that "knows" what content is all about.) They are fairly good starting points. Many still need to find a "voice" to pinpoint what they want to offer their users. Many also need to master the fine art of reviewing and annotating and incorporating other material into their presentations in addition to or instead of simply hyperlinking to other sites. Remember too, that this is an ever-evolving environment, and tomorrow the sites will have something they did not have today. Still, many sites do have considerable content on specific conditions and therapies; a very few of those (see the Bookmark section for more) are represented here.

Note: Unless otherwise specified, all content within this section, including the workshops, hyperlinked sites, educational programs, publications, clinical documents, and consumer information, is related to alternative medicine, natural healing, or complementary practice.

DIRECTORIES, GUIDES, AND CATALOGS

The Alternative Medicine Homepage
Provided by Charles B. Wessel, M.L.S., Falk Library of the Health Sciences, University of Pittsburgh

LINKS

Address: *http://www.pitt.edu/~cbw/altm.html*
Cost: No charge.

This is, of course, a totally unbiased review from a medical librarian. One of the best places to start looking for alternative medical sites was developed by a librarian, Charles Wessel. There are six sections on The Alternative Medicine Homepage, one called the *OAM, Office of Alternative Medicine* from the National Institutes of Health, one called *Mailing Lists and Newgroups,* one each about regional, commercial, and related resources, and the treasure, *Internet Resources.* Briefly annotated and listed alphabetically, the 70-some sites, although not exhaustive, are noteworthy for their breadth and inclusion of catalog-type sites that invariably lead the user to the multitude of other alternative sites available. From sites on acupuncture to homeopathy, to Reiki and vegetarianism, this is the place to initiate your journey into the world of alternative health care on the Internet.

Dr. Bower's Complementary and Alternative Medicine Home Page
Provided by Peter J. Bower, M.D.

LINKS   **Address:** *http://galen.med.virginia.edu/l~pjb3s/ComplementaryHomePage.html*
Cost: No charge.

Dr. Bower and the Dogwood Institute provide a marvelous starting point, as well as a viable point of return. There are six main areas on the home page. The *Complementary Practices TOPICS* lists therapies alphabetically by discipline, for example, aromatherapy, herbal medicine, and life extension. Each section has Listservs noted, if available, and numerous sites for hyperlinking. The sites are not annotated (some annotation would be welcome), but they seem to have been chosen with relatively substantial content in mind, as they generally possess descriptive or authoritative information. The *Other Comprehensive Complementary Medicine Links* include all the items that could not be categorized into the previous topics. Mostly directories are listed, and they're good ones at that. The practice registry and the *Commercial Stuff in my [Dr. Bower's] humble opinion worth looking at* are rather sparse but worth visiting. Dr. Bower has recently reorganized some of the topical information into *Treatment of Specific Disease Entities.* This is an inspiring feature and one that shows the philosophy behind the site. Only two diseases are presented so far. The cancer section has hyperlinks not only to sites such as the Gerson Institute and Burzynski's work but also to bibliographies of peer-reviewed articles on alternative therapies and National Cancer Institute articles on unproved cancer treatments. Allowing for both sides of a therapeutic issue is a feature of Bower's that should be nurtured here and emulated by other sites.

Health Action Network Society (HANS)
Provided by Health Action Network Society, Canada

LINKS   **Address:** *http://www.hans.org/*
Cost: No charge.

HANS, an interesting site, offers "…reliable information on current health issues and alternative medicines, treatments, and practitioners." The *Master Index* is an interesting blend of therapies, such as acupuncture, chiropractic, massage, and homeopathy and health-related issues, such as disease, fluoride, food, pesticides, vitamins, and water. Each category contains essays on the political nature of the subject matter, practitioner lists (for Canada), facts and fallacies about a subject, and videos and books about alternative therapies (many about cancer) that can be purchased. There is a distinct agenda here, but it does not overburden the basic information on the subjects.

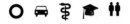

HealthCare Information Resources: Alternative Medicine (HCIR)
Provided by Health Sciences Library, McMaster University, Ontario, Canada

LINKS, SEARCH

Address: *http://www.~ hsl.mcmaster.ca/tomflem/altmed.html*
Cost: No charge.

Dr. Bower's list is more visible, Wessel's list is often cited, and Bastyr University's site is probably more "alternative," but HCIR is *annotated* and might well be more comprehensive. What an accomplishment! From the *General Resources in Alternative Medicine,* which include many reviewed herein, to *Specific Resources in Alternative Medicine,* which include disciplinary categories, such as Ayurvedic and naturopathy, the authors detail the basics of the site in a way that no other site reviewed here does. Almost all sites are American. Those marked with a tiny flag are Canadian. There is a helpful section on locating a practitioner. And, there are icons at the bottom of this entire list with links to the parent site, HCIR, that include voluminous listings (not annotated) on illness and wellness sites (such as the *Merck Manual,* Dietetics Online, nursing, physical therapy, and self-care). This is much like MedWeb's general index but with Canadian additions. *Bookmark* this site!

> ### ⚡ POWER TIP
> If a site does not have a search engine, and the list of resources is lengthy, use the *edit* menu and then the *find* function on your browser. Enter a subject, such as reflexology, and within the site, you will find any references.

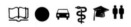

Internet and On-line Resources
Provided by Bastyr University

LINKS

Address: *http://www.halcyon.com/libastyr/netbib.html*
Cost: No charge.

Bastyr University is one of the most visible educational institutions that offers a curriculum in alternative therapies and complementary practice. The university library-produced Web site is top notch. As with so many directories, it is not annotated, but it is helpfully categorized. Beginning with Listservs or mailing lists, many are listed in alphabetical order. There's even one list devoted to drinkers of Kombucha tea. Newsgroups are next. The Listservs hyperlink; the

newsgroups do not. Other alternative sites make up the bulk of the categories and are presented in alphabetical order within the subjects of *Holistic Medicine, Diseases & Conditions,
Modalities of Treatment Publications, Institutions & Organizations,* and *Commercial &
Miscellaneous Sites of Interest.* Finally there is a list of Listservs assigned to "regular" areas of
medicine. This is a useful place to begin an Internet excursion into the world of alternative
health care.

Holistic Internet Community (HIC)

Provided by David Lazaroff

LINKS, SEARCH

Address: *http://www.holistic.com/welcome.html*

Cost: No charge.

HIC wants to provide a place "…to exchange information and congregate" and has made a
fairly good start at it. The *HIC Learning Center* (Surprise! The muted green headings are actually
hyperlinks.) includes unpublished essays written by holistic practitioners, other authors, and service providers on subjects such as Bach flower remedies, ways to prevent a heart attack, and
homeopathy. The *HIC Directory* has a search engine in which you can enter, for example
Ayurvedic, and find a listed practitioner. As with so many other sites reviewed here, these directories are in their infancy, so the listings are fairly limited. HIC also offers *Holistic Professions
Situations Wanted* for holistic health professionals and *Other Internet Resources,* which
AMR'TA's shared with HIC. HIC has made a capable start, but as a community, it needs more
exchange with the masses and more content to help those visitors.

Mother Nature's General Store

Provided by The Sphere

LINKS, SEARCH

Address: *http://www.mothernature.com*

Cost: No charge.

It's more than a store. It's a mall, an information center, and a place to discuss treatment for
cancer and exchange vegetarian recipes. "Walking" down these "aisles" takes some time, as
there are 15 main areas of information. Many of them have search engines borrowed from
MedWeb or Starting Point, which are quite serviceable. The labels on the buttons could be a bit
more indicative of the content. For example, *Category Search* is the place to order diet products, herbs, natural cleansers, and the like. Why not call it *Shopping?* There is information on
aromatherapy, herbs and spices, a bookstore, explanations of the properties of herbs, and a vit-
amin chart. The information on therapies is not substantive, but it is fun to browse. The *Health
Library* is really a nicely delineated group of Internet resources. *Traditional Medicine, Alternative
Medicine, Homeopathy, Nutrition,* and other lists contain multiple links to sites reviewed in this
guide. The site is a fine integration of health care resources in an unexpected spot. And when
you shop, you use a comfy *knapsack,* not the utilitarian shopping cart of most sites. Such inventiveness can go a long way toward separating this site from the crowd.

MedWeb: Alternative Medicine
Provided by Emory University

LINKS

Address: *http://www.gen.emory.edu/medweb/medweb.altmed.html*
Cost: No charge.

For a full review of MedWeb, see the General Medicine section. One of MedWeb's interestingly constructed categories is *Alternative Medicine,* which is subdivided rather eclectically to include *Consumer Health, Electronic Publications,* and *Sites,* where the disciplinary sites, such as acupuncture, herbal, macrobiotic, and Tibetan medicine links reside. As with MedWeb's other categories, there are no annotations, but the subjects are wide ranging, the categories are easy to follow, and the inclusions are inspired. Included within a huge directory of "regular" medical sites, it represents an attempt to illustrate the complete American medical scene, a rich amalgamation of innovative approaches to health care.

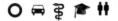

Wellness Zone
Provided by Stephen M. Powell, Santa Fe Online

LINKS

Address: *http://www.sfol.com/sfol/wellness/wellness.html*
Cost: No charge.

There are lots of local sites, and there are lots of sites devoted to individual practices or health centers. Some transcend their local heritage and offer an example of how it ought to be done. Wellness Zone is such a site. The schools and practitioners are local, but the links to *Aromatherapy/Herbs/Vitamins, Homeopathy, Bodywork/Energy/Chinese Medicine,* and *Consciousness/Transpersonal Psychology* (an unusual section among the reviews published here), and the list of frequently asked questions (FAQ) for herbs, homeopathy, and the like seem carefully selected. A few newsgroups are also included. Stephen Powell's spin on alternative therapy, referred to once as ramblings, offers interesting food for thought.

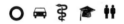

Natural Medicine, Complementary Health Care and Alternative Therapies/IBIS
Provided by Alchemical Medicine Research and Teaching Association (AMR'TA)

LINKS, SEARCH

Address 1: *http://www.teleport.com/~amrta*
Address 2: *http://www.teleport.com/~amrta/health.html*
Cost: No charge.

AMR'TA is producing an ambitious site; its purpose is "reuniting the art of healing and the science of medicine." The straightforward table of contents on the home page leads to a well-maintained *What's New* feature. One of the most welcome is a section on regular medical schools that have courses on alternative medicine. *Upcoming Events* includes conferences, seminars, and workshops, and *Internet Medical and Health Resources* consists of an unannotated alphabetical list of interesting sites. AMR'TA's sections on organizations, educational institutions, and training programs are particularly user friendly. In addition to the cursory address-type information, there are hyperlinks to sites such as Bastyr University. *Health Information and Tools for Wellness* needs augmented content, but the pieces that are there—diet and nutrition, shark cartilage, and homeopathy—are useful. Other promising features are the *Paracelsus* mailing list, where health care professionals can communicate, and hyperlinks to information about professional journals (no full text) and recommended books and magazines, which could use some annotation. The most interesting feature, especially in relation to other alternative sites is *IBIS,* the *Interactive BodyMind Information System,* the development of which is pending. Designed for health care professionals, educators, and researchers, it will feature hundreds of common medical conditions and offer treatments from more than 12 "systems" of alternative and complementary therapies. It will invite users to add their own data to the growing information on the program, as well as offer a "materia medica" of thousands of foods, herbs, remedies, and the like. Learn about further developments at http://www.teleport.com/~ibis/.

Health Trek
Provided by Health Trek

LINKS   **Address:** *http://www.healthtrek.com/*
Cost: No charge.

Health Trek wants you to "Explore the Alternatives!" To facilitate such a journey, it provides a *Shopping Mall* of products, a *Doctor's Office* where you can consult (for a fee) a naturopathic physician, and the *Newsletter* that includes articles by Health Trek. The *Message Board* includes inquiries from readers, the *Botanical Reference* offers numerous plant remedies and their applications, and the *Learning Center* lists the addresses and phone numbers of schools. The *Treatment Library* offers alternative remedies for diseases including asthma, bronchitis, and hypertension. The basic information about botanicals, naturopathy, and homeopathy is quite well done. The *Spotlight* highlights political news. As with most of the sites that are somewhat of a cross between a directory and guide, Health Trek could use more of everything, which will come as sites develop and grow.

ShareGuide
Provided by ShareGuide

LINKS   **Address:** *http://shareguide.com/mag/index.html*
Cost: No charge.

The ShareGuide publishes *Holistic Health Journal & Directory* quarterly. It is also a Web site. The articles on complementary medicine, massage and body work, somatics, and other topics are serviceable. The *Holistic Health Directory* is fairly limited so far. The *Links to other Holistic Web Sites* are a tidy sampling of what is available on the Internet. Briefly annotated, they are listed alphabetically by site name. Share Guide has the potential to evolve into an oft-visited site with additional directory listings and subsequent, annotated site listings.

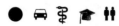

WorldWide Wellness
Provided by WorldWide Wellness and DoubleClick'd Publications

LINKS

Address: *http://www.doubleclickd.com/wwwellness.html*
Cost: No charge.

Among its options are *Online Resources,* which are fairly typical of the other sites reviewed here: a nice calendar of workshops and events and directories of practitioners and products that are evolving in content. The *Online Articles* are the reason to stop by. This interesting hodge-podge has on-line articles on rolfing, shamanism, the men's movement, colonics, and massage. The interviews with notables such as Daniel Redwood, a writer and member of the editorial board of the *Journal of Alternative and Complementary Medicine,* and Candace Pert, Ph.D., a pioneer in neurological aspects of the relationship between emotions and disease, are an exciting way to bring otherwise provocative or difficult subjects to the reader's attention.

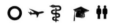

Yahoo!
Provided by Yahoo!

LINKS, SEARCH

Address: *http://www.yahoo.com*
Cost: No charge.

Briefly annotated and alphabetical by title of site (so fairly alphabetical by subject), Yahoo!'s hyperlinks are not embedded in a large search or difficult to find if you have forgotten to use a *bookmark.* The *Health: Alternative Medicine* section is part of the larger *Health* section. The table of contents lists topics such as Acupuncture, Conferences, Holistic, and Oriental Medicine. If you just want to browse the list, you will find all the basics. That's the beauty of Yahoo!. Start here and you can't go wrong.

INDIVIDUAL THERAPIES

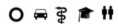

Acupuncture.com
Provided by Al Stone and Maximized Online

LINKS

Address: *http://www.acupuncture.com/*
Cost: No charge.

It is a pleasure to see what Al Stone has wrought. The table of contents suggests numerous traditional oriental therapies, among them, acupuncture, herbology, and Tui Na and Chinese massage. Within each group are consumer, student, or practitioner levels of information. Each level has content appropriate to the level of expertise. The consumer level is general, encyclopedic stuff, the student level includes more on diagnosis, and the practitioner level has more about further investigation into particular disease entities. *Consumer Resources* includes the listings of individual practitioners throughout the world, research on the use of oriental therapies for specific conditions that has been published in peer-reviewed medical journals, and individual testimonials. *Practitioner Resources* includes industry news and political concerns as they relate to traditional Chinese medicine. There is a constant posturing between alternative and conventional health care practice, and they make a good job of conveying how the dialog is progressing. There are also student resources, including information on certification and laws regarding practice. A *Marketplace* of software, well-chosen books, and the like is also available. This is a thoughtful, well-presented site. They should keep up the good work. For a more international flavor, try the Medical Acupuncture Web Page, address: http://antigoni.med.auth.gr/~karanik

Alexander Technique

Provided by North American Society of Teachers of the Alexander Technique (NSTAT)

LINKS

Address: *http://www.life.uiuc.edu/jeff/alextech.html*
Cost: No charge.

At this orderly site you will find information about NSTAT, the Alexander Technique (a body work therapy) which is the Australian counterpart to NSTAT, and a directory of teachers of the technique throughout the United States. The NSTAT journal, *Direction,* is highlighted, although there are no full text articles. The site includes a bibliography taken from *Wilson Periodicals* on the technique; this could be augmented with some other literature searches. The content is not voluminous, but it is a good illustration of an information site about an individual therapy and its professional organization. Another practical site in this regard is one on the Feldenkrais technique at http://www.usc.edu/hsc/neuroprotection/feldenkrais/faq.html

Perhaps it's that "body work-equals-psychological-wellness" ethos. It makes for helpful Internet sites.

Algy's Herb Page

Provided by Algy

LINKS, SEARCH

Address: *http://www.algy.com*
Cost: No charge.

There is so much here—*Catalogs* (11 different ones, one of them medicinal herb seeds), *Herbs* (ornamental for gardening and crafts and herbs for cooking), *Seed Exchange* with like-minded "herb" people, and *Discussion* about herbs— it boggles the mind. If all that were not enough, a *Bulletin Board,* on which you can ask questions and get answers about herbs (but not medical advice) is included. For our purposes, there is a voluminous section, *Medicinal Herbs* and links to alternative and complementary practice sites. It is all lovingly organized (in full screen or frames), illustrated, and presented. And with all of that, sites are even briefly annotated with short, often personalized, notes. However, when you are "the [W]eb's first and most comprehensible index and archive of herb information" sometimes it takes an awfully long time to load all that material. And as long as it is the most comprehensive, let's add some scientific literature. Could Algy offer bibliographies of literature from MEDLINE and similar databases on clinical trials being conducted using herbs? And could Algy come to our homes and help us set up our botanical herb knot garden? What I really like about Algy is the acknowledgment of related sites, like the ever-useful Henriette's Herbal Homepage by Henriette Kless, at http://sunsite.unc.edu/herbmed/ and the site for medical herbalists, Herbal Hall at http://www.crl.com/robbee/herbal.html. There is also the large and serious Herb Web, of which Algy says, "doesn't list me so it can't be that good." But it didn't keep this most diplomatic of sites from including *it*. This is one site where, besides the bulletin boards and such, the links are so well chosen and themselves link to consistently substantial sites that Algy's Herb Page gives the impression of actually having the content. Now *that* is clever. It's so rich, it's so fine, you must go visit and stay awhile.

Get Well
Provided by Russell Setright, Spurnarp Pty. Ltd.

LINKS

Address: *http://www.moreinfo.com.au/getwell/default.html*
Cost: No charge.

Naturopathy places a substantial emphasis on the influence of nutrition, water, light, and heat on the well-being of its patients. This interesting site is authored by an Australian naturopath who has done a commendable job of passing on useful information about basic health care to the public. There are informational pieces on a number of conditions, such as arthritis and constipation, that offer common-sense advice and treatment. The books are all written by Setright, and the distributors of vitamins and herbal medicines are all Australian, but two particular sections have broader appeal. Information in *Herbal Medicine* is quite sparse, but the inclusions there are nicely done. *The Latest Clinical Studies* (of which there are only a handful; one is on folic acid and heart disease) have summaries of recent peer-reviewed articles. This is an effective feature that should be supplemented regularly. Some generic information on what a person can expect from a naturopath in treating various conditions would be desirable.

Homeopathic Education Services (HES)
Provided by Dana Ullman, M.P.H., and Internet Health Resources

LINKS

Address: *http://www.ihr.com/homeopat/*
Cost: No charge.

Dana Ullman's content has found a new home on Internet Health Resources (http://www.ihr.com/ihrhome.html). In the midst of moving the page to a new location, HES manages to maintain its substantial transference of homeopathic information. Following some comprehensive pieces on modern homeopathy, the history of homeopathy, the international status of homeopathy, and common questions about the discipline, there is a range of articles by Ullman on specific uses of homeopathic therapy for conditions such as AIDS, pregnancy, and sports injuries. There is also a review of the clinical and laboratory research using homeopathic medicines, some tips on the pragmatic concerns of finding a homeopath, and a bit on training programs. Although the site is a tad Ullman centered, it shows the degree to which a subject can be covered both in a complementary and allopathic manner, and how strong content makes for a valuable site. For a more British spin with multiple hyperlinks, try the *Homeopathic Internet Resources List* at http://antenna.nl:80/homeoweb and the Homeopathy Home Page at http://www.dungeon.com/~cam/homeo.html

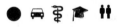

Aesclepian Chronicles
Provided by Synergistic Health Center (SHC)

LINKS

Address: *http://www.forthrt.com/~chronicl/homepage.html*
Cost: No charge.

In the spirit of all that is good and multifaceted on the Internet, here's a keeper. *Aesclepian Chronicles* is an electronic magazine (e-zine), available only at this site. Copies from 1995 to present are archived. The articles, on topics such as shamanism and transpersonal psychology, are thought provoking, illuminating, and occasionally, instructive. The SHC, located in North Carolina, is devoted to bringing the best of complementary and allopathic health care together, and it does an admirable job. The table of contents in the *Indices of Complementary and Allopathic References* is nicely delineated and includes links to all the usual sources (as seen in the directories included in this section) plus other e-zines, newgroups, and the like. Aesclepius himself would find this amalgamation of information and healing quite fascinating.

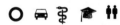

Massage Therapy
Provided by Mark Sincock, L.M.T., Northeastern Massage Therapy

LINKS

Address: *http://www.lightlink.com/massage/*
Cost: No charge.

Here at Mark Sincock's fine Web site, you can learn about massage. Educational aspects, a directory of massage therapists, related links on the Internet, resources, and even *Items for Sale*, are part of this well done site. Articles on the use of massage in carpal tunnel syndrome, during pregnancy, and for other purposes are included. Some information on the various types of massage (such as Swedish and Shiatsu) would be helpful. For a British variation, and one of the most charming logos around see Southampton University Massage Club at http://www.soton.ac.uk/~ktakeda/massage/massage.html

Music Therapy
Provided by Dirk Cushenbery

LINKS

Address: *http://falcon.cc.ukans.edu/~dirkcush/*
Cost: No charge.

The Internet environment is about sharing, and no one does it in a kinder spirit than does Cushenbery. This site, and that of Byung-Chuel Choi (http://falcon.cc.ukans.edu/~memt/mt.html) talk about the University of Kansas Music Therapy program, but more than that, they offer a music therapy Listserv. They link you to music therapy friends in Canada, Brazil, and Germany. They include hyperlinks to sites about the populations (such as Alzheimer's disease and adolescent psychology) that are served by music therapy. There are hyperlinks to other music sites. Succinct pieces are available on the various types of music therapy. A bibliography of published articles and abstracts of the research done on music therapy's role in various conditions would be a fine addition to this inspired collection. In short, if you have the slightest interest in this innovative approach to therapy, this is where you want to be.

BUSINESS AND POLITICS OF HEALTH CARE

Medical Source
Provided by Medical Alliances, Inc.

Address: *http//www.medsource.com/index.html*
Cost: No charge.

This is a fun and informative place to be. *Doctor Net Rater* gives you reviews of more than 500 medical Web sites. If you are getting frustrated searching the Web on your own, Medical Source puts it together for you. If you are interested in the business of health care or need tips for negotiating managed care and capitation contracts, there are new resources for these. Of particular interest is the article "The Future Isn't Just Primary Care—It's Multispecialty Networks." The information is cutting edge, positive, and unbiased.

National Information Center on Health Services Research
Provided by U.S. National Library of Medicine

LINKS

Address: *http://www.nlm.nih.gov/nichr.dir/nichsr.html*
Cost: No charge.

This department within the National Library of Medicine was developed in 1993 to assist health services researchers. In a textual but highly readable format, the collection, storage, analysis, retrieval, and dissemination of information on health services research, clinical practice guidelines, and assessment of health care technology can be found here. This will be of little interest to the general medical reviewer, but is highly valuable to anyone pursuing a master degree in public health, or otherwise engaged in health services research. The National Library of Medicine can be accessed through this site.

NIH Grants and Contracts
Provided by National Institutes of Health

SEARCH

Address: *http://www.nih.gov:80/grants/*
Cost: No charge.

This is your pathway into the NIH. The text is much more readable than the usual paper documents from the government. Here are complete applications and instructions for many different NIH grants, along with career opportunities ranging from high school to postgraduate education. Any recent newsletter from the NIH is also available. Reviewing this section was surprisingly pleasant.

AMSO Bio

Provided by American Specialty Organization, Inc. (AMSO)

SEARCH

Address: *http://www.dataslam.com/amso/amso.bio.html*
Cost: No charge.

Are you a specialist frustrated by managed care? Do you see the future as bleak? AMSO was formed to provide the medical specialist community with services to survive in a managed care world. AMSO provides a forum for dialogue, many resources, and a connection to a wide variety of management services relevant to managed care. For primary care physicians, the tenor of the information is very constructive and positive.

AMSO Capitation: An Open Forum

Provided by American Medical Specialty Organization, Inc.

Address: *http://www.dataslam.com/amso/capitation.html*
Cost: No charge.

This is where a specialist can ask questions or vent frustrations about managed care and get a response. Forum topics include health care reform and legislation, ethics of managed care, and cost-cutting ideas. There is an open forum on capitation. Any physician, but especially a specialist, getting involved with managed care will find this forum a marketplace of ideas.

AAHP Online

Provided by American Association of Health Plans (AAHP)

Address: *http://www.aahp.org*
Cost: registration; No charge.

This is an on-line service for members of AAHP, an organization representing the managed care industry. Accessing any information requires registration, and a limited amount of information is available to the public. The registration process is a bit tedious, and the information is very general. If you work for a managed care organization, see if it is a member of AAHP, and get level III services.

Health Policy Central

Provided by New Prospect Inc., Electronic Policy Network

Address: *http://epn.org/idea/health.html*
Cost: No charge.

This exciting electronic magazine provides excellent reviews of current health care legislation and issues in managed care. The editor is Paul Starr, author of Pulitzer prize winning *The Social Transformation of American Medicine.* This is the most sophisticated electronic magazine yet, and the format is inviting and easy to use. The first issue was published in January 1996, and there have now been three issues. This definitely looks like a winner.

Intergovernmental Health Policy Project

Provided by George Washington University (GWU)

Address: *http://www.gwu.edu/ihpp/*
Cost: No charge.

Interested in state health care policy? This project at GWU in Washington, DC, has been operating for 16 years and is the definitive source for information about state health care policy, proposed legislation, and health care research. Since national health care reform faltered in 1994, attention has been focused on the states, and this effort at GWU has been the definitive source. This Web site on the GWU home page has all of the textual information from this project in a highly organized and readable form.

NewsPage—Health Insurance & Managed Care

Provided by Individual, Inc.

SEARCH

Address: *http://www.newspage.com/NEWSPAGE/cgi-bin/walk.cgi/NEWSPAGE/info/d16/d4/*
Cost: No charge.

This is a good central source for newspaper articles. Knight-Ridder collects articles from newspapers throughout the country that discuss health insurance and managed care, with subtopics such as worker's compensation and what is happening to specific companies such as Blue Cross/Blue Shield. If you want to keep an eye on newspaper articles and are not looking for significant depth, this would be a good source.

DIAGNOSTICS, DRUGS, AND DEVICES

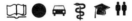

University of Kentucky College of Pharmacy Home Page

Provided by University of Kentucky College of Pharmacy

LINKS, SEARCH, JOURNALS

Address: *http://kerouac.pharm.uky.edu/default.html*
Cost: No charge.

This multimedia Web site includes several fun, downloadable sound clips. Multiple interesting subpages are referenced. These include an informational *Home Test Kits* page, a description of the department's high-tech teaching technique, and *Wave of the Future,* an electronic journal written on-line about chemistry and spectroscopy subjects. This site is exemplary in its demonstration of the educational applications of new Internet technology.

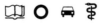

MEDMarket Virtual Industrial Park

Provided by MEDMarket, Inc.

SEARCH, REQUESTS
NETSCAPE

Address: *http://www.medmarket.com/medmarkt.html*
Cost: No charge.

This is the home page of MEDMarket, Inc., the managing organization behind the MEDMarket Virtual Industrial Park. MEDMarket is "the one-stop information source on the Web for the healthcare manufacturing industry." There buyers, sellers, manufacturers, and inventors alike can interact business-to-business as they exchange information on medical goods and ideas. Although it is somewhat wordy and tedious to navigate, this site is valuable for businesses and entrepreneurs as it provides the opportunity to interact globally.

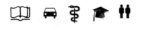

Diagnostic Test Information Server

Provided by William Detmer (University of California, San Francisco)

SEARCH

Address: *http://dgim-www.ucsf.edu/testsearch.html*
Cost: No charge.

This site is an Internet version of *Pocket Guide to Diagnostic Tests* (Detmer WM, McPhee SJ, Nicoll D, Chou T; Appleton & Lange, 1992). The resource provides a searchable index of virtually any diagnostic laboratory evaluation. Results of searches include normal values, causes of abnormal values, associated disease processes, and scientific references as information sources. The site is an excellent application created by UCSF's Division of General Internal Medicine.

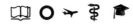

The ANNDEE Homepage

Provided by Austrian Research Institute for Artificial intelligence

LINKS

Address: *http:www.ai.univie.ac.at/oefai/nn/anndee*
Cost: No charge.

ANNDEE stands for Enhancement of EEG-based Diagnosis of Neurological and Psychiatric Disorders by Artificial Neural Networks. In short, this is an informational site describing the work being conducted in Austria at the Institute for Artificial Intelligence. This is an interesting new technology that will aid neurologists and non-neurospecialists as they attempt to classify diseases by EEG (electroencephalographic) findings. New breakthroughs and references are available to investigators on this easily navigated site.

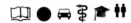

Pharmaceutical Information Network Homepage
Provided by VirSci Corporation

LINKS, SEARCH

Address: *http://pharminfo.com*
Cost: No charge.

This is the place for information about the pharmaceutical industry. This award-winning site has nine major categories to choose from. They are *Disease Centers, Drug Information, Meeting Highlights, Discussion Groups, Publications, Pharmacy Mall, Pharmacy Corner, Pharmacy Links,* and *Gallery.*

One powerful tool found within this site is *Drug Database,* a searchable database with information about nearly any drug. Several generic and trade name pharmaceuticals were searched and multiple references about each were found. This is an excellent reference for professionals and laypersons alike. It may replace heavy textbooks as users turn to the Internet for free information.

Another excellent subpage is the *Discussion Groups* page. This references Internet sites where patients, scientists, clinicians, and other groups can meet to exchange information and ideas. The *Patient Information Resources* page is particularly useful. Here one can find step-by-step "how-to" instructions on locating clinical trials, specific newsgroups, and other patient care associations.

A third subcategory, the *Gallery* provides Web surfers with selected, uncommon medicine-related works of art. This is an interesting section that may appeal to the casual browser and the serious collector.

Pharmaceutical Information Network is a first-rate site and a "must have" bookmark in anyone's virtual library.

DISEASES, DISORDERS, AND DISABILITIES

AIDS AND HIV

HIVNALIVE
Provided by Positively HIV

LINKS

Address: *http://www.hivnalive.org*
Cost: No charge.

Here's a colorful and award-winning site that provides information and links to advocacy groups for persons with human immunodeficiency virus (HIV) along with lay medical information.

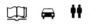

HIVNET
Provided by Hivnet/GENA

LINKS

Address: *http://www.hivnet.org*
Cost: No charge.

This is a Gopher menu and text with links to sites of interest to patients with HIV.

ALLERGY

Pfizer/Zyrtec Allergy Information Page
Provided by Pfizer Labs, manufacturer of Zyrtec

Address: *http://www.allergy-info.com*
Cost: No charge.

A patient-oriented site with excellent interface. The graphic point-click maps tour the outside and in-house environments as you are educated about common allergens. Questions and answers, allergy games, a library of information, and helpful hints are among the surfing options provided for the interested individual. Finally, a lengthy information subpage about Zyrtec introduces patients and health care providers to this drug. This page is an exemplary demonstration of multimedia advertising that provides a highly informational Web site.

ALZHEIMER'S DISEASE

Alzheimer Web Home Page
Provided by David Small, Department of Pathology, University of Melbourne, Australia

LINKS

Address: *http://werple.mira.net.au/~dhs/ad.html*
Cost: No charge.

Primarily for researchers, this site has links to more than 20 laboratories actively involved in Alzheimer's disease research. Space for "position wanted" ads is offered along with a list of relevant books in neuroscience, including abstracts for some. Information for laypersons is also available, including a movie tour of a brain affected by Alzheimer's disease; unfortunately it contains a significant amount of scientific jargon.

Alzheimer's Association
Provided by Alzheimer's Association, Inc.

LINKS, SEARCH

Address: *http://www.alz.org/*
Cost: No charge.

The recommended starting place for people with Alzheimer's disease and their caregivers. The site offers on-line versions of easy-to-read brochures and fact sheets. It also includes caregiver resources, a reading list, news of recent clinical trials, an archive of media releases and position statements, lists of conferences and other events, and information about public policy initiatives, research grants, and the Green-Field National Alzheimer's Library.

Users can click on a map of the United States to find the nearest local chapter, including its address and telephone number. A section of medical information is under construction. It will include excerpts from the association's newsletter for health care professionals and its newsletter for laypersons that explains the latest scientific research. The search engine has concise instructions that are appropriate for novice users.

Alzheimer's Disease Resource Page
Provided by University Alzheimer Center, Case Western Reserve University

LINKS

Address: *http://www.cwru.edu/orgs/adsc/intro.html*
Cost: No charge.

This site is about equally divided between resources for laypersons and those for researchers. Many of the lay resources come from the Alzheimer's Association (see the previous review), but there is wide ranging additional information on such topics as provisions for wills, congregate living, and emotional support networks. Resources for researchers include a list of National Institute on Aging (NIA)–funded sites, lists of trials in progress, and links to discussion groups, laboratory home pages, and neuroscience databases. This site won a 1995 National Information Infrastructure Award.

Alzheimer's Disease Review
Provided by Sanders-Brown Center on Aging, University of Kentucky, with commercial sponsorship

LINKS, JOURNALS

Address: *http://www.coa.uky.edu/ADReview/*
Cost: Subscription; no charge.

A new electronic peer-reviewed quarterly journal that began publication in the spring of 1996. It is designed for use with Netscape 2.0 and Adobe Acrobat (optional), both of which can be downloaded from this site. Each issue includes four to six review articles accompanied by commentaries. Links include access to the tables of contents, abstracts, or full text of a number of relevant print journals and the archives of other electronic journals.

Research on Alzheimer's Disease
Provided by National Institutes of Health (NIH)

SEARCH

Address: *http://cos.gdb.org/best/fedfund/nih-select/alzheimer.html*
Cost: No charge.

This searchable database of NIH grants for Alzheimer's disease research allows Boolean searches of the project number, institution, principal investigator, state, zip code, fiscal years left in the grant, title, abstract, key words, and amount. Extensive instructions with examples are given. From here users can access the NIH Grants Database, which in turn is part of the Community of Science Databases.

ANESTHESIA

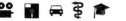

LINKS, JOURNALS

GASNet

Provided by Keith J. Ruskin, M.D., Yale University Medical School

Address: *http://gasnet.med.Yale.edu*
Cost: No charge.

GASNet, a pleasant way station on the Internet, is composed of multiple suites including (1) abstracts, journals, and newsletters; (2) book and software reviews; (3) a reference area; and (4) a calendar of upcoming events. Its literature search capabilities provide a limited bibliography. It has nifty multimedia capabilities—for example, without much difficulty you can download a transesophageal echocardiogram frame of a contracting left ventricle. The journals available include the *Journal of Clinical Monitoring,* the *Journal of Neurosurgical Anesthesia,* and the *American Journal of Anesthesiology.* Additionally there was an effective review of biomedical statistics. Adobe Acrobat is necessary for several of the areas. The site also provides links to multiple anesthesiology-related Internet sites. Overall, GASNet is user friendly and a well-designed site.

LINKS, GERMAN

The Swiss Anaesthesia Server

Provided by the University of Basel

Address: *http://www.medana.unibas.ch/*
Cost: No charge.

In this impressive page, the provider goes to great lengths to give the visitor a combination of text with effective and detailed illustrations. For example, a detailed rendering of the University of Basel is included on this site. What makes this site a "must visit," however, is the time spent to create a comprehensive list of links. Provided here is a "must see" list, an alphabetical list of all the important anesthesia sites around the world, and the "picks of the month." Additionally, this site has educational benefits and can be a great resource for residents. Visitors can obtain a list of lectures, educational activities at the university, and research papers. It also provides the "Resident's Redbook." Finally, an "Ask the Expert" section covering topics from malignant hyperthermia to ICU cost benefit is provided to add to the breadth of this site.

ANXIETY

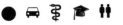

LINKS, SEARCH

Noodles' Panic-Anxiety Page

Provided by Steve in Murfreesboro, Tenn, Middle Tennessee State University

Address: *http://www.algy.com/anxiety/anxiety.html/*

Cost: No charge.

Here you'll get the lowdown on high anxiety. It covers all angles, definitions, medications, books, other sites, support groups, and more. The graphics are soothing and the site is easy to use for those with short attention spans.

ARTHRITIS

Arthritis Diagnosis, Differentiation, and Classification

Provided by Mallinckrodt Institute of Radiology; Washington University

Address: *http://kayla.wustl.edu/arthrit/ARTH_MAIN.HTML*

Cost: No charge.

This site presents rheumatologic diseases from a radiologic perspective. The information consists of good introductory medical material, mostly presented at a medical resident level. The radiographic images are extensive and are generally of high quality. The style is "bullet" outline form. This is one of the better basic expositions of rheumatic diseases for students, residents, or nonspecialist physicians. The Mallinckrodt Institute of Radiology has other related information on the Internet.

LINKS, SEARCH

Arthritis Foundation

Provided by Arthritis Foundation

Address: *http://www.arthritis.org*

Cost: No charge.

Brochures and fact sheets developed by the Arthritis Foundation for consumers, patients, and the lay public can be found at this site. It is quite basic and easy to understand. This would be of interest to the lay public or to physicians who want general information for their patients.

LINKS

Division of Rheumatology, University of Colorado Health Sciences Center

Provided by University of Colorado Health Sciences Center

Address: *http://www.uchsc.edu/sm/rheum/*

Cost: No charge.

This site offers some information about arthritis at a level appropriate to the lay public and some links to other sites. It also summarizes the interests of the rheumatology faculty at the

Mosby's Medical Surfari

Now available. Ask for it at your local bookstore.
Or you may order additional copies here.

Yes, I'd like to order **Mosby's Medical Surfari** (30461) $24.95.

❏ for myself ❏ for a friend

Billing information
❏ Please bill me
❏ Charge my American Express / Visa / MasterCard

Shipping address (if different from billing address)

Name

Name

Address

Address

City   State   Zip

City   State   Zip

Acct. No.   Exp. Date

Signature   Office Phone

E-mail address

Take a full 30 days to evaluate your purchase. If you want to return it, do so, and we'll cancel your invoice. All orders are billed for postage, handling and state sales tax, where appropriate. All prices subject to change without notice. If using a purchase order, please attach this card and send to Pat Newman at the Mosby-Year Book, Inc. address.

Or charge by phone
1-800-426-4545

Mosby's Medical Surfari

Now available. Ask for it at your local bookstore.
Or you may order additional copies here.

Yes, I'd like to order **Mosby's Medical Surfari** (30461) $24.95.

❏ for myself ❏ for a friend

Billing information
❏ Please bill me
❏ Charge my American Express / Visa / MasterCard

Shipping address (if different from billing address)

Name

Name

Address

Address

City   State   Zip

City   State   Zip

Acct. No.   Exp. Date

Signature   Office Phone

E-mail address

Take a full 30 days to evaluate your purchase. If you want to return it, do so, and we'll cancel your invoice. All orders are billed for postage, handling and state sales tax, where appropriate. All prices subject to change without notice. If using a purchase order, please attach this card and send to Pat Newman at the Mosby-Year Book, Inc. address.

Or charge by phone
1-800-426-4545

University of Colorado. This could be of value to someone who wants specific information about rheumatologists at the University of Colorado.

Duquesne University, Study of Rheumatoid Arthritis
Provided by Duquesne University

Address: *http://www.duq.edu/PT/RA/Tableof Contents.html*
Cost: No charge.

Only a simple monograph on rheumatoid arthritis is presented here. Although it does not provide more diverse or comprehensive information, the content level is appropriate for patients or students. Similar information, as part of more comprehensive presentations, is available at other Internet sites.

BRAIN

The Whole Brain Atlas
Provided by Department of Radiology and Department of Neurology, Brigham and Women's Hospital; Harvard Medical School

LINKS
Address: *http://www.med.harvard.edu/AANLIB/home.html*
Cost: No charge.

This outstanding on-line atlas of correlative CT and MR brain anatomy is sponsored by Brigham and Women's Hospital and Harvard Medical School. You can quickly switch between the CT image and various MR sequences for any brain section level, with or without anatomic labels. Admittedly, the interface can be a bit clunky or confusing at times, but it is still a great idea that is decently executed. In addition to the atlas of normal anatomy, several pathological cases add to the high value of this site.

BREAST

Breast Lecture
Provided by Dr. William H. Wolberg, M.D.

LINKS
Address: *http://www.biostat.wisc.edu/surgery/Wolberg/breast.html*
Cost: No charge.

This site contains a lecture intended for medical students that includes anatomy, physiology, and pathology with selected abstracts from journal articles. The graphics are good, although they are a trifle slow. This is a good review for any women's health care provider, and there is valuable information for patients as well. There is also a link to a page by Dr. Wolberg on breast problems and frequently asked questions (FAQs) for patients that addresses such problems as breast pain and lumps, abnormal mammograms, and breast cancer treatment options.

CANCER

General

American Cancer Society

Provided by American Cancer Society

LINKS

Address: *http://www.cancer.org/*

Cost: No charge.

Get ready to use our bookmark. This is the home page of the American Cancer Society, and the original material that has found its way onto many Web sites comes from here. Although mostly directed at patients, it also contains content directed at professionals including grant application information and some professional meetings. A list of links to other important Internet sites is supplied. Information about regional offices is posted as well. Information is updated regularly, and although there is no obvious search engine, the resource is well organized and content is easily located.

The Gray Lab CancerWeb

Provided by the Gray Laboratories in the UK

LINKS, SEARCH, JOURNALS

Address: *http://www.graylab.ac.uk/cancerweb.html*

Cost: No charge.

This well-organized resource contains cancer information directed at patients and professionals. Most content comes from the National Cancer Institute's CancerNet resource. Links to support groups and other sites are also provided. Content is updated monthly for the CancerNet statements.

Medicine On Line

Provided by UltiTech Inc. and supported by pharmaceutical corps.

LINKS, SEARCH

Address: *http://www.meds.com/*

Cost: No charge.

Medicine On Line provides quality content directed at professionals and consumers with a focus on leukemia and lung cancer. The information ranges from discussion groups to professional peer-reviewed manuscripts on a variety of topics. The MEDLINE search for Molecular Biology Subset Records is available. Links to other important resources are also posted. Some content requires registration to view.

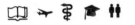

LINKS, SEARCH, JOURNALS

M.D. Anderson Cancer Center

Provided by M.D. Anderson Cancer Center

Address: *http://utmdacc.uth.tmc.edu/*
Cost: No charge.

M.D. Anderson Cancer Center is a "Comprehensive Cancer Center" as designated by the National Cancer Institute. This Web site has information about the facilities and functions as an Internet site and an Intranet resource. Content is directed toward the center's own patients, as well as its employees and regional physicians. There is both professional and patient-directed information. Numerous well-organized links to outside facilities exist. Poetry and essays written by patients have been placed on-line, along with photographs. The substantial original content includes *Conquest Magazine,* the center's quarterly publication. Information is updated at least monthly.

SEARCH, JOURNALS, SPANISH

National Cancer Institute

Provided by National Cancer Institute

Address: *http://www.nci.nih.gov/*
Cost: No charge.

This really is a spectacular site! It contains a wealth of information that is ultimately the source for much of the cancer-related Web material being posted. Included are comprehensive cancer statistics (NCI Fact Book), CancerNet (from the International Cancer Information Center), meeting announcements, patient information brochures, legislative information related to the NCI and the National Institutes of Health, and grant information. There really is much more, and it is extremely well organized given the vast content. Patients and professionals should consider this site a "must see," and should bookmark it. Updates are frequent!

LINKS, SEARCH

Oncolink

Provided by The University of Pennsylvania Cancer Center

Address: *http://Oncolink.upenn.edu/*
Cost: No charge.

Here's a perfect combination of information for the health care professional and the patient. Without a doubt, a person interested in oncology could get lost in this page for hours. To help guide visitors in the right direction, Oncolink has even started an experimental audio guided tour of the page! Time on this page will certainly be well spent.

The University of Pennsylvania Cancer Center effectively uses graphics to enhance this site. Right after the text material like user statistics, a disclaimer, and the request for on-line submissions, the visitor sees an area entitled "Confronting Cancer Through Art." The visitor can see the showcased art, but is also given information about this exhibit at the museum. By starting the page this way, the human side to this disease takes center stage. Other areas that focus on the human side on this page include psychosocial support and personal experiences, cancer FAQs (frequently asked questions), and medical supportive care for the patient.

On the professional side, physicians are able to link directly to intact published medical journals, search CNN and the *Mayo Clinic Health Letter,* and look up conferences, meetings, and the latest in clinical trials. They can also click on the *Editor's Choice Awards* and see what top providers of cancer-related information over the Internet have to say—each article receiving an award can be accessed. The professional can even use a number of search engines provided on this page in case certain information has not been provided. After visiting this page, however, it is hard to imagine that there is any related information on the Web that has not been linked to this page!

Oncology Online
Provided by Medical Services Online, LLC

SEARCH, JOURNALS

Address: *http://medserv.com/*
Cost: No charge.

Directed at medical professionals, this site requires the user to provide a DEA number to register. It contains content found on many other sites that do not require registration (e.g., PDQ and CancerLit, *The Journal of the NCI*), as well as quality internal content ("Dialog With The Experts" and "This Week in Oncology," for instance). Free MEDLINE searches through PaperChase, which work nicely through a Telnet client, are a real plus. News from outside services and internal news is updated daily.

TeleSCAN: Telematics Services in Cancer
Provided by Netherlands Cancer Institute

LINKS, FRENCH, DUTCH, SPANISH, GERMAN, ITALIAN

Address: *http://telescan.nki.nl/*
Cost: No charge.

This is the European Web-based cancer information resource. It contains U.S. CancerNet statements and links to many other resources. Cancer meetings are posted.

Breast Cancer

Breast Cancer Information Clearinghouse
Provided by the New York State Education and Research Network

LINKS, SEARCH

Address: *http://nysernet.org/bcic/*
Cost: No charge.

Information for breast cancer patients and their families is provided here. The site contains patient-directed information mostly from other sources and virtually all concerning the detection, diagnosis, and treatment of breast cancer.

Life Time Online –Breast Cancer
Provided by Lifetime Entertainment Services

SEARCH

Address: *http://www.lifetimetv.com/HealthNutrition/BreastCancer/brhome.html*
Cost: No charge.

This resource contains comprehensive breast cancer information directed toward patients. Much of the content originates from the National Cancer Institute. A chat forum is also sponsored.

Self Breast Examination and Mammography
Provided by Internet Advisor Communications, Inc.

Address: *http://www.net-advisor.com/mammog/*
Cost: No charge.

Although the site places a lot of emphasis on hawking the author's book, it does offer detailed useful information to patients about breast self-examination. However, information about mammography can *only* be received by buying the advertised book.

Y-Me National Breast Cancer Organization
Provided by Y-Me National Breast Cancer Organization

LINKS

Address: *http://www.y-me.org/*
Cost: No charge.

This is an excellent, patient-directed resource. It is well organized with content ranging from contact information for breast cancer resources to a "Kid's Corner," where original essays written by patients' children are posted. The site seems to be updated at least monthly. Most of the content is original. This one is a real winner!

Gynecologic Cancer

Gynecologic Oncology
Provided by University of Washington, Dr. Hisham K. Tamimi, M.D.

LINKS

Address: *http://gynoncology.obgyn.washington.edu/*
Cost: No charge.

This site has tutorials for practicing physicians and medical students, as well as reference materials for cancer patients. The tutorials cover the spectrum of gynecologic malignancies and include pathology reviews and treatment options. There are links to other oncology information sites including the University of Washington Library with some on-line accessible references. The graphics are very good and the information is well organized and well presented.

Pediatric Cancer

St. Jude Children's Research Hospital
Provided by Bioinformatics Unit, St. Jude Children's Research Hospital

LINKS

Address: *http://www.stjude.org*
Cost: No charge

Awarded "4 Stars" by NetGuide, this site is an excellent example of a professional presence on the Web. From maps of the St. Jude complex to reviews of many childhood cancers written for patients, this site has it all. Research efforts are profiled as are educational services for fellows. The story of St. Jude and The American Lebanese Syrian Associated Charities is presented as well. Links to other useful sites on the Web are available. Interface design is elegant and intuitive.

Skin Cancer

Melanoma Research Project
Provided by: Melanoma Research Project, Hamburg, Germany

Address: *http://ourworld.compuserve.com/homepages/mrp/*
Cost: No charge.

Learn how to identify those frighteningly common and deadly melanomas, along with other skin cancers. "What's New?" in therapy and research summaries for physicians are continually updated. Visitors can ask a simple question for free or receive a detailed consultation for a fee.

The Mole Hill
Provided by: University of Florida Health System

LINKS

Address: *http://www.hsc.ufl.edu/hs/molehill.htm*
Cost: No charge.

From the University of Florida come pictures of normal and abnormal moles, melanoma, and other skin cancers. With our alarming rate of increase in melanoma diagnoses, we simply cannot have too much information out there! The site has links to a list of sites where you can ask medical questions.

CARDIOLOGY

Cardiology Compass
Provided by the Section of Medical Informatics, Washington University School of Medicine, Washington University Medical Center

LINKS

Address: *http://osler.wustl.edu/~murphy/cardiology/compass.html/*
Cost: No charge.

The number of links on this site makes it invaluable to anyone who deals with heart patients. The creators of this site provide and maintain an unbelievable list of on-line resources—there is even a list of sites once believed helpful, but that are now no longer active! The clinical trials section offers the visitor a searchable database of trials! The education section is also worth a visit, because it provides detailed images of complex interventions and three-dimensional reconstructions. Also offered are listings of newsgroups, on-line journals and publications, including ACLS (advanced cardiac life support) guidelines and relevant general medical resources. Cardiology Compass can direct you to sources to meet all your information needs.

Heartweb
Provided by Amadeus Multimedia Technologies, Ltd.

LINKS, SEARCH

Address: *http://webaxis.com/heartweb/*
Cost: No charge.

Heartweb offers physicians three main areas to access: departments, features, and databases. Those venturing into the department area can read abstracts from *Pacing and Clinical Electrophysiology*, list their thoughts in an open forum, read comments by the editors, or check the employment board. The features section offers original contributions, case reports, and two dimensional motion echocardiography demonstration, with EKG puzzles to be up soon. A real asset to this site is the database section. Visitors can choose from the following: pulse generator, lead, and historic pulse generator. This is an informative site worth a visit.

CROHN'S DISEASE

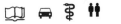

Welcome to the Crohns Disease Ulcerative Colitis Inflammatory Bowel Disease Pages
Provided by Bill Robertson

LINKS

Address: *http://qurlyjoe.bu.edu/cduchome.html*
Cost: No charge.

Here is an excellent index of patient resources for inflammatory bowel disease (Crohn's disease and ulcerative colitis). Its well-formatted, attractive home page provides links to support groups, medical institutions, government agencies, and a useful message board. Text in some of the links looks typewritten and is hard to read, but the information is up to date and balanced. You will find what you want about inflammatory bowel disease by starting here!

CYSTIC FIBROSIS

Cystic Fibrosis
Provided by Rob Calhoun at MIT

LINKS

Address: *http://www.ai.mit.edu/people/mernst/cf/*
Cost: No charge.

This Web site is a growing collection of cystic fibrosis (CF)-related information that seems primarily directed toward patients and the public because it includes definitions and the medically related information is easy to digest. For the physician, there are several reference areas to current molecular research. Furthermore, there is an excellent antibiotic and infectious disease reference section from the University of Wisconsin. Lists of support groups and lots of Web links are available for those interested in this troubling genetic illness.

DERMATOLOGY

General

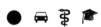

Departemt of Dermatology - University of Iowa
Provided by Department of Dermatology-University of Iowa

LINKS

Address: *http://tray.dermatology.uiowa.edu/home.html*
Cost: No charge.

This cool Web site for patients and health care professionals interested in dermatology has loads of valuable links (also available at the American Academy of Dermatology site) and the usual departmental information. The bright spots of this Web page are the original contributions, which include a "dermpath" tutor that covers basic concepts with text and images, an illustrated "Intro to Derm" lecture, a section correlating morphology and differential diagnosis, and 140 of the University's own clinical images.

Dermatology-Mie University School of Medicine HomePage
Provided by Mie University School of Medicine

LINKS, JAPANESE

Address: *http://www.medic.mie-u.ac.jp/derma/index.html*
Cost: No charge.

See electron microscopic images of skin structures and several viral infections. This is a mirror site for the University of Erlangen's Dermatology Online Atlas. There is a special section on skin diseases seen mostly in Asia and Japan—a neat idea.

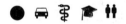

Dermatology in the Cinema
Provided by Vail Reese, M.D.

LINKS

Address: *http://itsa.ucsf.edu/~vcr/Dermcin.html*
Cost: No charge.

This is an entertaining, unique look at the use of skin conditions as tools of expression in the cinema and a list of your favorite stars' skin problems. Find out what that brown patch is on Richard Gere's frequently bared back. The links are both dermatologic and cinematic.

The Language of Dermatology

Provided by Peter Odland, M.D., and Gregory J. Raugi, M.D., Ph.D., Division of Dermatology, University of Washington

LINKS

Address: *http://www.hslib.washington.edu/education/derm/*
Cost: No charge.

The basics of dermatologic lexicon have been made simple. Intended as instructional support for second year medical students at Washington University, this vocabulary lesson is a valuable stop for all health care providers who want to sound skin smart!

Matrix Dermatology Resources

Provided by University of California (UC) at Davis

LINKS, SEARCH

Address: *http://matrix.ucdavis.edu/index.html*
Cost: No charge.

Powerful stuff from UC Davis! Listen in as dermatologists discuss a long list of clinical problems and their treatments on *RxDerm Archives.* This is invaluable to practicing dermatologists and interesting to patients with specific diseases. Links are available to *Dermatology Online Journal* and a tutorial, on skin tumors with hundreds of good clinical examples, for second year medical students.

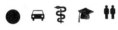

National Skin Centre, Singapore

Provided by National Skin Centre (Singapore)

LINKS

Address: *http://biomed.nus.sg/nsc/nsc.html*
Cost: No charge.

This is a good source of public and patient information with easy-to-understand discussions of common skin conditions. Information about meetings, other dermatologic professional organizations in Singapore, and a bulletin board are also included.

Project Dermatology Online Atlas (DOIA)

Provided by University of Erlangen, School of Medicine, Department of Dermatology, Germany

SEARCH

Address: *http://www.uni-erlangen.de/docs/FAU/fakultaet/med/kli/derma/bilddb/db.htm*
Cost: No charge.

The ultimate dermatologic image database! This project comes from the University of Erlangen and has mirror sites in Japan and Italy. This growing collection of more than 1,600 images is accessed with a search engine and database query interface. It has *Fantastisc* pictures and is a great idea. All of the diagnoses are listed in German.

LINKS, JOURNALS

Yale Dermatology Home Page
Provided by Yale University Department of Dermatology

Address: *http://info.med.yale.edu/dermatology/Welcome.html*
Cost: No charge.

The Energizer Bunny must have collected the links for this university department Web site. They just "keep going and going" and include just about every skin-related site on the Web. The resource guide has links to the full texts of the *Archives of Dermatology, Current Opinion in Dermatology, Dermatology Online Journal,* and *Medical and Surgical Dermatology.*

Birthmarks

LINKS

Birthmarks aka Port Wine Stains
Provided by Michael D. Steffano

Address: *http://www.fc.net/~msteffan/birthmark.htm*
Cost: No charge.

Stork bite central! This site was created from one man's desire to share his experience and insights about having a disfiguring vascular birth mark. It is loaded with personal anecdotes and resource information, particularly about laser treatments.

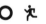

LINKS

PanAmerican Society for Pigment Cell Research
Provided by PanAmerican Society for Pigment Cell Research

Address: *http://lenti.med.umn.edu/paspcr/*
Cost: No charge.

If you already know that "Interpig" means International Pigment Database, this net site is for you. It's mostly for experts. Information is included on membership, newsletters, and meetings of the PASPCR.

Cutaneous Disease

Skin Deep
Provided by Health Press

Address: *http://www.grossbart.com/*
Cost: No charge.

The mind and body come together in this electronic book written by a well-qualified clinical psychologist. Read about the psychogenic components of common skin conditions and learn how most cutaneous disease is more than just "skin deep."

Cutaneous Reactions

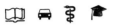

SEARCH

Cutaneous Drug Reaction Database
Provided by Jerome Z. Litt

Address: *gopher://gopher.Dartmouth.EDU:70/00/Research/BioSci/CDRD*
Cost: No charge.

A wonderful resource for the informed browser that is updated yearly. It includes references for cutaneous reactions to a long list of medications but doesn't attempt to judge the usefulness of each report. The site is fast and very easy to use.

Infections

Advances in Therapy—Skin Infections
Provided by Neil H. Cox, B.Sc., MB, Ch.B., F.R.C.P., F.R.C.P. (Ed)

Address: *http://www.dundee.ac.uk/meded/webupdate/skin/skin.htm*
Cost: No charge.

Updates on five categories of skin infections where new therapies are available. This site offers a nice concise review of new treatments for bacterial, viral (other than warts), warts, scabies, and fungus infections from the British perspective on available drugs and cost of these newer drugs.

LINKS

Medical Mycology Research Center, Galveston, Texas
Provided by Medical Mycology Research Center, Galveston, Texas

Address: *http://fungus.utmb.edu/myco.html*
Cost: No charge.

The place to go to find fungus! This site includes loads of information about this comprehensive mycology reference laboratory. Ongoing fees for service activities are detailed, along with mycologic and pharmacologic research and some basic fungal facts. The beginnings of what will be a fantastic resource for images is the Herbarium and Fungus culture collection. The site currently has more than 60 images, many of excellent quality. This is the ultimate "fungus head's" favorite destination!

Hypersensitivity

LINKS

The Skin Channel
Provided by The Chronicle of Skin and Allergy

Address: *http://www.chronicle.org/skin.htm*
Cost: No charge.

This is an electronic version of the *Chronicle of Skin and Allergy,* a Canadian publication with lots of pharmaceutical company support. It is intended for medical practitioners.

Psoriasis

LINKS, SEARCH

The National Psoriasis Foundation
Provided by National Psoriasis Foundation (NPF)

Address: *http://www.psoriasis.org/*
Cost: No charge.

Primo foundation page! This site is dedicated to helping patients with psoriasis. At this easy-to-navigate site you can sign up with the NPF to receive the latest information by conventional mail or e-mail. Access a wealth of factual information about the nature of the disease and its treatment and read about ongoing research projects, recent discoveries, foundation activities, and opportunities to volunteer. Up-to-date information for psoriasis sufferers can be found here, like warnings about antimalarial medications given to travelers going to some parts of the world. Mail order pharmacies with discounts for NPF members and detailed, easy to understand explanations of the confusing morass of psoriasis therapies are two more jewels in the crown of this foundation page. The site also has links to psoriasis-related journal abstracts on the Web, research links, and links to psoriasis newsgroups. Summary fiscal information is presented about where your money goes if you give to the NPF—public education (mostly), research and administration, and fund raising. The links are extensive!

Vitiligo

LINKS, SEARCH, JOURNALS

National Vitiligo Foundation, Inc.
Provided by University of Texas Health Center at Tyler

Address: *http://pegasus.uthct.edu/Vitiligo/index.html*
Cost: No charge.

There is still so much construction going on here you can almost hear the workmen. See pictures of people with vitiligo, learn some basic facts about this disease, and read the foundation's newsletter.

LINKS

V.I.P.-the Vitiligo Information Pages
Provided by Ludger Solbach, Hamburg, Germany

Address: *http://goofy.ti6.tu-harburg.de:80/vitiligo*
Cost: No charge.

Everything you ever wanted to know about vitiligo is here. The style is straightforward, and the site loaded with content (e.g., personal experiences, new and alternative treatments, and updates on current research). The vitiligo newsgroup is archived here, and there is a growing researcher's page. You can sign up for the Vitiligo Support and Information Group (VSIG) mailing list at no cost.

DIABETES

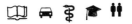

American Diabetes Association
Provided by ADA

LINKS

Address: *http://www.diabetes.org/*
Cost: No charge.

This is obviously a very credible source. The site offers an on-line diabetes risk test. Every state in the United States has a chapter of the ADA, and the ADA home page provides links to each. The ADA newsletter, *The Diabetes Advocate,* is on-line here. This is a place for diabetics to become politically active to protect their interests. The latest diabetes research and new product information are presented. The site is kept current and is well organized.

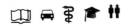

Children With DIABETES
Provided by Castle Web

LINKS, SEARCH, JOURNALS

Address: *http//www.castleweb.com/diabetes/*
Cost: No charge.

Rated as being in the top 5% of all Web sites, this is the on-line information source for children with diabetes. A searchable index makes locating information a breeze. This page contains an exhaustive list of on-line resources: endocrinologists willing to answer your questions, a list of camps for children with diabetes, cookbooks, a diabetes dictionary, information on glucose meters and accompanying software, lists of on-line magazines, chat rooms, and information for teachers. The list goes on and on. Of course, there are numerous links to related Web sites—all part of the index. Castle Web has done an excellent job with this site; the awards are well deserved.

Diabetes Monitor
Provided by Midwest Diabetes Care Center, Inc.

LINKS, SEARCH, JOURNALS

Address: *http://www.mdcc.com/*
Cost: No charge.

As the name suggests, this page is monitoring cyberspace for any useful information about diabetes to provide you with one-stop access. Web pages here are bursting with information on all aspects of diabetes, subdivided by topic. These include general (e.g., overview, standards of care, and glossaries), types of diabetes, complications, coping (e.g., diabetes organizations, lifestyle changes, and support groups), management, medications, and research. The site is so well organized that most information is available in less than three clicks of the mouse. It provides links to an enormous number of related Web sites that are also organized into intuitive groups for ease of use. The diabetes monitor is a "must bookmark" for anyone interested in this disease.

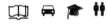

NIDDK Home Page (National Institute of Diabetes and Digestive and Kidney Diseases)
Provided by National Institutes of Health

LINKS

Address: *http://www.niddk.nih.gov/*
Cost: No charge.

Diabetes is just one of the diseases covered at this site, but it is covered extensively. Pages contain well-written patient information documents covering the *Diabetes Control and Complications Trial,* all the major complications of diabetes, and gestational diabetes. Information about research being conducted at the NIDDK, news releases, and links to other sources of U.S. Government health information are available.

Virtual Diabetes
Provided by University of Notre Dame

Address: *http://www.nd.edu/~hhowisen/virtual.htm/*
Cost: No charge.

This site offers a humorous game, the object of which is to get Derwood the Diabetic through an adventurous day without ending up in the hospital. This game teaches the basics of insulin therapy in a lighthearted and enjoyable format.

DIAGNOSTICS

MRI

MRI Patient Information
Provided by William H. Wright, M.P.A., R.T. (R) (MR)

Address: *http://waterw.com/~Wstuff/mri.html*
Cost: No charge.

Written by an MRI technologist in his spare time, this is a pithy one to two pages of FAQs (frequently asked questions) for those about to have an MRI. It is perfect for downloading, printing, and handing out to your anxious patients. FAQs are among the best things on the Internet—concise, informative, well organized, and to the point, with no unnecessary bells or whistles. This site is a perfect example of this.

Radiology

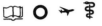

Biomedical Imaging Conferences

Provided by Image Processing Group, United Medical and Dental Schools of Guy's and St. Thomas' Hospitals

Address: *http://www-ipg.umds.ac.uk/~cb/ipg/conferences.html*

Cost: No charge.

This site lists biomedical imaging conferences ranging from radiology and MRI to radiation oncology and basic science and technology. The site is not very comprehensive at this time, but it's a great idea, and it allows users to submit details about upcoming conferences. It is very simple in appearance and respectably organized.

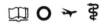

Brigham RAD

Provided by Brigham and Women's Hospital, Department of Radiology, Harvard Medical School

Address: *http://www.med.harvard.edu/BWHRad/*

An excellent resource from a premier institution. The unknown cases are well illustrated, not only with imaging examples, but also with microscopic and gross pathology in some instances. From pediatric to adult, the areas of interest cover all organ systems. Multiple modality imaging is included. This is an excellent teaching resource that also carries a "Finding-the-Path" module. Brigham RAD is highly recommended.

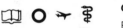

Collaborative Hypertext of Radiology (CHORUS)

Provided by Department of Radiology, Medical College of Wisconsin (MCW)

SEARCH

Address: *http://chorus.rad.mcw.edu*

Cost: No charge.

Maintained by Charles Kahn, M.D., and his colleagues at the MCW, CHORUS is intended to be a quick reference to radiology. In many ways, it is like Dähnert's *Radiology Review Manual*—very pithy flash card–style outlines of factoids and mnemonics, in a spartan, easy-to-process format. (In fact, readers of Dähnert may find some of these flash cards extremely familiar.) However, no topic is explored in-depth, as CHORUS aims to be broad.

CHORUS is the Internet successor to a very similar database system, which Dr. Kahn set up in 1990 at the University of Chicago, called FactFile. When there was the threat of an impromptu quiz from an attending, radiology residents there counted on FactFile to give them a 5-second rundown on the topic of interest. CHORUS can be used in a similar manner. Entries can be found by searching for a key word or by using the index (which is sorted by organ system). Everyone on the Internet is invited to submit entries (which are posted after being checked by one of MCW's staff members), demonstrating the only partially realized collaborative potential of the World Wide Web.

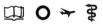

HealthWeb: Radiology

Provided by Ruth Lilly Medical Library, Indiana University

LINKS

Address: *http://www.medlib.iupui.edu/cicnet/rad/radnetho.html*
Cost: No charge.

A pretty good index to many radiology Internet sites, with decent organization and presentation. However, it is less comprehensive (or less intimidating, depending on your point of view) than other "links list" sites like MedWeb.

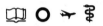

Indiana University Department of Radiology

Provided by Department of Radiology, Indiana University Medical Center

LINKS, SEARCH

Address: *http://www.indyrad.iupui.edu/homepage.htm*
Cost: No charge.

Indiana University and its clinical and research programs are discussed in this standard WWW site. One unique feature is its searchable database of grants and research funding opportunities.

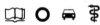

The Medical Radiography Home Page

Provided by WorldNET

LINKS

Address: *http://web.wn.net/~usr/ricter/web/medradhome.html*
Cost: No charge.

This is a very comprehensive index to radiology resources in a simple yet attractive interface. It's similar to Yahoo! in its excellent hierarchical organization, which makes up for the absence of a search engine. Another plus is that it seems to be updated more frequently than other similar sites.

The site is maintained by a radiologic technologist (RT), and a fair amount of the site is geared toward RTs (for example, the continuing education links list). But make no mistake, it is still extremely useful for radiologists and other health care professionals.

For those of you just beginning your search for radiology-oriented sites on the Web, this is a great place to start. Evidently others think so as well, because it has two mirror sites to handle the user load.

Radiology Web Server

Provided by University of Washington (Seattle), Department of Radiology

Address: *http://www.rad.washington.edu/*
Cost: No charge.

This Radiology Web Server contains radiology teaching files with full discussions, as well as *quickie cases.* These have no discussions, but represent typical imaging findings and are highly effective. The *virtual case* of the week is up-to-date and the previous weeks' cases are included. Pediatric cases from the University of Hawaii are represented. This resource has versatility and the images look good.

Virtual Hospital
Provided by Department of Radiology, University of Iowa, College of Medicine

Address: *http://indy.radiology.uiowa.edu/*
Cost: No charge.

Two aspects of this resource are especially attractive. *Physiological imaging* provides information from researchers, physicians, and technical staff and contributes to learning about such modalities as electron beam CT, MRI, and positron emission tomography. The Paediapedia is an imaginative imaging encyclopedia of pediatric diseases (see review in Pediatrics). It is presented well and is relatively comprehensive. Examples of the images are cleverly and graphically illustrated in miniature in the text links to the larger radiographic images. The Virtual Hospital is a leading resource on the Web for morphologic and functional imaging.

The Visible Human Project
Provided by National Library of Medicine

LINKS, SEARCH

Address: *http://www.nlm.nih.gov/research/visible/visible_human.html*
Cost: No charge.

The National Library of Medicine decided that an atlas of the anatomy of a normal male and a normal female, with exact correlation of transverse CT, MRI, and cryosection cadaver images made shortly after death, was needed for the electronic medical library of the future. Thus the Visible Human Project was born, which made national headlines when a condemned murderer donated his body to the project for use immediately after his execution.

The Visible Human Project site is well organized, attractive, and very interesting, with a lot of background information about the Project and the scores of research groups developing applications using the Visible Human data sets. Sites featuring sample images abound, but the most obvious thing that you would be looking for—live WWW access to the images—is not there, since the massive data sets are actually only for sale.

Ultrasound

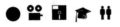

Obstetric Ultrasound
Provided by Dr. Joseph S. K. Woo, OB/GYN, Hong Kong

LINKS

Address: *http://www.hkstar.com/~joewoo/joewoo2.html*
Cost: No charge.

What a *wonderful* page. This site has been awarded three stars by Magellan and listed in the top 5% of Web sites by Point Survey. Once you visit, it will not be hard to understand why this site garners raves. This is a multimedia site using Java, RealAudio, and Quicktime to show some of the best collection of ultrasonography (including some of the new three-dimensional stuff) anywhere. Included are tables of measurements and links to other sites with supportive information.

There is a wealth of information including an explanation of how ultrasound works and the types of abnormalities that it can detect. This site is highly recommended to practicing physicians and medical students as a resource on the current capabilities of ultrasonography, as well as to the patient for a more thorough explanation of this technology and its capabilities.

X-ray

The X-Ray Century
Provided by Department of Radiology, Emory University

LINKS   **Address:** *http://www.cc.emory.edu/X-RAYS/century.htm*
Cost: No charge.

Original reports and publications of x-ray and radiation discoveries from 100 years ago are reproduced in this site. It is updated monthly so WWW surfers can follow the progress of science as it happened in "the good old days," exactly one century ago. Sure, the site is not useful, but it is interesting, well designed, well organized, and great for history of science buffs.

DIGESTIVE DISEASES

Patient Info Documents on Digestive Diseases
Provided by NIDDK

Address: *http://www.niddk.nih.gov/DigestiveDocs.html*
Cost: No charge.

Although there are no graphics or color, this site has straight-talking, patient-oriented information on many disorders of the gastrointestinal system. There are no links, but each heading has a good annotated list of additional resources with citations, addresses, and phone numbers.

DYSPHAGIA

Dysphagia Resource Center
Provided by P. Palmer

LINKS   **Address:** *Http://www.dysphagia.com/*
Cost: No charge.

Overall, this is a good basic source for dysphagia, with easy access to several related topics by alphabetical listing. The site includes case studies, anatomy, book reviews and references, research information, and tutorials. Also, it provides extensive links to general otolaryngology, as well as to other medical topics (e.g., history taking). A large amount of information is contained in this site, but sometimes a large amount of mouse clicking is required to reach it. Graphics are adequate but legends are sometimes lost when pictures are enlarged. Videostroboscopy samples are available if the computer has Quicktime. There are so many links that at times it is easy to get lost. Overall, this a good Web site for dysphagia and otolaryngology.

EMERGENCY MEDICINE

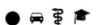

LINKS, SEARCH, JOURNALS

The Emergency Medicine and Primary Care Home Page
Provided by Ash Nashed, M.D., and Glenn Fink, M.D.

Address: *http://www.njnet.com/~embbs/*
Cost: No charge.

Keep this site at the top of your favorites list! With over 300,000 visits logged in just 1 month, it seems that Internet users are flocking to this gold mine. It was awarded the Physician's Choice award for top Internet sites and is one of the Top 5% of All Web Sites. It is the most comprehensive emergency medicine area out there, and it can keep you entertained for hours. Look through the radiology, CT, medical photography, and ECG file rooms for great graphics, which are easily downloadable for use in presentations. If you are looking for a challenge, try out the ACLS (advanced cardiac life support) and PALS (pediatric advanced life support) Megacode simulator or browse through the file of challenging emergency medicine cases. You can pick up the latest information from the *Toxicology corner, Clinical Reviews,* or *Pearls from Academic Emergency Medicine.* You will find extensive links to other sites of interest, and this site's user-friendly setup and relatively quick loading times make it a breeze to use.

Finding the Path
Provided by Brigham and Women's Hospital

Address: *http://www.med.harvard.edu/BWHRad/*
Cost: No charge.

Twenty-seven problem-based patient cases that represent common diagnostic problems in the emergency department can be found here. The simulations allow you to choose from several options for diagnostic imaging in each of the scenarios, and an algorithm for diagnostic imaging of each clinical presentation is offered. You can also access algorithms for radiographic confirmation of a particular problem by clicking on any of 23 different diagnoses. Overall, this is a good review for proper use of radiographic studies in the emergency department.

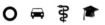

Clinical Reviews in Depth
Provided by Robin Hemphill

Address: *http://www.njnet.com/embbs/cr/cr.html*
Cost: No charge.

This site contains two case reviews that go into considerable depth on the topics presented (toxicity of alcohol and renal failure). The reviews are presented in an easy-to-use format with different sections for *Case Presentation, Goals and Objectives, Discussion, Diagnosis,* and *Treatment.* Each also contains a bibliography. These are exceptional cases that are great for individual review or for use in teaching situations. Quality definitely supersedes quantity in this case.

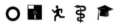

Global Emergency Medicine Archives
Provided by John Ellis, M.D.

SEARCH, JOURNALS

Address: *http://gema.library.ucsf.edu:8081/*
Cost: No charge.

An on-line emergency medicine journal with a wide variety of articles, which also contains interactive cases, clinical simulations, simulated patients, and an interactive forum. Clicking on *EMED-L* will get you a list of current topics in emergency medicine, and clicking any topic will give you the current discussion and an opportunity to put in your two cents worth. This site is a recipient of the Physicians' Choice Award and is in the Top 5% of All Web Sites. Two particulars worth checking out are an article on emergency medicine and the Internet (under original publications) and an ultrasound demo (you'll need Quicktime software to view this).

EMERGING INFECTIOUS DISEASES

Outbreak
Provided by Pragmatica

LINKS, SEARCH, JOURNALS

Address: *http://www.objarts.com/cgi-outbreak-unreg/dynaserve.exe/index.html*
Cost: No charge.

A very useful site that provides up-to-date information on emergent diseases. The site is divided into several heavily linked sections: *The Latest News, Welcome* (which includes FAQs), *General Information,* and *In Depth Coverage.* The last section currently covers bovine-spongiform encephalitis, dengue, Ebola, hantavirus, malaria, and yellow fever. Although parts of this site are still under construction, links in In Depth Coverage are extensive, including plans to develop searchable databases. Quotes and statements from experts in the field, as well as important news statements are included. This is a very useful site for physicians who wish to keep abreast of emerging infectious diseases.

FAMILY MEDICINE

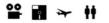

Family Health
Provided by Ohio University College of Osteopathic Medicine

Address: *http://www.tcom.ohiou.edu/family-health*
Cost: No charge.

You will find 2-minute patient education audio sound bites—lots and lots of them. The material is useful, but slow to download (average 1.2 MB per file). The same kind of advice is often available on telephone information lines in many major cities.

Journal of Family Practice Online
Provided by Appleton & Lange

LINKS, SEARCH, JOURNALS

Address: *http://www.phymac.med.wayne.edu/jfp/jfp.htm*
Cost: No charge.

This full-text "journal club" includes reviews of articles and has a search utility for archives (ditto software reviews). A couple of hundred medical Web links are usefully organized and regularly updated. Handy instructions are included on subscribing to family medicine–related Listservs.

FIBROMYALGIA

MARRTC Fibromyalgia Page
Provided by Missouri Arthritis Rehabilitation Research and Training Center

LINKS

Address: *http://proteus.mig.missouri.edu/fibro/*
Cost: No charge.

Here's some basic patient- and physician-oriented information about fibromyalgia.

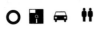

National Fibromyalgia Research Association (HTML document for the World Wide Web)
Provided by National Fibromyalgia Research Association

LINKS

Address: *http://www.teleport.com/~nfra/*
Cost: No charge.

This is a resource for patients, with descriptive and promotional information about the association. Organizations and journals are listed. Quality information about fibromyalgia is provided by Dr. Rob Bennett, a recognized authority.

Sheri's Fibro Page
Provided by Sheri Graber

LINKS, SEARCH

Address: http://prairie.lakes.com/~roseleaf/fibro/index.html
Cost: No charge.

Sheri has fibromyalgia. She has really done a nice job of collecting extensive and useful patient-oriented information. Humor, sex, poetry, meditation, books, links, resources, other patients' stories, Sheri's picture, and recent updates—think what you might about a fibromyalgia patient's home page, this is a commendable and useful effort. Indeed this is the best site on fibromyalgia.

GENETICS

Alliance of Genetic Support Groups
Provided by The Alliance of Genetic Support Groups

Address: http://medhlp.netusa.net/www/agsg.htm
Cost: No charge.

If there is a support group, this site has it listed—everything from cystic fibrosis to muscular dystrophy, fragile X syndrome to breast cancer. The site offers quick access to national genetic voluntary organizations with their services, phone numbers, and addresses.

Information for Genetic Professionals
Provided by University of Kansas Medical Center

LINKS

Address: http://www.kumc.edu/GEC/prof/geneprof.html
Cost: No charge.

Comprehensive and a *bookmark must.* Designed for the medical genetics professional, this site is equally useful to the practicing physician who wants information on specific genetic disorders, genetics resources and centers, or patient care. This user-friendly site with a table of contents of 14 items gets you in and out fast. It links to authoritative review articles, research protocols, commercial companies, government agencies, and university programs. This is the best site for one-stop shopping in medical genetics. As new genetics resources are developed, this site will find them for you. The site has links to all the other genetics sites reviewed herein.

National Center for Human Genome Research
Provided by National Center for Human Genome Research - NIH

LINKS, SEARCH

Address: http://www.nchgr.nih.gov/
Cost: No charge.

You can't think about medical genetics without access to the Human Genome Project. This is where molecular biologists access tools and databases to do their work. Physicians will want to use the key word search engine to find the latest genome research available on specific diseases. Also, there is information on how to apply for a National Institutes of Health grant or fellowship.

Online Mendelian Inheritance in Man (OMIM)
Provided by National Center for Biotechnology Information - Johns Hopkins University

LINKS, SEARCH

Address: *http://www3.ncbi.nlm.nih.gov:80/Omim/*
Cost: No charge.

Now the *number one authority* where geneticists go for up-to-date, complete information on more than 8,000 genetic diseases. This is also an easy-to-navigate resource for the neurologist or pediatrician and for other clinicians as well who want information on any genetic disease from alpha 1-antitrypsin deficiency to Melas syndrome. Simple queries by disease name give from one to 50 pages of text, pictures, and references on the disease searched and all other disorders with the disease name in the OMIM entry. This provides information for a differential diagnosis of related disorders. In addition to the complete OMIM article, a clinical synopsis gives concise, clinically pertinent information. Copious references, MEDLINE links to abstracts and full length articles, and "neighbor" article searches allow fast and complete access to the world's literature on any disease. The medical geneticists and researchers will find quick access to the current human gene maps and the National Institutes of Health DNA sequence database.

HEPATITIS

Brian's Chronic Hepatitis Home Page
Provided by Brian G. Arenas

LINKS

Address: *http://ourworld.compuserve.com/homepages/HEPA/*
Cost: No charge.

This chatty resource provides a patient perspective on liver diseases but does not have much original information. Start first at the American Liver Foundation (ALF) page.

Hepatitis B Foundation Home Page
Provided by The Hepatitis B Foundation

Address: *http://www.libertynet.org/~hep-b/*
Cost: No charge.

Many practical questions are covered here and information for patients with hepatitis B. The graphics are excellent and the text is readable. A list of expert physicians can be obtained.

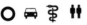

Hepatitis C Info and Support
Provided by Planet Maggie

LINKS

Address: *http://planetmaggie.pcchcs.saic.com/hepc.html*
Cost: No charge.

This patient-oriented site has current, well-written, balanced technical information on hepatitis C and links of interest to both patients and providers.

Hepatitis Weekly
Provided by CW Henderson, Publisher

Address: *http://www.holonet.net/homepage/1h.htm*
Cost: No charge.

Geared to hepatologists, this site provides truncated abstracts of the very latest technical publications in hepatitis. For full text, a subscription is necessary.

IMPOTENCE

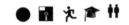

Successfully Treating Impotence
Provided by Pharmacia & Upjohn

LINKS

Address: *http://www2.impotent.com/caverject/home.html*
Cost: No charge.

This page is created by the company that manufactures Caverject, a form of intracavernous injection therapy for impotence. With a beautiful appearance, valuable information regarding the product and brief descriptions of the pathophysiology and evaluation of erectile dysfunction, are provided. The internal links to this frequently visited site are well constructed. The quiz and myths about impotence section add further appeal to this site. Treatment alternatives are, however, quite biased toward the product.

INFERTILITY

Atlanta Reproductive Health Centre; Infertility, IVF, Endometriosis Homepage
Provided by Dr. Mark Perloe, M.D.

LINKS

Address: *http://www.ivf.com*
Cost: No charge.

This is the mother of all obstetric and gynecology home pages, figuratively and, in a number of cases, literally. This award-winning page has been the inspiration for a number of offspring (no pun intended). The wealth of information available here encompasses the body of the subspecialty of reproductive endocrinology and is directed at everyone from the new infertility patient to the practicing obstetrician. There is an on-line book with information about infertility and how to deal with the physical and emotional problems associated with the medical treatment for the patient and her spouse. There are also numerous links to sites with information about such topics as in vitro fertilization, endometriosis, and menopause as well as FAQ (frequently asked question) lists for all topics. This page is a multimedia extravaganza using Java, RealAudio, and video. It is highly recommended for all and suitable for anything from light Web surfing to detailed information gathering.

Spermatology Home Page
Provided by Murdoch University, Veterinary Medicine

LINKS

Address: *http://numbat.murdoch.edu.au/spermatology/spermhp.html*
Cost: No charge.

For the sperm enthusiast and male infertility patient or couple, this site provides non-peer–reviewed information, pictures, and gossip. A busy home page offers related Web links. A plus is access to numerous fertility related journals, Androlog and Reprendo mailing lists, and job placements.

KIDNEY DISEASE

Hypertension, Dialysis, and Clinical Nephrology (HDCN): Renal Diseases Electronic Journal
Provided by Medtext, Inc.

LINKS

Address: *http://www.medtext.com/hdcn.htm*
Cost: No charge.

This is the best resource for nephrologists interested in end-stage renal disease therapies and clinical nephrology. Here, physicians can find answers to frequently asked questions, pointers to recent review articles, and summaries of hot new hypertension, dialysis, and nephrology papers, abstracts, and meeting presentations. The site also provides information about medical products, devices, services, and drugs. A list of links to relevant organizations, medical provider networks, and databases is available. The information presented is reviewed by a distinguished editorial board composed of specialists. A weekly update section tells what has been added. The CME site of the week shows a new *Nephrol* thread or *Ask the Prof!* material. Articles are listed quarterly by topic. American Medical Association press releases and those from American Heart Association can also be accessed.

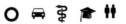

RENALNET
Provided by Gamewood Data Systems, Inc.

LINKS

Address: *http://www.gamewood.net/RENALNET.html*
Cost: No charge.

RENALNET is an excellent site for information relating to renal disease. It is a clearinghouse for information on the cause, treatment, and management of kidney disease and end-stage renal disease (ESRD). RENALNET uses the vast resources of the Internet to open avenues of communication among individuals and organizations involved in the care of patients with renal disease. This information is used for education, research, and treatment, and is freely available to interested individuals; it is hoped that it may raise public awareness about this common, life-threatening disease. Features of RENALNET are categorized in several sections. *What's new on RENALNET* provides a link to several useful renal resources for the general public and health professionals. *Conference room* is an on-line discussion forum for nephrologists, nurses, dietitians, and administrators. *Jobmart* posts open positions in nephrology. A dialysis unit search may be done by city, state, or country. The site also provides an e-mail service.

LINKS

Starting Point for Nephrology, Renal Pathology, and Transplantation Home Pages
Provided by University of Alberta

Address: *http://fester.his.path.cam.ac.uk/big/synapse/000p0035.htm*
Cost: No charge.

This site is very user friendly and good for beginners. It provides access to a vast amount of nephrology resources, as well as to information about renal pathology and transplantation. You will find access to home pages of the American Society of Transplant Physicians, the International Society of Nephrology, the Renal Pathology Society, and the International Society for Peritoneal Dialysis and photos and papers from the Third Banff Conference on Allograft Pathology. *Centerspan* is a communication tool for members of American Society of Transplant Physicians and American Society of Transplant Surgeons.

Topics in Primary Care: Nephrolithiasis
Provided by University of Chicago Primary Care Group

Address: *http://uhs.bsd.uchicago.edu/uhs/topics/nephro.html*
Cost: No charge.

As one of a series of sites on topics in primary care, Nephrolithiasis provides brief information about kidney stones. It has good resource material for the general public and physicians. It may even be a useful quick review for candidates taking tests.

LIVER DISEASE

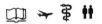

American Liver Foundation Homepage
Provided by American Liver Foundation

Address: *http://sadieo.ucsf.edu/alf/alffinal/homepagealf.html*
Cost: No charge.

Here's an excellent source of information and support for patients with liver disease. Sponsored by a respected national organization for patients, the site also includes up-to-date information for health care professionals, particularly on hepatitis C. It contains a table of ongoing clinical research but doesn't provide links.

Atlas of Liver Pathology

Provided by University of Iowa (Frank A. Mitros, M.D.)

Address: *http://indy.radiology.uiowa.edu/Providers/Textbooks/*
    LiverPathology/Text/TitlePage.html

Cost: No charge.

This site is an on-line atlas of liver pathology, a subsite of The Virtual Hospital. Many chapters are still text only, but the text is easy to follow. The format to access photos is very usable (mini-photo icons are pasted into text) and allows the user to easily select photos for expanded viewing. The subject matter is very useful for the resident level on up.

Diseases of the Liver

Provided by Columbia University

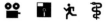 **LINKS**

Address: *http://cpmcnet.columbia.edu/dept/gi/disliv.html*

Cost: No charge

Start here for patient and provider information about liver disease. The site contains concise, current summaries of the diagnosis of and therapy for many hepatic disorders. For a site with many references and links to National Library of Medicine citations, the page is curiously drab. There are abundant links to related sites and a superb, lucid section on "current papers" by Dr. Howard Worman.

Dr. Greenson's Gastrointestinal and Liver Pathology Homepage Extravaganza

Provided by University of Michigan Dept. of Pathology (Joel Greenson, M.D.)

Address: *http://www.path.med.umich.edu/users/greenson/home.htm*

Cost: No charge.

A "case of the month" section was once part of this site, but the author no longer has time to update the cases monthly. Cases are, however, high quality and challenging. Download the movie about *Helicobacter*—it is the best cartoon depiction of organisms since those venereal disease films of the 70s with the dancing gonococci!

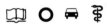

Hans Popper Hepatopathology Library
Provided by University of Michigan Department of Pathology

LINKS

Address: *http://zapruder.path.med.umich.edu/users/hepatopath/*

Cost: No charge.

Primarily a jumping-off point for resources in liver and gastrointestinal pathology, with useful links to the Atlas of Gastrointestinal Pathology (described elsewhere in this section) and Dr. Greenson's Gastrointestinal and Liver Pathology Homepage Extravaganza (see the previous review). An on-line protocol for conducting a polymerase chain reaction test for hepatitis C is also available. The target audience is most likely gastroenterologists, hepatologists, and hepatopathologists.

LUPUS

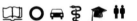

Lupus Home Page
Provided by Hamline University, St. Paul, MN

LINKS

Address: *http://www.hamline.edu/lupus/index.html*

Cost: No charge.

A reasonably extensive compilation of medical and lay material, conferences, symposia, abstracts, links, news updates, and other resources for lupus is presented at this site. A physician, patient, or layperson would probably find what they want to know about lupus here.

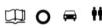

Systemic Lupus Erythematosus (SLE/Lupus)
Provided by MedicineNet by Information Network, Inc.

LINKS

Address: *http://www.medicinenet.com/mainmenu/encyclop/article/art_s/syslupis.htm*

Cost: No charge.

This is one page of MedicineNet, an extensive medical reference site. It is a basic description of lupus for the nonphysician. Whoever titled this should consider changing the spelling in the URL from "lupis"(sic) to the correct spelling, "lupus."

LYME DISEASE

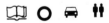

American Lyme Disease Foundation
Provided by American Lyme Disease Foundation

Address: *http://www.w2.com/docs2/d5/lyme.html*

Cost: No charge.

This fair and fairly basic information for laypersons relates mostly to ecologic and environmental issues. Those seeking more about clinical Lyme disease— symptoms, management, treatment, or recommendations—should look to other sites.

MARFAN SYNDROME

National Marfan Foundation

Provided by National Marfan Foundation

LINKS

Address: *http://www.marfan.org/*

Cost: No charge.

The National Marfan Foundation is an example of one of the hundreds of single gene disease foundations that raise money for research, disseminate information to patients and professionals, and support families and patients. This site is an excellent source of resources for patients and introductory information for physicians.

NEUROLOGY, NEUROSCIENCE, AND NEUROSURGERY

General

MGH Neurology

Provided by Massachusetts General Hospital, Neurology

LINKS

Address: *http://neuro-www.mgh.harvard.edu/*

Cost: No charge.

This winner of three stars is a noncommercial, nonmoderated *Gateway to Neurology.* The contents include WEB-FORUM, an on-line interactive open platform between patients and their families and the MGH neurologists, makes a good review of clinical neurology topics through personal case histories, and *What's New,* with a wealth of information for patients and professionals on several neurologic disorders, is an excellent resource place that is continually updated. The site has medical links to Hospital Web (the master list of hospitals on the Web), government resources (the Centers for Disease Control and Prevention), National Institutes of Health resources, and Boston medical libraries.

Mass General Hospital Department of Neurosurgery

Provided by Massachusetts General Hospital (MGH)

LINKS, SEARCH

Address: *http://neurosurgery.mgh.harvard.edu*

Cost: No charge.

This is one of the premier institutional home pages and is part of the much larger Harvard home page system. You could spend days reading all of the subpages. The site is divided into two sections.

The Clinical Units section includes 12 neurosurgical subspecialty home pages. Each of these provides journal-quality updated informational text about the subject, complete lists of links to related Web sites, and telephone numbers with names of individuals at MGH to contact for more information.

The Clinical/Educational Resources section is equally impressive. Introductions to the individuals and their work at MGH draw the clinicians and patients alike to this fine resource. Furthermore, there is information about MGH history and conferences and courses in the neurosurgery department. This site is exemplary in its demonstration of institutional use of the World Wide Web.

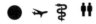

The UNC-Chapel Hill Division of Neurosurgery

Provided by University of North Carolina at Chapel Hill

LINKS

Address: *http://sunsite.unc.edu/Neuro/uncns/home.html*

Cost: No charge.

This home page is replete with organized, frequently updated, useful information for interested laypersons and professionals. There is a table of contents that directs you quickly to the various facets of the site and offers general information about faculty, residents, research interests, and case presentations. But, where else on the Web have you seen full-color, quick-to-load, high resolution images of real cadaveric dissections. The Internet Grand Rounds with Louisiana State University, Massachusetts General Hospital, and New York University and their respective links gives the site a sense of Internet community spirit. Resident neurosurgeons may wish to consult the Resident Online Handbook now and then for practical clinical pearls. It is easy to see why this academic site has received nearly 10,000 "hits" since January 1996 .

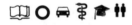

Neurosciences on the Internet

Provided by Neil A. Busis, M.D.

LINKS, SEARCH

Address: *http://www.lm.com/~nab*

Cost: No charge.

A reference site that includes search engines and "site roulette" as it presents a complete list of links to almost every imaginable area of neurologic interest. Neurobiology, neurology, neurosurgery, psychiatry, psychology, and cognitive science sites and information on human neurologic diseases are covered. No fewer than 26 subjects are indexed, and these are merely the tip of the neurologic iceberg. There is no doubt that neurospecialists and patients alike will use this page to readily find the information they need.

NeuroSource

Provided by Cybermed, LLC

LINKS, SEARCH, JOURNALS

Address: *http://www.neurosource.com.*

Cost: No charge.

Here's one of the "biggies." It has tables of contents, and the target audience is mainly neuromedical specialists. The site is extremely well organized. Three mouse-clicks will get access to *Digital Library,* which includes articles, atlases, books, and manuals. The first on-line journal,

Alzheimer's Disease Review, is available in full text. The medical students and neurology residents can review neuroanatomy, neuropathology, and neuroradiology in their respective teaching files. *Disorder Directory* has tons of information from national and international contributors. Neurosource is a powerful site where physicians and patients can find the information they seek. Usually updated daily, this site is a pleasure to use.

NEUROSURGERY://ON-CALL

Provided by American Association of Neurological Surgeons

LINKS, SEARCH, JOURNALS

Address: *http://www.neurosurgery.org*
Cost: No charge.

Enter through the operating room doors to NEUROSURGERY://ON-CALL, a site principally for members of The American Association of Neurological Surgeons. A membership fee, registration, and password are required to access some of the services and information. The site has simple graphics but they are attractive, and some are animated. An organized index directs the user to information on socioeconomic topics, an outcomes database, meetings and CME, AANS membership information, bulletin boards, a marketplace, and a resource that teaches coding of operations. Further, there is a Topic search engine with Boolean operators, lots of links, and a library with a searchable database of more than 275 neurological surgery–related periodicals and meeting abstracts.

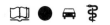

Robert's Neurology Listings on the Web

Provided by Case Western Reserve University

LINKS, SEARCH, JOURNALS

Address: *http://medinswww.meds.cwru.edu/dept/neurology/robslist.html*
Cost: No charge.

This is a very good Web site. It is well organized and full of useful material. Laypersons and professionals will find it helpful. Category I addresses general medicine and health care issues. The American Medical Association's home page has information about 7,400 fellowships and residencies. You can learn about a specific program by state and region. There is even an opportunity to use a "family medical guide" CD ROM. Abstracts from the *New England Journal of Medicine, British Medical Journal, Stroke, Nature, and Archives of Neurology* are worth checking out. Category II, Neurology for Physicians, has tons of information. For example, under epilepsy explore Albert Einstein's Comprehensive Epilepsy Center and learn about investigational drug trials and how to get into one. Read descriptions of epileptic syndromes. Category III, Neurology for the General Public, is very graphic and a winner of three stars; "eldercarweb," is a collection of resources available on the Web for the elderly and their caregivers. There is information available on almost every neurologic disorder.

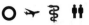

Welcome to the Department of Neurosurgery at NYU
Provided by New York University Department of Neurosurgery

LINKS

Address: *http://mcns10.med.nyu.edu*
Cost: No charge.

What is neurosurgery? Look at the NYU Department of Neurosurgery home page that boasts some 13,000 "hits" since December 1995! Obviously, some people were curious. This site is judiciously balanced with information for patients and professionals, as well as information about the residents and faculty, interesting cases, and fellowship information. The icon-based table of contents is simple and direct. An electronic neurosurgical consultation service is also available, as are links to other neuro sites and services.

Child Neurology

MGH/Child Neurology
Provided by: Massachusetts General Hospital/Neurology

Address: *http://neuro-www.mgh.harvard.edu/neurowebforum/childneurologymenu.html*
Cost: No charge.

This site is primarily for families with children who have neurologic problems. Physicians practicing in the neurological sciences will find this to be a good educational experience. MGH/Child Neurology provides an interactive, on-line forum for real people with real problems. Feel free to post your problem or solution to the problem.

OPHTHALMOLOGY

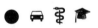

Arkansas Children's Eye Clinic
Provided by University of Arkansas Department of Ophthalmology

LINKS

Address: *http://www.ach.uams.edu:80/services/ophth/*
Cost: No charge.

The Arkansas Children's Eye Clinic is a very eye-catching stop on the Internet tour. Sections detail physicians and current eye research, along with photos of recent cases in pediatric ophthalmology. The site has a very nice layout with links to other universities and pages devoted to vision care. It is a great starting point for navigating the ophthalmology roadways.

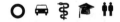

Cyberspace Hospital Ophthalmology Department
Provided by National University of Singapore

LINKS, SEARCH, JOURNALS

Address: *http://ch.nus.sg/CH/ch.html*
Cost: No charge.

The National University of Singapore has created a cyberspace hospital. This is an intensive Web link system not only to ophthalmology sources, but also to recent medical news and journals.

Ophthalmology links from this page include that of NASA vision group, Ophthalmic Photographers' Society, The Glaucoma Foundation and Ophthalmic Nursing Care, just to name a few. You will be able to link to the National University of Singapore Visible Human Project and even download information and files needed to view the 3D Cyberspace Hospital. This is a welcome map to the information superhighway.

Digital Journal of Ophthalmology
Provided by Massachusetts Eye and Ear Infirmary

LINKS, SEARCH, JOURNALS

Address: *http://www.meei.harvard.edu/meei/DJOhome.html*
Cost: No charge.

Definitely a "must see." This is a well-organized page with a multitude of interesting subpages. Included are Java script, JPGview, and Quicktime files covering basic information for patients on cataracts, retinal detachment, glaucoma, and floaters and flashes, just to name a few. Areas for those working in the field of ophthalmology, from the weekly updated grand rounds presentations, to recent publications, to a section detailing the attending and resident physicians are also at this site. It will not take long to become enthralled and consumed by this Internet site. The style and presentation are inviting and easy to use. It also includes a list of other WWW sites, Gopher sites, and e-mail response capabilities. This page definitely lives up to the Harvard reputation.

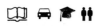

National Eye Institute
Provided by Federal Government National Institute of Health

LINKS, SEARCH

Address: *http://www.nei.nih.gov/*
Cost: No charge.

Another system of links to recent publications and clinical studies. Bonuses include search engines such as Yahoo! and Gopher. It is not a "must see," but it is a comprehensive page provided by our government.

University of California-San Diego Shiley Eye Center
Provided by University of California-San Diego Department of Ophthalmology

LINKS, SEARCH, JOURNALS

Address: *http://eyesite.ucsd.edu/*
Cost: No charge.

A basic home page with outstanding pictures. Included are links to sources covering not only vision-related topics, but also general medical information sites, journals, and even general information about traveling to San Diego. The site also provides access to search engines including Webcrawler and Infoseek. This is a thorough page for establishing links to whatever your query involves.

University of Missouri-Columbia Department of Ophthalmology

Provided by University of Missouri-Columbia

LINKS

Address: *http://www.hsc.missouri.edu/hospital/ophthalmology/*

Cost: No charge.

This basic page provides detailed descriptions of the department, including services provided and details about the faculty. Listings of upcoming events and available CME conferences are provided along with a brief description of the residency program and its members. Recent news releases about treatment modalities are also included. The site provides a simple but efficient description of the department with links to the University of Missouri home page.

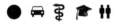

Wilmer Eye Institute

Provided by Johns Hopkins University - Wilmer Eye Institute

LINKS, SEARCH, JOURNALS

Address: *http://www.wilmer.jhu.edu/*

Cost: No charge.

Now *this* is a home page. One of the best eye institutes in the country certainly lives up to its reputation. This well-designed and graphically enhanced page lists detailed information about the institute—specifically services, training, research, and patient information. MPEG movies are provided, and the viewer is also available to download them. Extensive links to journals, such as the *Journal of the American Medical Association (JAMA), Digital Journal of Ophthalmology (DJO),* and *Archives of Ophthalmology,* as well as links to the American Academy of Ophthalmology and the American Medical Association are available. Links to other universities and search engines (e.g., Yahoo!) will allow for easy navigation. Thoughtfully included is a help section that provides a WWW guide and an HTML programming guide. No corners were cut in developing this site—a must see!

ORTHOPEDICS

"Bones are Us"

Provided by Charlotte Orthopedic Specialists (COS)

LINKS

Address: *http://www.cosortho.com*

Cost: No charge.

Designed to provide patients with background information on a number of orthopedic disorders, this site has a very effective skeleton graphic that allows individuals to point and click on a specific bone for which they want to obtain information. For the less adventurous, a text list is also provided. The general descriptive information is provided about COS and its doctors, as expected, but this page is actually a source of information, not a plug for the COS. The Common Orthopedic Questions and Sports-Related Problems sections provide excellent explanations complete with definitions, common symptoms, causes, diagnosis, and treatment where applicable. To get any information from this page, a disclaimer must be read and the visitor must click an "I understand" icon. This is a very informative site and could be recommended to patients in search of additional information

Southern California Orthopedic Institute Home Page
Provided by SCOI

LINKS

Address: *http://www.scoi.com/*
Cost: No charge.

A good source for patients with general questions. It offers an introduction to basic anatomy, sports injuries, and orthopedic procedures. Additionally, there are sections on pediatric orthopedics and joint replacement. An especially helpful feature is the list of frequently asked questions. The SCOI page allows visitors to make appointments, ask sports medicine–related questions of their doctors, and chat with physicians through America Online (AOL). For non-AOL users, transcripts of these conversations can be obtained through the Internet interface. The page ends with a list of what is coming soon to entice users to revisit the site. It also offers an extensive list of links that alone justifies a visit.

OSTEOPOROSIS

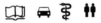

Clinical Trials: Osteoporosis/Specific Disease Category Listing (111)
Provided by CenterWatch Clinical Trials Service

LINKS

Address: *http:www.centerwatch.com/CAT111.HTM*
Cost: No charge.

CenterWatch, a Boston publishing company, has posted this listing of clinical trials relating to osteoporosis. Patients and physicians seeking this type of information would find it here.

National Osteoporosis Foundation
Provided by National Osteoporosis Foundation

Address: *http://www.nof.org*
Cost: No charge.

The National Osteoporosis Foundation has prepared a nice, comprehensive, and informative site. It offers general information on a wide variety of osteoporosis-related topics, practice guidelines, and cutting edge information. Patients, laypersons, physicians, or health professionals seeking information about osteoporosis would be satisfied with this offering.

LINKS, SWEDISH

Osteometer HomePage
Provided by Osteometer

Address: *http://www.osteometer.se/osteometerhomeeng.html*
Cost: No charge.

Because this site begins with the Swedish flag and the words "Swedish version," one would presume this is a Swedish effort. Osteometer, however, is located outside of Copenhagen, Denmark. (However, Osteometer has Swedish and Norwegian subsidiaries and is represented in other countries.) This company makes bone densitometers; this is probably the reason it uses this Web site to provide some basic information about osteoporosis. From the perspective of measuring bone density, there is some good general information about osteoporosis.

LINKS, SEARCH

Osteoporosis - Doctor's Guide to the Internet
Provided by P/S/L Consulting Group Inc.

Address: *http://www.pslgroup.com/osteoporosis.htm*
Cost: No charge.

Offered here in an engaging manner is reasonable broad and diverse information about osteoporosis, including medical news and alerts, disease information, therapeutic information, discussion groups, newsgroups, links to a number of other sites, and information about new developments. Users have an opportunity to be notified by e-mail of updates to this site. This is a useful feature and it would be valuable to those who want to be informed about osteoporosis.

SEARCH, JOURNALS

Osteovision
Provided by the European Foundation for Osteoporosis and Bone Diseases (EFFO) Health Council on Osteoporosis

Address: *http://www.sams.ch/osteovision/*
Cost: No charge.

This specialty site provides a wealth of information for physicians and scientists interested or specializing in osteoporosis. A worthwhile feature is the "aim of the site," which is written by the editor. He explains what he envisions this site becoming and of note is his intent to provide visitors with negative results of studies. He notes that an electronic arena provides a great forum for this type of information because it can be disseminated quickly and at low cost. Print journals do not have this luxury. For the print fans, an electronic version of *Advances in Osteoporosis* is provided. An address database of osteoporosis professionals and the option to sign up for a Listserv are also included. Finally, visitors are provided with a literature-based search section that makes this an attractive site for the busy professional.

OTOLARYNGOLOGY

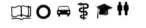

Grand Rounds Archive

Provided by Baylor College of Medicine, Department of Otorhinolaryngology and Communicative Service

LINKS

Address: *http://www.bcm.tmc.edu/oto/grand/grand.html*

Cost: No charge.

Grand Rounds Archive is a tremendous source for those reviewing or preparing presentations on topics in otolaryngology. Sources are well documented and topics include laryngology, neoplasms of the head and neck, otology and neuro-otology, pediatric otolaryngology, facial plastic and reconstructive surgery, and rhinology. These date back to July 1991. Beyond this section, there are also several interesting links to everything from computer shopping to sites devoted to classic television series. This site is a good source for students and physicians.

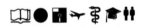

JHU Center for Hearing and Balance

Provided by Johns Hopkins University

LINKS

Address: *http://www.bme.jhu.edu//labs/chb/*

Cost: No charge.

THE site for vestibular abnormalities and research. Case studies, poster presentations with images, quizzes, and a glossary of terms are an excellent source of information for professionals and students. The site is quite user friendly. One of the strong areas of this site is its set of links to other Web sites. The Meniere's page at Washington University (St. Louis) is a great example. This provides rapid access to additional information about vestibular maladies. *Frequently Asked Questions* is an area of interest for patients about balance abnormalities, and it is quite useful. Overall, an excellent site.

Otology Online

Provided by The Shea Clinic

LINKS, SEARCH

Address: *http://www.ears.com/*

Cost: No charge.

There is a lot at this site for physicians and patients. It is easy to access UTMB (University of Texas Medical Branch) Grand Rounds in Otolaryngology. Also, patients can connect with the Shea Clinic for information on various otologic disorders. Overall, the site requires many clicks to reach the end point, but it is worth the effort. The on-site search engine makes researching a specific topic much quicker. Electronic otolaryngology text, grand rounds, and mini-monographs are likewise available and make this an invaluable source for student or physician. There are extensive links to otolaryngology-related areas. Meniere's Club meetings on-line and special recipes are but a sampling of what is available for the public. There is also a short clip on electrode insertion in cochlear implantation that can be viewed if the terminal has Quicktime. This is an excellent site for otology and general otolaryngology.

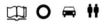

The Vestibular Disorders Association
Provided by VEDA

SPANISH

Address: *http://www.teleport.com/~veda*
Cost: No charge.

A great source for patients with vestibular problems. It offers a variety of types of assistance and an on-line discussion group. Also, there is a directory of local support groups for patients with balance disorders. The site has some information in Spanish as well. Patients and their families would be well advised to visit this site on the Web for lots of useful information. It also offers the opportunity to view several brochures from the American Academy of Otolaryngology–Head and Neck Surgery.

PAIN AND PAIN MANAGEMENT

Pain Net
Provided by Pain Net, Inc.

CME

Address: *http://painnet.com/*
Cost: No charge.

Pain Net, Inc., was developed by physicians, educators, and business professionals to provide educational and support services to health professionals, primarily physicians. This site will be most useful to medical professionals, although there are a few exceptions. For patients, there is a Patient Bill of Rights, a list of practitioners by state, free resources on pain, and other resources such as books and videos. A particularly interesting feature is the list of questions patients should ask when seeking treatment for pain. For physicians, lists of continuing education activities in areas such as medical pain management and certification is included. And there are several courses on pain topics, such as migraine pain and reflex sympathetic dystrophy available on-line with CME credit. These courses seem very cost-effective. A newsletter is available, but a table of contents or index was not included. The *Question and Comments* section promotes dialog among site users.

Talarian Index
Provided by University of Washington

Address: *http://www.stat.washington.edu:80/TALARIA/indexn.html*
Cost: No charge.

This outstanding resource for information on pain, with a special emphasis on cancer pain, includes 103 pages of information on a variety of topics ranging from conscious sedation for procedures to ablation to observation of children in pain. The information reflects recommendations from federal guidelines and cites findings from recent research. Patients and professionals will find this encyclopedia of information on pain very helpful. Topics are listed alphabetically. Tables and a comprehensive bibliography are available.

PARKINSON'S DISEASE

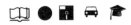

National Parkinson Foundation
Provided by National Parkinson Foundation

LINKS

Address: *http://www.parkinson.org*
Cost: No charge.

This is the home page of the National Parkinson Foundation. Its missions of research, education, and service are well stated with the pledge to "improve the quality of life for both patients and their caregivers." Current news and events, a library of information, links to centers and programs, and conferences and help groups, as well as information about receiving and providing financial support are the indexed topics. This site provides a very thorough, up-to-date, and easy-to-use resource for those whose lives are affected by Parkinson's disease.

PARASITES

American Society of Parasitologists
Provided by American Society of Parasitologists

LINKS, JOURNALS

Address: *http://www-museum.unl.edu/asp*
Cost: No charge.

A great page for students of parasitology. It is heavily linked to photos and movies about parasites. The main purpose of the page is to provide information to Society members. The guidelines for authors are included in the journal link.

PATHOLOGY

Armed Forces Institute of Pathology Home Page
Provided by Armed Forces Institute of Pathology (AFIP)

LINKS, CME

Address: *http://www.afip.mil/*
Cost: No charge.

An excellent site for pathology CME credit from a well-known and respected source of pathology expertise, as well as a variety of other services. This physically attractive and easy-to-use site includes information about the various AFIP departments, consultation services (including telemedicine consultations), information on ordering the newest edition of the *Atlas of Tumor Pathology* series (the "AFIP Fascicles" known and loved by pathologists worldwide), and the National Museum of Health and Medicine (a "must see" when visiting the metro Washington, DC area). Back issues of the *AFIP Letter* are also available. Radiologists will find the site useful to register for the popular radiology course that the AFIP offers.

CME information includes on-line registration and brochures for many popular AFIP workshops and courses, as well as on-line CME credit in a variety of pathology, veterinary pathology, and radiology topics. A year-long list of AFIP weekly seminars is also available for pathologists and scientists in the Washington, DC, area (another source of CME credit).

University of Alberta Department of Laboratory Medicine and Pathology
Provided by University of Alberta Department of Laboratory Medicine and Pathology

LINKS

Address: *http://fester.his.path.cam.ac.uk/big/synapse/000p0025.htm#12*
Cost: No charge.

This site differs from the usual university pathology department home page because it includes a number of photographic and text contributions by Dr. Ed Uthman of Houston, Tex, who has a real talent for putting pathology terms in lay language. His text files entitled *The Routine Autopsy* and *The Biopsy Report* are "must reads" for the public, because they delineate the pathologist-patient interface in a non-threatening way. The file, *An Introduction to Photography in General … And Gross Specimen Photography in Particular,* should be required reading on the basics of gross specimen photography for first year residents. Other titles, *Hematologic Infections, Diffuse Infiltrative Lung Disease Including Selected Pneumoconioses,* and *Red Cell and Anemia* are good general reviews for all levels of medical expertise.

University of Michigan Pathology Handbook
Provided by University of Michigan Department of Pathology

Address: *http://pathweb.pds.med.umich.edu/handbook/index.htm*
Cost: No charge.

Because this is essentially an on-line version of the University of Michigan Hospital's laboratory handbook, some items here are purely of internal interest (such as the days that particular tests are performed). An excellent reference resource of the standard offerings available at most university hospital laboratories or medium to large-sized reference laboratories, however, is provided. Collection requirements, dietary restrictions, and reference ranges are covered in detail. Also available at this site is a comprehensive list of brand name and generic drugs and abbreviations and symbols used in the handbook.

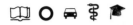

University of Washington Department of Pathology WWW Server

Provided by University of Washington Department of Pathology

LINKS

Address: *http://www.pathology.washington.edu/*

Cost: No charge.

The Cytogenetics Gallery, a nice basic resource for abnormal karyotype images for those who have not read karyotypes in a while, is featured here.

PEDIATRICS

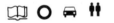

The Children's Hospital Online Information Resource (C·H·O·I·R)

Provided by The University of Missouri-Columbia Hospitals and Clinics, The Children's Hospital, Ambulatory Division

Address: *http://www.choir.missouri.edu*

Cost: No charge.

C·H·O·I·R is an excellent example of a combined "intranet" and Internet site. With access to information about the Children's Hospital, this site provides links to all electronically accessible faculty via electronic mail and sets the standard for electronic consultation via the Internet. Links to all schedules and residency information are direct and intuitive. Educational multimedia cases are available at the practitioner-resident level of expertise. Advanced HTML 2.0+ features and frames are used extensively here, so be sure to have the latest browser software available. This site sets a new standard of innovation in education and organization for pediatric sites on the Web. A "must see."

Drs4Kids

Provided by Dr. Frederic Suser

LINKS, SEARCH, JOURNALS, CME, LANGUAGE

Address: *http://www.drs4kids.com*

Cost: No charge.

Dr. Suser has created a children's Web page focused on pediatric illnesses. The *Topics* page offers information on two common infectious problems, chickenpox and fever. The *Ask Dr. Suser* page includes the Virtual Pediatric Office that permits direct submission of questions. This is a very nice site for children and their parents.

The Hypertextbook of Pediatric Critical Care

Provided by Barry P. Markovitz, M.D., Carl Weigle, M.D., and Steve Pon, M.D.

LINKS

Address: *http://pedsccm. wustl.edu/hypertext/hpccm_toc.html*

Cost: No charge.

Drs. Markovitz, Weigle, and Pon envision this site as an evolving series of links to resources of interest to the pediatric critical care specialist. As part of their comprehensive site, this "hyper-textbook" provides links to sites local and distant. Topics range from airway management and cardiovascular physiology and support to poisonings and ethics. Although it is geared for the critical care specialist, this site serves as an excellent educational resource for all pediatricians. It is best viewed with Netscape 2.0 or an HTML 2.0+ compliant browser.

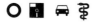

LINKS

The Johns Hopkins Hospital Virtual Children's Center

Address: *http://www.med.jhu.edu/peds/pedspage.html*
Cost: No charge.

Largely under construction, this site has the potential to become one of *the* stopping points for pediatrician Web surfers. Arranged in an icon-driven interface, the site offers links to clinical information, announcements, research, family information, helpful medical software, and per-haps most notable, simply the most comprehensive listing of pediatric Internet sites available. (See Pediatric Points of Interest, profiled elsewhere in this publication.) The only major drawback is that most of the links lead to disappointing "Under Construction" messages. Yet, The Virtual Children's Center promises to be an interesting site and is worthy of regular visits to keep up with developments. Be advised, tables are used extensively at this site, an HTML 2.0+ compliant browser is recommended.

LINKS

The MedAccess Site

Provided by MedAccess Corporation

Address: *http://www.medaccess.com*
Cost: No charge.

This is a consumer-oriented site. The site page contains detailed information about most child-hood infections, as well as links to immunization schedules.

SEARCH

Paediapedia: An Imaging Encyclopedia of Pediatric Disease

Provided by Michael P. D'Alessandro, M.D., Pediatric Radiology Section, Department of Radiology, University of Iowa College of Medicine

Address: *http://indy.radiology.uiowa.edu/Providers/TeachingFiles/PAP/PAPHome.html*
Cost: No charge.

As part of the Virtual Hospital (developed and maintained by Electric Differential Multimedia Laboratory, University of Iowa College of Medicine), this site lives up to the fine standards set by its predecessor. Although limited to neonatal radiographs at present, this site has been excel-lently crafted by Dr. D'Alessandro to provide an excellent reference on pediatric imaging. The collection of cases is comprehensive with explanations of imaging modalities. Unknown cases are presented to test your skills. The selected images are professionally rendered, and text has been presented to maximize download time without sacrificing quality. Interface design and navigation is direct yet elegant. Search facilities are most comprehensive for a site-specific engine. This definite "must see" is worthy of a bookmark.

PEDBASE Homepage
Provided by Atlantic Connect PEI

Address: *http://www.icondata.com/health/pedbase/*
Cost: No charge.

Dr. Alan Gandy has produced an excellent reference for the practicing pediatrician and the resident. This site consists of a database of more than 500 pediatric diseases ranging from common illnesses treated by the generalist to rare genetic and metabolic disorders. Each disease is reviewed in a straightforward outline format for easy review. Data transfer is fast, given the almost complete text-based structure of the site. If you like, you can download a shareware version of the database for a "try before you buy" trial. Downsides are the lack of navigation icons or links at the bottom of the pages and the absence of a search engine. You will need to rely on the "forward" and "back" keys of your browser to navigate the site. To search the database, use the "find" feature of your browser. This is a "must add" for your bookmark file.

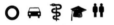

Pediatric Points of Interest
Provided by Johns Hopkins University, Dr. Christoph U. Lehmann

LINKS, SEARCH, JOURNALS, CME

Address: *http://www.med.jhu.edu/peds/neonatology/poi.html*
Cost: No charge.

This is simply the ultimate jump point to explore pediatric sites on the Web. More than 700 links are catalogued here and arranged in logical groups. Jumping to a set of links is facilitated by an excellent table of contents at the beginning of the page. A site-specific search engine is provided with links to several popular search engines on the Web. Links to professional organizations, resources for children and parents, journals and newsletters, professional opportunities, software, and electronic consultation are just a few of the points of interest listed. New entries can be added by using a simple entry form (no mail system needed on your end!). Dr. Lehmann has set the bar one notch higher for those seeking to provide the "ultimate" pediatric site on the Web. Every physician, student, and nurse caring for children should have this site listed first in their bookmark file. Simply excellent.

PEDINFO: A Pediatrics Web Server
Provided by Andy Spooner, M.D., and University of Alabama Birmingham

LINKS

Address: *http://W3.LHL.UAB.EDU/pedinfo/index.html*
Cost: No charge.

Dedicated to the dissemination of on-line information for pediatricians and others interested in child health, Dr. Spooner's site provides links to institutions (educational and professional), educational resources, medical software, and parenting resources. Included is a link to join the PED-INFO mailing list to stay abreast of medical informatics developments in pediatrics. Graphic content is slim, so page loading is fast even on a 14.4 K line. This is a fantastically organized jumping point to valuable sites on the Net.

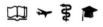

Vanderbilt Pediatric Interactive Digital Library
Provided by Dr. Bob Janco

LINKS   *Address:* *http://www.mc.vanderbilt.edu/peds/pidl/*
Cost: No charge.

This site offers a nicely developed library of monographs on various pediatric diseases. Links from the home page lead to text pages that load fairly quickly. Disease reviews are concise. Although it is still under development, the site has tremendous potential to become a valuable educational reference site on the Web. It lacks graphical navigation icons and links are text based. Graphics that would better convey concepts are conspicuously absent. No search engine is available; use the "find" feature of your browser or search using wide-area information server (WAIS). Links to the more prominent pediatric sites on the Web are provided.

PLASTIC AND RECONSTRUCTIVE SURGERY

Plastic Surgery Info Service
Provided by the American Society of Plastic and Reconstructive Surgery (ASPRS) and the Plastic Surgery Educational Foundation (PSEF)

LINKS   *Address:* *http://www.plastic.surgery.org/*
Cost: No charge.

It seems that this site is designed to be equally useful for the professional and the patient. Although most of the professional side is still under construction, the site offers a "what's new" section (updated regularly), an overview and tips section complete with mission statements and a president's message, and links to other relevant sites. The invaluable side of this site, however, is its patient resources. A section entitled "Finding a Plastic Surgeon" is included, and by choosing a geographic area, a patient can find a physician. Because the information is provided by the ASPRS, a potential patient can find out if a physician is board certified; this may be important for insurance purposes. Also provided is a list of insurance and finance options and the procedures that the surgeon performs. Additionally, this site provides explanations of topics that range from total patient care to the psychological aspects of cosmetic surgery. Finally, cosmetic procedures are explained in detail, covering everything from what to think about when considering surgery to your new look, complete with color illustrations. The ASPRS and the PSEF have spent a lot of time making sure this site is comprehensive, and they have certainly succeeded.

LINKS

Plink
Provided by the Dutch Association of Plastic Surgery (NVPC)

Address: *http://www.nvpc.nl/plink*
Cost: No charge.

This site is an excellent resource for anyone interested in plastic and reconstructive surgery. The home page lists 17 subjects from departments in plastic and reconstructive surgery to related societies and organizations. In each department, a list of related sites is presented, complete with a small graphic and a one-sentence comment about the site. These comments are helpful and range from telling the visitor to visit a certain site for the desired information to whether a particular site is difficult to access. The goal of this page is not to answer questions about plastic and reconstructive surgery, but to provide enough links that no matter what you ask, by using this page you will be able to find applicable information.

POISONS

Poison Control

List of Poison Information Resources
Provided by University of Pittsburgh, School of Medicine

LINKS

Address: *http://www.pitt.edu/~martint/pages/poisres.htm*
Cost: No charge.

Many U.S.- and non–U.S.-based poison control centers are listed here. Links are provided to many resources dealing with toxins, and poisons, including venomous creatures and treatments. Unfortunately, this site lacks focus.

Plants

Guide to Poisonous and Toxic Plants
Provided by US Army Center for Health Promotion and Preventive Medicine

LINKS

Address: *http://chppm-www.apgea.army.mil/ento/plant.htm.*
Cost: No charge.

A nice resource for identification of plants and their toxic effects. It is referenced by type of plant (e.g., house or garden) and alphabetically, along with common names. Some pictures of plants are presented. This area is being updated. It offers a nice (nontechnical) reference for professionals, as well as students and nonprofessionals.

Most Commonly Ingested Plants

Provided by Kids Source Online, American Association of Poison Control Centers Toxic Exposure Surveillance System

Address: *http://www.kidsource.com/kidsource/content/ingested.html*
Cost: No charge.

Descriptions of the 20 most frequently ingested plants as compiled by the American Association of Poison Control. It gives information about common names of plants, active toxins, and symptoms. General reference material is offered.

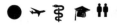

FRENCH

Poison Ivy, western poison oak, poison sumac

Provided by Agriculture and Agri-Food Canada, Product Development Unit

Address: *http://res.agr.ca/brd/poisivy/title.html*
Cost: No charge.

A brief review of these wicked weeds is given from the Canadian perspective. Reasonable recommendations for prevention, treatment, and eradication are included.

Snake Bites

LINKS

Medical Herpetology, Snakebite and Wilderness Med

Provided by Unknown

Address: *http://www.xmission.com/~gastown/herpmed/med.htm*
Cost: No charge.

A fantastic page for all you snake lovers, with current information about snake bites, including venoms, antivenoms, and treatments. The site is well organized, but has limited graphics. A link to a wilderness emergency medical services Web site is provided.

POLIO

LINKS

Polio Survivors Page

Provided by Unknown

Address: *http://www.eskimo.com/~dempt/polio.htm*
Cost: No charge.

Dedicated to polio survivors and patients with postpolio syndrome, this page is full of useful links for patients: a review and link to a book written by a survivor, a link to a textbook, and links to other polio survivor pages. The graphics on this page are dynamic.

The Rollin' Rat

Provided by Richard Spear

LINKS

Address: *http://www.indirect.com/www/rspear/rollin.html*

Cost: No charge.

This patient-oriented site has lay explanations of the disease, links to polio survivor groups, and plans for support group newsletters. This is a useful reference site for patients with postpolio syndrome and for physicians who care for these patients.

PSYCHIATRY AND MENTAL HEALTH

American Psychiatric Press, Inc.–The Prime Site for Insight

Provided by American Psychiatric Press, Inc.

SEARCH, JOURNALS

Address: *http://www.appi.org/*

Cost: No charge.

A site that is both giving and hawking. It's clutter-free, easy to use, fast, and attractive. Useful information about the American Psychiatric Association is made available.

Dr. Bob's Mental Health Links

Provided by Robert Hsiung, M.D., University of Chicago

LINKS, SEARCH, JOURNALS

Address: *http://uhs.bsd.uchicago.edu/ bhsiung/mental.html*

Cost: No charge.

An attractive site that provides almost 200 links that range widely, but selectively, including journals. This is a great site. If you have any tendencies for obsessive-compulsive disorder, you may never leave your PC screen even long enough to be told to "get a life."

Internet Mental Health

Provided by Internet Mental Health, Vancouver, Canada

LINKS, SEARCH

Address: *http://www.mentalhealth.com*

Cost: No charge.

This Canadian site has a good list of links to other sites and makes available texts on medications, disorders, definitions (from the *Diagnostic and Statistical Manual* and the *International Classification of Diseases, 10th Revision*), and various articles.

LINKS, SEARCH

Mental Health Infosource
Provided by CME, Inc. and Psychiatric Times

Address: *http://www.mhsource.com/*
Cost: No charge.

This commercial site is good for support group information, as well as articles and continuing education opportunities from the *Psychiatric Times.*

LINKS, SEARCH

Prevline: Preventions Online
Provided by National Clearinghouse for Alcohol and Drug Information

Address: *http://www.health.org/*
Cost: No charge.

Tax dollars are spent well here. The format is clear, nonbureaucratic, and works at the speed of a New York City taxi meter. The site throws a broad net of offerings, including many fact sheets, voluminous government statistics not easily available elsewhere, kits, conferences, and even President Clinton's drug abuse and prevention goals.

LINKS, SEARCH

Psych Central
Provided by John M. Grohol, M.D.

Address: *http://www.coil.com/~grohol/*
Cost: No charge.

This is an excellent site for finding all the right data in all the right places. The site is particularly strong for Usenet groups (in excess of 100). *DSM IV* and book reviews are available. Dr. Grohol notes which links he personally likes best.

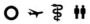

LINKS, SEARCH

WPIC Library Mental Health Resources
Provided by WPIC Library

Address: *http://wpic.library.pitt.edu/psychiat.htm*
Cost: No charge.

This site has the format of point and shoot at the first letter of the category of data for which you wish to search. This is a site-of-sites and especially good in providing information not readily available from publishers and libraries.

Psychopharmacology

LINKS, SEARCH

Psychopharmacology Tips

Provided by Robert Hsiung, M.D., University of Chicago

Address: *http://uhs.bsd.uchicago.edu/ bhsiung/tips/tips.html*
Cost: No charge.

Devoted to psychopharmacology, this site consists of experts' tips in a chat group format. The viewer must definitely do a bit of sorting, but there are enough pearls to be found to make this site a keeper.

RADIATION

LINKS

DOE Office of Human Radiation Experiments

Provided by Office of Human Radiation Experiments (OHRE), Department of Energy

Address: *http://www.ohre.doe.gov/*
Cost: No charge.

Information from the newly-created Office of Human Radiation Experiments is available here. As the main page states, the OHRE "leads the Department of Energy's efforts to tell the agency's Cold War story of radiation research using human subjects." Although this topic probably is not of direct practical value to most of us, this is nevertheless, a fascinating place to visit. Recently declassified federal documents have been directly scanned as images on the site. These, combined with the archive of photographs contemporary to the experiments, give the site a richly historical flavor, as if you are really digging through a long-forgotten file cabinet in the basement of a government building. Overall, this is a well-organized, well-designed site.

LINKS, SEARCH

Radiation and Health Physics Home Page

Provided by University of Michigan Student Chapter of the Health Physics Society

Address: *http://www-personal.umich.edu/~bbusby/*
Cost: No charge.

Lots of useful and interesting information about radiation, with separate sections geared toward laypersons and toward professionals. This site is very well organized and surprisingly comprehensive, and its appearance is simple and functional. This site is a good place to start for those of you interested in this topic.

RESPIRATORY DISORDERS

International Lung Sounds Association

Provided by Hans Pastercamp, University of Manitoba

Address: *http://www.umanitoba.ca/medicine/pediatrics/ILSA/index.html*
Cost: No charge.

This forum for physicians, physicists, and engineers who study respiratory acoustics is complete with the important peer reviewed journal citations and an extensive (although not reviewed) bibliography. This site would be worth a regular visit. Hear! Hear!

Medical Matrix Pulmonology

Provided by Slack Incorporated/Medical Matrix

LINKS

Address: *http://www.slackinc.com/matrix/SPECIALT/PULMONAR.HTML*
Cost: No charge.

Medical Matrix Pulmonology presents multiple links to Internet sites emphasizing pulmonary medicine. It is one of several medical specialties included in Medical Matrix, which provides a significant number of pathways on the information superhighway. Emphysema, sleep apnea, pneumonia, pulmonary thoracic surgery, asthma, and radiation oncology are informative locales to visit. Most were text interspersed with a few graphics. Furthermore, its descriptions of a number of procedures and pulmonary diseases could be valuable as patient teaching information.

Respiratory Disorders

Provided by University of Washington

Address: *http://weber.u.washington.edu/~conj/resp/respir.htm*
Cost: No charge.

Respiratory Disorders is a multimedia site from the University of Washington covering an extensive array of pulmonary pathology. Although not as extensive as a textbook, there is enough substance for most medical students. It has multimedia with CT scans and chest x-ray films, as well as excellent (and visible) histopathology slides. Although lacking in references, it is worth a look.

RHEUMATOLOGY

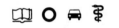 ### *General Rheumatology*

Medical Matrix - Rheumatology
Provided by HealthtelCorp.

LINKS   **Address:** *http://www.slackinc.com/matrix/SPECIALT/RHEUMAT.HTML*
Cost: No charge.

Resources, comments, documents, and guidelines are listed here. The presentation is topical and somewhat diverse. It is similar to, but not superior to, other sites. This may be of interest to laypersons or medical individuals seeking general information about rheumatology.

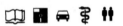 **National Institute of Arthritis and Musculoskeletal and Skin Diseases**
Provided by National Institutes of Health

Address: *http://www.nih.gov/niams*
Cost: No charge.

This *seems* to be the NIAMS home page—with a description of the institute; news and events; some health information; fact sheets and brochures; the institute's scientific resources; a listing of grants, contracts, requests for applications, requests for proposals, and program announcements; clinical studies; and reports. Although it is an obviously complete and informative description of NIAMS, this is not the place for physicians or nonphysicians to find general information about arthritis, osteoporosis, or other rheumatic and musculoskeletal diseases.

 Rheumatology, Criteria and Other Resources
Provided by Dr. Ivan Shim

LINKS   **Address:** *http://www.shim.org.sg/rheumatology/*
Cost: No charge.

A variety of criteria and guidelines developed by the American College of Rheumatology. These are available at other Internet sites as part of more comprehensive presentations. This site lists some cross-references and links. This might be of value to someone with a specific question pertaining to rheumatologic guidelines and criteria.

Rheumatology Resources
Provided by Fred Tempereau

LINKS   **Address:** *http://www.crl.com/~fredt/rheum.html*
Cost: No charge.

Fred Tempereau provides an extensive source list, index, and repository of other sites on the Internet pertaining to rheumatology. Although there was no unique or original information at this site, it was one of the most comprehensive. This would not be an unreasonable place for rheumatologists, other physicians, or laypersons to begin seeking rheumatologic information. Although this site may not provide specific information, it offers other appropriate sources.

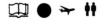

Sources Index
Provided by Department of Orthopaedics, University of Washington

Address:

http://www.orthop.washington.edu/Bone%20and%20Joint%20Sources/Sources.idx.html
Cost: No charge.

The nice presentation of this site begins with an alphabetical index of rheumatologic and musculoskeletal topics for selection. Information presented is fairly basic and oriented toward patients and laypersons.

Pediatric Rheumatology

Pediatric Rheumatology Home Page
Provided by Thomas J.A. Lehman, M.D.

LINKS

Address: *http://www.wp.com/pedsrheum/home.html*
Cost: No charge.

A respected pediatric rheumatologist has prepared good basic information for patients and families and for physicians treating children with arthritis. This site offers appropriate information on a variety of childhood arthritides that is presented in a personal and effective manner. The information is relatively easy to access, and several links are provided to other sites that are more extensive (such as the Rheumatology Resources Page).

SURGERY

Laparoscopy.com
Provided by Gabriel Medical, Alex Gandsas, M.D., and Mark Pleatman, M.D.

LINKS

Address: *http://www.laparoscopy.com/index.html*
Cost: No charge.

Laparoscopy.com is a Magellan four-star site! The providers (Gabriel Medical, Alex Gandsas, M.D., and Mark Pleatman, M.D.) have created a simple, graphic table of contents to direct you to the case of the week, a meetings list, articles, links, laparoscopic photos, and more. This site is clearly on the growing edge of Web site technology as it offers quality pictures, music, and laparoscopic videos. All that is lacking is the popcorn.

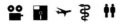

McGill General Surgery Home Page

Provided by McGill University

LINKS, FRENCH

Address: *http://www.mcgill.ca/surgery/mgshp.htm#toc*

Cost: No charge.

This one is for patients and professionals—and it will leave you impressed! Although this site provides general academic information about the faculty, residents, alumni, upcoming events, and teaching rounds, it particularly shines in organization (table of contents), and it is pleasing to the senses. There is also an inviting section on Montreal. The quick loading graphics are atypical (coffee beans background), but quite appealing! Take a look. Within 30 seconds of arriving at the site you should be comfortably browsing while you are entertained by pleasant music. A password is required to access some of the information on-site, but useful links are available to other sites and services. Updates are done biweekly (the first and 15th of each month).

TOXICOLOGY

Medical, Clinical, and Occupational Toxicology

Provided by University of Pittsburgh, School of Medicine

LINKS

Address: *http://www.pitt.edu/~martint/welcome*

Cost: No charge.

Access to other Web references related to toxicology is provided here. It also features professional certification information for physicians and nonphysicians, and provides a list of dates and locations of continuing education conferences in toxicology.

MedWeb Toxicology

Provided by Emory University Health Sciences Center Library

LINKS

Address: *http://www.gen.emory.edu/medweb/medweb.toxicology.html*

Cost: No charge.

This is the *most* comprehensive Web site pertaining to toxicology. Areas included in this page are case studies, clinical practice, conferences and calendars, consumer health databases educational resources, electronic publications, emergency medicine, family medicine, health sciences societies and associations, institutes and agencies, lists of Internet resources, microbiology and virology, the National Library of Medicine, neurology, occupational health and safety, oncology, pediatrics, pharmacy and pharmacology, and public health. This is a well-organized page with everything you need to research your interest. If all Web pages provided this much information, life would be excellent. The only thing that is missing from this page is a search engine.

Selected Cases in Toxicology from the Rocky Mountain Poison Control
Provided by Richard Dart, M.D., Ph.D., Director Rocky Mountain Poison and Drug Center, Associate Professor, University of Colorado Health Sciences Center, Denver

Address: *http://www.medconnect.com/finalhtm/dart/dart21.htm*
Cost: No charge.

This page provides interactive education as it presents selected cases in toxicology and then discusses diagnoses and treatment protocols. It allows for interaction between peers with a discussion page for the presented case.

Toxikon: Medical Toxicology On-Line
Provided by University of Illinois at Chicago

LINKS

Address: *http://www.uic.edu/~crockett/default.html*
Cost: No charge.

Toxikon presents virtual toxicology cases, with detailed histories and therapeutic plans. The site is under construction, but the provider plans to provide more interesting topics. Antidotes to common toxins is coming soon; also featured is the toxin of the week. This site is entertaining and informative. Emergency room physicians who enjoy being challenged by the virtual cases should visit this site. Research topics and links are provided.

TRAUMA

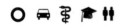

Trauma Org

LINKS

Address: *http://www.trauma.org/*
Cost: No charge.

Although the graphics are initially impressive, attempting to get useful information from this site is a daunting task. Many of the listed information categories are simply links to other Internet sites, and although the information you seek may be out there, it may be 10 clicks down the road. Set aside a large chunk of free time if you plan to explore this site.

University of Texas Health Sciences Center - San Antonio Trauma Page
Provided by University of Texas Health Services Center–San Antonio

LINKS

Address: *http://rmstewart.uthscsa.edu/*
Cost: No charge.

If you look beyond the very clever graphic at the top of this site, you will find some great educational materials. The site is full of trauma prevention and treatment, including materials appropriate for patient education. You will find in-depth information on specific topics, several brief yet complete patient presentations with photographs and radiographs included, and links to several other related sites.

TUBERCULOSIS

The People's Plague Online
Provided by PBS, WMHT Educational Telecommunications

Address: *http://www.pbs.org/ppol/*
Cost: No charge.

The People's Plague is a historical chronicle about tuberculosis in the United States. Aesthetically, it is very pleasing. This is a first rate product and subjectively informative. The site has a multimedia in design and e-mail to interact with experts in tuberculosis and the authors of this site. From a pulmonologist's perspective, there is not a lot of medical detail, but the vivid presentation of this Net site is excellent.

UROLOGY

LINKS, JOURNALS

Digital Urology Journal

Address: *http://www.dju.com*
Cost: No charge.

The *Digital Journal of Urology* (DJU) is a free, primarily text-based site, with a peer-reviewed journal format. It is readily accessible and has an average response rate. Although some areas are still under construction, the foundation seems solid. The pleasant home page provides easy access to a variety of general urology topics appealing to the urologic professional and interested patient. Based primarily out of the Harvard-Longwood urology program in Boston, the editorial board composition is varied, with respected authorities including Drs. Clayman, Lue, Raz, Retik, and Richie.

The DJU home page allows you to select from several interlinking options. *Grand Rounds* reviews interesting cases and is formatted to allow submissions. *Original Articles,* still in the conceptual phase, provides standard criteria for article submission. A particularly useful option is the *List of Meetings* that presents upcoming events and their points of contact. A similar, but more limited choice is the *New Frontier* that details grant specifications and deadlines. *Employment Opportunities* are very limited here, but presumably job postings for physicians, researchers, and allied professionals are solicited. The *Patient Information* section provides basic, encyclopedic, explanations of common urologic problems. Audience participation is requested for the *Urology Olympics,* in which submissions are taken for the case-of-the-week diagnosis. A survey feedback form is available. Links to other medically related Web sites are included.

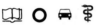

PEYRONIE DISEASE
Provided by National Center for Biotechnology Information
Online Mendelian Inheritance in Man (OMIM) Home Page

Address: *http://www3.ncbi.nlm.nih.gov/htbin-post/Omim/dispmim?171000*
Cost: No charge.

This site is part of the home page of OMIM, which has a specific interest in the genetic and inherited basis of diseases. Edited by Dr. Victor A. McKusick and colleagues at Johns Hopkins and elsewhere, a brief description of the genetic basis of Peyronie's disease (most commonly believed to be traumatic in origin) is presented with references. This one paragraph review with six references is intended to complement a larger body of work on genetics, and not to provide a comprehensive understanding of the disease process.

Peyronie's Disease
Provided by NIDDK Home Page

LINKS

Address: *http://www.niddk.nih.gov:80/Peyronie'sDisease/Peyronie'sDisease.html*
Cost: No charge.

A well-organized and succinct overview of Peyronie's disease for the patient and nonurologist. This National Institutes of Health publication from May 1995 provides an up-to-date, easily accessible description of the disease process and potential treatments from a reputable source. Entirely consisting of text, this page provides an informative introduction with addresses of other sources for more information.

VIROLOGY

The Irish National Virology Reference Laboratory Home Page
Provided by University College, Dublin

LINKS, SEARCH, JOURNALS

Address: *http://hermes.ucd.ie/~virusref*
Cost: No charge.

This site is run by the Irish Viral Disease Laboratory. The diagnostic virology service links to a series of pages that provide summary information for the clinical and laboratory diagnosis of a variety of viral syndromes. The news section provides current information about viral outbreaks in Ireland. Moreover, this site has extensive links to a number of Web sites of interest to infectious disease physicians and other specialists: the Centers for Disease Control and Prevention (CDC) site, the World Health Organization site, and communicable disease surveillance sites in the UK and France. Under epidemiology, the site links to the CDC Epi-Info Freeware site and to the WWW Virtual Library on Epidemiology. Several search engines are included, as well as a link to the on-line version of the *British Medical Journal*.

The "Virtual" Medical Center Pathology and Virology Center
Provided by Jim Martindale

LINKS   **Address:** *http://www-sci.lib.uci.edu/~martindale/MedicalPath.html*
Cost: No charge.

Although this site is a treasure trove of links, it is *very* slow. The site carries a wide variety of information, including World Daily Reports, Travel Warnings, Immunization guidelines, anatomy and biochemistry tutorials, pathology tutorials, and a few quality pathology images. The last time I tried to use this page, however, the pathology links had a "bug" in them that kept sending me back to the home page. I could not access the pathology images again.

WOMEN'S HEALTH

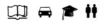

KKH Web Server - The International Obstetrics and Gynecology Resources
Provided by KK Infoweb

LINKS   **Address:** *http://biomed.nus.sg/kkh/foreign.html*
Cost: No charge.

This site is composed of a list of links, some of which are annotated. Most of them are self-explanatory. They are grouped in categories of interest, such as women's health, gynecologic oncology, maternal-fetal medicine, and midwifery. This is a good resource site but not much to look at because there are minimal graphics and none of the new multimedia effects.

Women's Medical Health Page
Provided by an anonymous medical student at University of California, San Francisco (UCSF)

LINKS   **Address:** *http://www.best.com/~sirlou/wmhp.html*
Cost: No charge.

Abstracts of recent journal articles concerning women's health issues are presented at this site. Archives of previously listed articles are also available. Links to numerous sites of medical interest, including the UCSF digital library, World Health Organization home page, and MEDWEB are available. The page is text only, but is very well done for a personal page. This page was awarded a Magellan four-star award; it is easy to see why. The site is highly recommended as a browsing page or a jumping-off point for a search.

DIVERSE HEALTH DISCIPLINES

CHIROPRACTIC

LINKS, SEARCH, JOURNALS

American Chiropractic Association Chiropractic Online
Provided by American Chiropractic Association (ACA)

Address: *http//www.cais.net/aca/*
Cost: No charge.

The ACA has produced a comprehensive and informative Web site, with information useful for practicing chiropractors and interested patients or consumers. The site is graphically attractive and provides the reader information on chiropractic care for back pain (including the most recent findings from researchers in a variety of fields) and for headache. The site provides a review of research pertaining to the profession, information on what chiropractors do in a clinical setting, and information on the training necessary to become a chiropractor. There are links to a reference library, as well as to the *Journal of the American Chiropractic Association* and to a variety of medical and health-related Web sites. A search engine is provided. This is a thoroughly useful site containing a wealth of information.

LINKS

Chiropractic Resources Referral Directory
Provided by Chiropractic Resources Referral Directory

Address: *http://www.mtii.com/chiro/*
Cost: No charge.

This site provides a lengthy glossary of chiropractic terms that may help patients to better communicate with their chiropractors. In addition, each term is referenced to current literature, and avoids taking any particular philosophical slant. This is a plus. There is also a list of chiropractic colleges. The scope, presentation, and usefulness of the site are modest.

Chiroweb
Provided by Web Ventures One

LINKS

Address: *http://chiroweb.com*
Cost: No charge.

Here's a relatively plain referral service that allows the reader to enter a city or state location and obtain a list of chiropractors. There is also a section entitled *All About Chiropractic* that provides general information and links to a variety of sources about the chiropractic profession. It is possible to access some research findings through this site, but the depth of coverage is rather shallow. There are links to other alternative medicine sites, too.

LINKS

Chiropractic Health for Washington State
Provided by Washington State Chiropractic Association

Address: *http://www.chirohealth.org/*
Cost: No charge.

The aim at this site is to aid the public and health decision makers in learning more about the art and science of chiropractic. Therefore, general information about the profession, a compendium of current chiropractic news, information about the Washington State Chiropractic Association and its members are provided. It offers a service to help the reader locate a practitioner. The news section is especially well presented and informative, and it is regularly updated. The general information section about chiropractic is quite comprehensive, with numerous links to more information. This is a well done and professional site.

LINKS

New Jersey Chiropractic Page
Provided by Dr. Joseph Garolis

Address: *http://www.chiro.org/states/nj/*
Cost: No charge.

This site offers a compendium of legislative information about the practice of chiropractic in New Jersey. In addition, there are links to national legislation (federal level) and state and county societies and an explanation of the scope of a chiropractic practice. It is possible to obtain synopses on recent chiropractic research. One of the most appealing components of this site is the section on case reports. Interested doctors can submit case reports for distribution and dissemination; a set of rigorous guidelines is posted, and the cases reviewed were thorough and interesting. Cases covered head and cervical region, thoracic spine, lumbar spine, upper and lower extremity, and organic conditions. These cases, although mostly all text, were well done. This site is a fine mixture of professional and consumer interests. There are numerous links to other related sites.

OPTOMETRY

LINKS

Contact Lens Council
Provided by Contact Lens Council

Address: *http://www.iglobal.com/clc/*
Cost: No charge.

Concise, easy-to-read information about contact lenses and related topics, primarily for patients. The provider, the Contact Lens Council, is a consortium of contact lens manufacturers, but the limitations of contact lenses are discussed along with the benefits. The site provides links to manufacturer Web sites, as well as links that will be of most interest to professionals, such as those to optometry colleges and professional societies.

Optometric Computing

Provided by Optometric Computing

LINKS **Address:** *http://www.webcom.com/optcom/*

Cost: No charge.

Too many Web sites simply provide facsimiles of printed pages. At this excellent site, optometrists can get information that is not available except through computer technology, such as *Digital Grand Rounds, John Warren's Topography Class,* and bulletin-board style discussions on low vision, contact lenses, ocular disease, managed care, and other topics. Perhaps the most interesting feature is a link to *The Adventures of Superdoc,* a clinical self-assessment tool that was developed by the Southern College of Optometrists.

Other resources include *Jobsite* (for both providers and seekers), *Marketstreet* (a place to buy or sell equipment), downloadable software, links to state optometry associations and other optometric sites worldwide, and a link to the *Southern Journal of Optometry.*

PODIATRY

A Foot Talk Place on the Net

Provided by Ron LeDoux, D.P.M.

LINKS **Address:** *http://www.foottalk.com/*

Cost: No charge.

The good information, mostly for patients, found here is not easily accessible for anyone who is just beginning to explore the Web. It is impossible to know exactly how to proceed from the *Welcome* screen, because the icons are labeled with cryptic pictures instead of words (e.g., one is labeled with a forward arrow, one with a caduceus). Once the user selects a topic, icons labeled with words appear, but these are vague (e.g., a file of frequently asked questions is labeled "Podiatry").

This problem aside, the information for patients is clear enough, and some topics are illustrated. The links range from professional resources (e.g., the American Podiatric Medical Association) to commercial sites (e.g., shoe manufacturers).

Podiatric Medical Educational Network

Provided by American Association of Colleges of Podiatric Medicine

Address: *http://www.podiatry.org/podiatry.html*

Cost: No charge.

For students and prospective students, this site provides information about the profession of podiatry, residency and licensing requirements, a weekly newsletter, and a placement bulletin for fourth-year students. However, posting of both publications was 6 months behind at the time of this visit. For educators, there is a calendar of events, and two files are under construction: an *Alert Center* for news about podiatric medical education, and *The Academy* for downloading monographs.

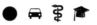

California College of Podiatric Medicine
Provided by California College of Podiatric Medicine

LINKS, CME

Address: *http://www.ccpm.edu/*
Cost: No charge.

CME credit is to be available on-line from this site, although only one course was available in July 1996. At that time, a tutorial with photographic images was being offered as a free demo. The tutorial included a 7-question quiz to be submitted by e-mail, and results were available immediately. No information was available about future charges or a system for awarding credits.

Besides the CME program, this site is largely a public relations vehicle for the college. However, it links to the Foot and Ankle Web Index (http://www.footandankle.com/), a commercial site that claims to link to "all known podiatry information on the WWW," patient and professional.

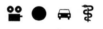

Podiatry Quick Reference
Provided by Todd Haddon, podiatric medical student

LINKS

Address: *http://pages.ripco.com:8080/~haddon/*
Cost: No charge.

Among the 35 links in this collection, the most fun is *The Interactive Ankle,* an imaging program that lets users select various anatomical layers of the ankle to view and read about (e.g., bone, muscle, or nerve). There are excellent podiatry-related links, notably to Podiatry Online (http://www.netrunner.net/%7Efootman/pdonline.html), and excellent general medical resources, such as disease-specific on-line tutorials and the *Antibiotic Index,* a resource for prescribers compiled by the Medical College of Wisconsin. There are also links to schools, medical societies, and publications. The downside is that the user must scroll up and down through a grid that lists all 35 options in random order.

MIDWIFERY

Marilyn's Midwifery Page
Provided by Marilyn Greene

LINKS

Address: *http://frank.mtsu.edu/~mhgreene/marilyn.html*
Cost: No charge.

This site includes an excellent annotated bibliography on midwifery, including journals and Internet sites. In addition, there's a current calendar of upcoming national and international continuing education, current political and legislative hot topics, and consumer awareness information about drugs, the "system," and choosing midwives and physicians. The extensive index includes topics on parenting, pregnancy, birth, nutrition, alternative health remedies, and drug safety. Links are available to pregnancy- and birth-related organizations.

MIDIRS (Midwives Information and Resource Service)
Provided by MIDIRS (Midwives Information and Resource Service)

Address: *http://www.gn.apc.org/midirs*
Cost: No charge.

This newly developed site from Great Britain was scheduled to be fully on-line by June 24, 1996. The *MIDIR DIGEST* is a quarterly international digest. The site will provide on-line articles pertaining to midwifery and birth issues.

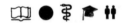

Goals of Midwives Alliance of North America (MANA)
Provided by Donna Dolezal Zelzer

LINKS

Address: *http://www.efn.org/~djz/birth/add695/managoals.html*
Cost: No charge.

The goals of the umbrella organization for all midwives in North America are described at this site. Links to regional contacts and other midwifery- and birth-related resources are available.

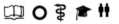

Online Birth Center Midwifery, Pregnancy, Birth and Breastfeeding
Provided by Donna Dolezal Zelzer

LINKS, SEARCH, JOURNALS

Address: *http://www.efn.org/~djz/birth/birthindex.html*
Cost: No charge.

A juicy site for those interested in independent, apprentice-trained or direct entry midwives. It includes many references to and from the popular periodical, *Midwifery Today.* The site has been rated among the top 5% of all sites on Internet by Point Survey. A collage of articles and information address topics such as midwifery education, conferences, clinical problems, networking information, and birth stories. Nutrition information and alternative health resources are also available. Color contrasts make some listings difficult to read.

A Potpourri of WWW Sites of Interest to Midwives
Provided by Kate Weber Brown

LINKS, SEARCH

Address: *http://www.islandnet.com/~browns/homebirth/wwwsites.html*
Cost: No charge.

What an outstanding site! It includes comprehensive index links to Internet sites for virtually all pregnancy-, birth-, and parenting-related topics. Links are available to excellent home birth information, including personal birth stories, literature review, statistics, and answers to common questions about home birth.

The American College of Nurse-Midwives
Provided by The American College of Nurse Midwives

LINKS, SEARCH, JOURNALS

Address: *http://www.acnm.org*
Cost: No charge.

This is the official resource about certified nurse-midwives (CNMs). Sponsored by their national professional organization, ACNM, it is comprehensive and well organized. A few broad topics are linked to detailed information. Consumers will be interested in how to find CNMs, descriptions and testimonials that differentiate their practice from that of obstetricians, answers to questions about educational preparation and programs, legal status, and outcome statistics. There are also links to other sites with similar interests, such as parenting chat groups and midwifery advocacy groups. Interview questions for the consumer are included. The choice of birth sites including home, birth center, and hospital, is addressed. Students and midwives from countries outside the United States can find out about nurse-midwifery schools, entrance requirements, curriculum, and credentialing requirements. Professionals will find links to midwifery-related journals (national and international) including *The Journal of Nurse Midwifery,* as well as to MEDLINE, the World Health Organization, and national legislative information.

WHO Midwifery Board
Provided by the World Health Organization

Address: *http://www.who.ch/programmes/nur/MIDWIFERY.html*
Cost: No charge. Registration and password after first visit as a guest.

The exchange of ideas and midwifery concerns are restricted to the group of registrants. This is a typical bulletin board of opinions and shared experiences. There is no guarantee that information is accurate.

PHYSICIAN ASSISTANTS

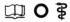

American Academy of Physician Assistants
Provided by American Academy of Physician Assistants

LINKS

Address: *http://www.aapa.org*
Cost: No charge.

This is the American Academy of Physician Assistants home page. The Academy boasts that it is the only organization representing PAs in all specialties and employment settings. Membership includes students and supporters of the profession and qualifying physician assistants. The site is divided into several subpages, which can be grouped into three categories.

The first category is general information. Material about the association, related organizations, products, and publications is provided and well organized to teach the user about this new and exciting field of medical care.

The second category is educational. Provided mainly for PA students, these subpages encourage individuals to join the Academy and become locally active. Information about scholarships and awards is included.

The final category regards current events. A *What's new* subpage shows recently posted news to keep professionals and the public abreast of topics in the field. A handy submission form allows individuals to be alerted by e-mail when the site is updated.

This is the place to begin searching for information about physician assistants. Whether you are looking for a history of the specialty or scholarship information, you will find answers and references here. The site is very fast and easy to navigate.

The National PA Student Page
Provided by Student Academy of the American Academy of Physician Assistants

LINKS

Address: *http://members.aol.com/medicjer/index.html*
Cost: No charge.

Written by PAs and students to benefit PA students, this home page is an excellent reference with many useful subpages. Main categories include directories of faculty and students, classified ads, connections, clinical challenges and pearls, resources and references, and a PA program locator. Graphics accentuate the site's colorful text scheme, and there are excellent links to other sites. If you're considering this field of medicine, this is the place to look.

The National PA Page
Provided by John Schira, P.A.-C

LINKS, JOURNALS, CME

Address: *http://www.halcyon.com/physasst*
Cost: No charge.

This is the National Physician Assistants' home page, "The Internet's first and foremost resource for and about the Physician Assistant profession." The site is aesthetically pleasing with multi-framed organization and motion graphics. Subpages are excellent and include free MEDLINE searches, a directory of PA e-mail addresses, professional and program information, and continuing medical education opportunity listings. Overall, this site is excellent as a resource for PAs, students, and health professionals, but also for interested individuals who appreciate first-rate applications of Netscape technology.

DENTISTRY

AAPD Online
Provided by American Academy of Pediatric Dentistry

LINKS

Address: *http://www.aapd.org*
Cost: No charge.

A must for parents with young children. It contains useful information about oral health care for children. The information in this site is clearly written, well organized, and from a reliable source. The links and indexes are easy to navigate, and the page designs are clean and the graphics are pleasing. Some formatted documents require Adobe Acrobat Reader to view after downloading. A dentist could print these documents and distribute them to patients. The site includes an excellent list of links to Web sites, as well as dental-related mailing lists and news-groups, a useful list of sites for parents, and a list of other health organizations, associations, and government agencies. There is an electronic newsletter for Academy members.

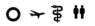

ADA Online
Provided by American Dental Association (ADA)

LINKS, SEARCH

Address: *http://www.ada.org*
Cost: No charge.

Of course this site is a must for every dentist, but there is a lot of patient information here as well. Patients and dentists can find the latest breaking news on a wide variety of topics in oral health care. There are news releases on legal and policy topics as well as updates on amalgam and on infection control in the dental office. The ADA maintains a long list of on-line publications and official position statements. For people interested in a career in dentistry, this site has fact sheets on dental hygiene, dental assisting, dental laboratory, and dental school admissions and education programs. The ADA Online server is fast, and the design is easy to use. Of course, there is an extensive list of links to other good dental Web sites. The search engine is a useful feature since this site contains so much information.

National Institute of Dental Research
Provided by the National Institute of Dental Research, National Institutes of Health

LINKS, SEARCH

Address: *http://www.nidr.nih.gov*
Cost: No charge.

Dental research is still alive and well in the United States, and this site provides information on federally funded oral health grants and contracts, publications, consensus conferences and meetings. It is a must for the budding oral health researcher, as well as for the established research scientist. This site also contains a link to National Oral Health Information Clearinghouse, a service of the National Institute of Dental Research, that provides oral health information for special care patients. The oral health database indexes materials such as fact sheets, brochures, videocassettes, newsletter articles, catalogs, and other educational resources for patients and professionals, but it does not contain full text articles.

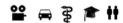

HKDA Online
Provided by Hong Kong Dental Association

LINKS

Address: *http://www.hkda.org*
Cost: No charge.

A great site that's maintained by another dental association. The access speed is a little slow, but you are crossing the Pacific Ocean. Most of the information on this site is for dentists, but there is a section where patients can submit questions to HKDA dentists and get some general information on oral health. There are monthly multimedia case presentations for dentists that can be used for informal continuing education. After reviewing a case, the dentist can read and post messages to an on-line case discussion group. Another innovative feature is that cases can be submitted to this site electronically. Of course, there is a list of links to other dental sites, but there is also an overview of MEDLINE, a glossary of terms, and a forms-based quiz on general oral health facts and terms. This site is updated monthly. Some links, like the member's newsgroup, are restricted to HKDA members, but this is the exception.

CDA Online
Provided by California Dental Association with assistance from Loma Linda University

LINKS, SEARCH

Address: *http://www.cda.org*
Cost: No charge.

This site is a pioneer from state dental associations. It contains a lot of information for patients and dentists. For the dentist, the site contains information on legislative and government issues, news, association calendars and events, and various hot topics for the dental practice. Patients can find information on a variety of topics ranging from "Baby Bottle Decay" to "Oral Health Care for Seniors." There is also information on CDA funded programs for dental care and scholarships. Free access to the *CDA Members/Subscribers Access* section has been extended indefinitely, but the ADA/CDA membership requirement may be enforced in the future.

Colgate-Palmolive Company
Provided by Colgate-Palmolive Company

Address: *http://www.colgate.com*
Cost: No charge.

To its credit, Colgate does not hide the fact that this is a commercial site. Most of the information is on general oral hygiene and is targeted to parents and children. There is an on-line

"Cavity Club" and coloring book for kids, plus some cute multimedia stories. Put a computer in the dental office, and this would be a great diversion while the kids are waiting for their appointments. Overall, it is a great design, but there is not a lot of content.

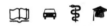

ITALIAN, GERMAN

Dentistry On-Line
Provided by Priority Lodge Education Limited (British)

Address: *http://www.cityscape.co.uk/users/ad88/dent.htm*
Cost: No charge.

An innovative use of Web-based publishing, this site's on-line publication for patients and professionals contains articles submitted via e-mail and reviewed by an international editorial board. There is a question and answer page arranged by topics, but the consumer should be aware that this is similar to a newsgroup. Anyone can submit information and there is no indication of peer review for the answers provided. There is a large international editorial board, but the qualifications of the board members are not listed. Overall this is a well-designed and organized site.

OSTEOPATHY

An Introduction to Osteopathic Manual Therapy: Diagnosis and Treatment of the Axial Skeleton
Provided by Peter J. Bower, M.D.

Address: *http://avery.med.virginia.edu/~pjb3s/Osteopathic_Intro.html/*
Cost: No charge.

Detailed and well organized, this introduction to Dr. Bower's Complementary and Alternative Medicine Home Page provides clinical procedures for those performing manual therapy (see review of Dr. Bower's page). Intending to expound on various types of manipulation and their contraindications, Dr. Bower faithfully follows the outline he creates at the beginning, making the information easy to comprehend. Useful, especially to the student, is his refresher course of basic anatomy, necessary for knowledge of manual therapy. Although the text-heavy page could benefit from some graphics or some three-dimensional figures (for those of us who need a visual, hands-on approach), his explanations are thorough and algorithmic enough to get the point across. In other words, you will get a lot of information from this site, even if it is not so pretty to look at.

LINKS, JOURNALS

The Source: The Osteopathic Medical Student Web Site
Provided by OMEGA

Address: *http://avicom.net/thesource/index.html*
Cost: No charge (although to access the *Education* links, users may be required to register for free).

This excellent resource for premedical and medical students with osteopathic medicine as their focus is maintained by medical students. It weaves lighthearted humor (and some self-promotion) into its bevy of information. In addition to basic facts—including a succinct definition of osteopathic medicine and a friendly message from the president of the American Osteopathic Association—the *Information* subheading provides addresses for and specialties of osteopathic medical schools and residency programs in the United States. One of the more useful features of the *Education* subheading is a page called *Dave's Bookshelf,* which lists some of the seminal texts for students wishing to pursue osteopathic medicine, as well as some recommended reading in various disciplines. The *Entertainment* section could be a useful tool for those who do not know exactly what they want from the field: the section includes an e-mail list of "guests" (previous visitors to the site), many of whom are doctors of osteopathy. Also included here are some links to student journals (free registration required). The student-creators of the page are surely benefiting their colleagues-to-be; their press release, promoting the page (and themselves!) indicates that maybe they know it.

PHARMACY

American Society of Health Systems Pharmacists Webpage
Provided by American Society of Health Systems Pharmacists (ASHP)

LINKS, SEARCH, JOURNALS

Address: *http://www.clark.net/pub/ashp*
Cost: No charge.

A great site with awesome and unlimited places to go, this is the "granddaddy" of links to many aspects of pharmaceutical practice. First and foremost, it links to all ASHP services, including product lines, publications, continuing education, newsletters, and meeting announcements. Additionally, it links with other pharmacy organizations, their publications, and direct e-mail access to organization leaders.

This site links to all national colleges of pharmacy with direct e-mail capabilities to the faculty members. Once the college of pharmacy is accessed, the user can link directly to the university's home page. The site also links directly to pharmaceutical manufacturers.

This site is easy to navigate and access, even as a beginning surfer. For those with advanced skills, there is plenty of information and access to multiple other sites. "Wow!" was the response to this site.

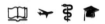

World Wide Web Virtual Library-Pharmacy
Provided by David Bourne, University of Oklahoma College of Pharmacy

LINKS, SEARCH, JOURNALS, CME

Address: *http://www.cpb.uokhsc.edu/pharmacy/pharmint.html*
Cost: No charge.

A site that eclipses the ASHP yellow pages site. There are regular updates and links to multiple pharmacy-related sites. It includes a pharmacy chat site, pharmacy world wide web sites, international pharmacy school sites, pharmacy organizations, pharmaceutical companies, and links to drug stores. There are easily accessible links to multiple journals. Databases and drug information centers links are quite handy.

The section entitled "unclassified" is a real find. This list includes Web sites for suppliers (whether for research supplies or pharmaceuticals), users groups, disease management groups, and many more. The sheer quantity of information available through this site boggles the mind. Fortunately, the site is well laid out in an easy to use format that even the neophyte can navigate. This site has it all and has the advantage of being updated frequently and routinely. If there was one site to know, this is it, especially for faculty and university-based practitioners. Although the information is not primarily oriented toward the public, there are links to patient-oriented information.

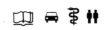

LINKS, SEARCH

RXList, The Internet Drug list
Provided by Neil Sandow, Pharm.D.
Address: *http://www.rxlist.com*
Cost: No charge.

The graphics are relatively plain, but the site is easy to access. It's primarily geared toward laypersons, and drug specifics are minimal. It does not support drug information questions other than indications and side effects. The information is not quantified (i.e., the percentage of patients having a certain side effect), nor is the information referenced. Links are available to several other continuing education and drug information sources. The best qualities are its straightforwardness and ease of use. The site is user friendly does not overwhelm the beginner with an enormous amount of information.

LINKS, SEARCH

American College of Clinical Pharmacy Home Page
Provided by University of Pittsburgh

Address: *http://www.pitt.edu:81/~gjb/accp.html*
Cost: No charge.

Although currently under construction, this site should be revisited. At present the background/set is somewhat goofy looking. A lot of space is used for pictures. Access to organization leader e-mail addresses is available. It also has a job placement link.

NUTRITION

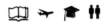

Ask the Dietitian
Provided by Joanne Larsen, R.D., in association with Hopkins Technology Nutrition and Health Products

Address: *http://www.hoptechno.com/rdindex.htm*
Cost: No charge.

Here is an opportunity to ask a registered dietitian with 24 years of combined hospital and clinical experience your questions about nutrition. In addition, there is a listing of informational topics ranging from alcohol, allergies, and anorexia to vegetables, vegetarians, and vitamins. Joanne Larsen serves up a smorgasbord of Q&A formatted nutritional dialogue. This site rates in the top 5% of all Web sites. There is also a collection of 94 on-line booklets and pamphlets covering topics such as nutrition, preventive medicine, fever blisters, gallstones, and peptic ulcer disease.

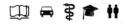

The Transporter
Provided by Mike Cochran

LINKS   **Address:** *http://www.pe.net/~paragon/transport.html*
Cost: No charge.

"Beam me up Scotty"—transport yourself to one of 89 useful food- and nutrition-related Web sites organized under four headings: Government, Schools, Protein, and Others. If you cannot find what you are looking for in this list, it probably does not exist.

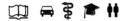

FDA Center for Food Safety and Applied Nutrition
Provided by Food and Drug Administration (FDA)

LINKS   **Address:** *http://vm.cfsan.fda.gov/list.html*
Cost: No charge

"The FDA regulates $1 trillion worth of products, which account for 25 cents of every dollar spent annually by American consumers." Any organization with this kind of clout ought to have a Web site to match. The FDA does not disappoint. This site is well organized and teeming with information about food- and nutrition-related topics. Major areas include consumer advice, material for educators, food borne illness, cosmetics, pesticides and chemical contaminants, seafood, and press releases.

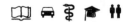

Food and Nutrition Information Center
Provided by U.S. Department of Agriculture (USDA)

LINKS, SEARCH   **Address:** *http://www.nal.usda.gov/fnic/*
Cost: No charge.

The name says it all. Here the USDA dishes out useful, credible information about nutrition and your health including dietary guidelines for Americans, food and nutrition software and multimedia programs, food service management, and how to plug into government programs, such as WIC (Women, Infants, and Children program). Nutritionists at this site "are willing to answer any questions related to food or human nutrition." Want to know how much fat is in hearts of palm? The answer is here. This site is well organized and searchable—an excellent resource.

HEALTH-RELATED INFORMATION

GENERAL MEDICINE

Directories or Catalogs

Achoo

Provided by MNI Systems Corp. Ontario, Canada

SEARCH, LINKS

Address: *http://www.achoo.com/*

Cost: No charge.

Achoo is a visionary directory that has given nearly 6,100 links an order. It includes broad categories like *Human Life, Business, Hospitals,* and *Practice of Medicine,* and each large category is divided into reliable, smaller divisions. Click on a division and browse the list, or use the search engine to find a needed topic. Additional features include *Healthcare Newsgroup Discussions* in a searchable database and *Healthcare Headline News,* which cleverly links to hundreds of headlines; you must subscribe to NewsPage (http://www.newspage.com) to get the whole story. Brief annotations and *Sites-of-the-Week* help you choose one or more treasures in this vast, although not entirely comprehensive, trove.

Diseases, Disorders, and Related Topics

Provided by Karolinska Institute

LINKS

Address: *http://www.mic.ki.se/Diseases/index.html*

Cost: No charge.

A simple, yet extensive index. The home page lists 21 disease categories. There is also a biomedical section and some interesting inclusions like *Nobel Prizes, Animal Diseases,* and *Forensic Medicine.* Perhaps it's the black and blue coloring and font shape—it's easy to read, easy to follow, and includes international and otherwise obscure listings. No annotations are given.

Hospital Web

Provided by Department of Neurology, Massachusetts General Hospital

LINKS

Address: *http://neuro-www.mgh.harvard.edu/hospitalweb.nclk*

Cost: No charge.

This site has an extensive (and continually growing) index of U.S. and world hospitals that are listed alphabetically by state or country. "Interesting Medical Site of the Week" links to new, annotated medical and medical school residency resources. The hospitals included are those with main Web servers, so there is generally substantial content. The site notes other Medical Lists (like ElNet Galaxy) on the Web.

LINKS, SEARCH

Medical Matrix
Provided by Slack Incorporated

Address: *http://www.slackinc.com/matrix/special.html*
Cost: No charge.

In this "Guide to Internet Clinical Medicine Resources," you know you are dealing with pros. The first thing you see is a full-site search capability that includes Boolean operators (AND/OR). Well-constructed subject delineations (from Disease, to Medical Electronic Journals, from Employment Resources to Biomedical Industry), with each division divided again into logical indices, sites, forums, and the like. This directory shines in organization and layout, although some of the inclusions, especially the disease category, could be heavily augmented. Within specialties there are links to such helpful items as Practice Guidelines, Journals, Clinical Cases, and Proceedings and Meetings. The search engine is available globally and within each division. Brief annotations of the sites allows for some measure of selection among all the choices. The breadth, layout, and clarity of vision make the visit worthwhile.

LINKS, SEARCH

MedWeb
Provided by Emory University Health Sciences Center Library

Address: *http://www.cc.emory.edu/WHSCL/medweb.html*
Cost: No charge.

Build a Web site and they will come. This "field of [Web] dreams" has a browsable table of contents that is categorized by specialty or discipline. Each category is then divided into multiple parts with a "book index" look and feel. The site has extensive hyperlinks to the biomedical community, from Anatomy to Disabilities, from Genetics to Mental Health, from Public Health to Telemedicine. Additional subjects include Consumer Health, Electronic Journals (!), National Library of Medicine, Societies and Associations, and Virtual Reality in Medicine. Search capability is available but not very evident. The overlap between categories is apparent, and that is a good thing. Minimal annotations are given, but the judicious inclusion of so many specialties and subjects makes MedWeb a tidy, logical place to start.

LINKS, SEARCH

Omni
Provided by Omni Consortiums

Address: *http://omni.ac.uk*
Cost: No charge.

It's British, and it's been done suitably. Search the United Kingdom sites or Worldwide sites, or both. You can browse the lists—they are divided into specialty areas (e.g., AIDS, forensic medicine, hospitals, and pathology)—or enter search terms in the interface to go directly to the sites. A more familiar category breakout might be warranted; for example, there is no cancer or oncology, but neoplasms is included. Annotations are cleverly used. A resource name is displayed; then you (1) click on the name for a short description or (2) click on the radio button to go directly to site. The content is not voluminous, but it's well executed.

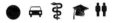

Jonathan Tward's Multimedia Medical Reference Library (MMRL)
Provided by Jonathan Tward

LINKS, SEARCH

Address: *http://www.med-library.com*
Cost: No charge.

MMRL has two versions: the Frames Version, which you see foremost, and the No Frames Version, which you must choose. The Frames Version holds you as a happy hostage within the voluminous content; wherever you link to, you always stay within MMRL. However, you cannot go "Back" with your browser within the provider's content; for that, you need the No Frames Version. Confused? Persevere, get past the tiny script on the tiny buttons, the bothersome color choices, the overt advertising, the constant scrolling down to content, and the busy layout. MMRL has free MEDLINE with a serviceable NLightN search engine. Among its *many* components, it links (or offers, depending on the version you have chosen) to medical curricula, medical school home pages, classified ads, medical software, full text of journals like the *Journal of the American Medical Association,* audio clips of heart sounds, hospital home pages, and a fairly comprehensive categorized disease list that provides government and private documents.

Professional Guides

BioMedNet
Provided by Electronic Press

SEARCH, JOURNALS

Address: *http://www.cursci.co.uk/*
Cost: Currently free; registration, cost initiates at the end of 1996.

The London-based BioMedNet is an ambitious "World Wide Club," covering biomedicine and medicine. Its content includes full texts of the biomedical publications from Rapid Science Publishers (such as the *Current Opinion* series); a shopping mall for software, equipment, services, and publications; and Mouse Knockouts, for data on laboratory mice. Discussion groups, meeting rooms, and a job exchange add to the community feel of this interesting service. Ignore the constantly reloading icons and look for this highlight—the search engine explores not only the clinical documents, but also the job exchange, the shopping mall, and the discussion groups. Put in DNA, and you get articles, employment opportunities in Britain, and banter from colleagues. MEDLINE is coming soon. You can search for other members of BioMedNet who might hold interests similar to yours. Special membership is required for libraries.

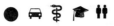

Cyberspace Telemedical Office (CTO)
Provided by Digital Media San Diego

LINKS, SEARCH, MULTILINGUAL

Address: *http://www.telemedical.com*
Cost: No charge; registration, some charges.

The iconographic and screen layouts make it a bit of a challenge to figure out the method behind this site's relative "madness." Professionals, patients, and medical students alike, can, among many other things, create personalized medical records, get drug information, link to clinical trials, search MEDLINE from HealthWorld (http://www.healthworld.com/), find information on diseases, enter a personalized Wellness Center, and consult with an on-line physician. Although CTO seems to be fashioning a novel way to access and gather medical information, it must, in a succinct manner, share with its audience just what it has in mind.

Medconnect–Information Services for the Medical Community
Provided by Medical Network, Inc.

CME

Address: *http://www.medconnect.com*
Cost: No charge for the Case of the Month; fee-based CME subscription services are available.

As part of Medconnect, a fee-based service, this monthly case is presented as a "learn as you go" presentation. Each component of the case presentation is followed by multiple choice questions. At the end of the case scenario, you are invited to share your opinions with colleagues through a built-in message entry window. The well-crafted interface as part of Medconnect provides an excellent educational service. This site offers a superior example of the future of interactive medical education.

Doctor's Home Page
Provided by Gary S. Nace, David P. Heller

LINKS

Address: *http://users.aol.com/drspage*
Cost: No charge.

Physicians, get your bearings here! This site has a compilation of links and other useful resources, including Patient Education Materials on the Web, Medical Sites on the Web (listed by specialty), Medical Humor, ICD-9 (International Classification of Diseases, 9th Revision) and DRG (diagnosis related groups) coding resources, A Collection of Other Doctor's Home Pages, and so on. It also includes a very nice piece on "How to Get Started on the Internet."

HOLA Information System (HETCAT, OnLine Activities)
Provided by South Central Region-University of Texas Health Science Center

LINKS, NEWSLETTERS

Address: *http://macorb.uthscsa.edu/rivas*
Cost: No charge.

Let's all make our Web sites as visually stunning as this one. HETCAT is a program to improve the supply, distribution, quality, and efficiency of health service providers attending Hispanics, especially along the United States-Mexico border. HOLA extends an on-line avenue for that assistance. HOLA offers a great guide to health careers (the information is not geographically limited), including links to continuing education for nurses, dentists, and physicians, and information on funding, research, and scholarships. It provides several publications in full text, including the *HOLA Newsletter,* and provides information about programs that HETCAT has completed and proposed that might be of use to other administrators. Well constructed and executed, this site should be visited by more than just the folks at the University of Texas.

LINKS, SEARCH

Doctor's Guide to the Internet
Provided by PSL Group

Address: *http://www.pslgroup.com/Docguide.htm*
Cost: No charge.

Its purpose is obvious; its content is exemplary. This one is a keeper. The site has a strong showing on medical news, new medical sites issued weekly, information about new drugs, medical conferences, clinics and medical centers, CME events, and a *Doctor's Exchange,* in which professionals from around the world can quibble and kibitz. Top it off with a comprehensive database of medical sites on the Web (although it is not obvious how comprehensive this section is) *and* resources to be recommended to patients, and you have one heck of a Web site. It has its own search engine, as well as links to Excite, Infoseek, McKinley, and AltaVista. It has a feature that other sites would do well to emulate: an icon that links to its sponsors, an understated but effective way to show support. The awards this site has received seem well deserved.

LINKS, JOURNALS, CME

Med Nexus
Provided by Amherst Publications, Affiliated Healthcare Systems

Address: *http://www.mednexus.com*
Cost: No charge; registration.

Med Nexus, "An Internet Medical Community," is a local site (New Hampshire's medical and nursing community) that is hitting the big time. Its on-line journal, *Nexus,* medical news, conference listings, newsletters, and medical forum make for a site that is of more than local interest. Forget the *Open Door* icon; its "Quick Guide" should be right up front, for it links to other Internet medical resources (Medical Link), job opportunities, slide preparation, a speaker's bureau, CME (on the horizon), and local, regional, and national medical organizations, as well as to *Fun Page* and *Politics and Medicine.* It even offers a "real librarian" that will perform searches for reasonable fees. It also offers PaperChase's MEDLINE through a Telnet connection. Add a site-based search engine, a little up-front reorganization, less "scrolling down," and the upcoming content-rich library, and Med Nexus will be a front runner.

SEARCH, JOURNALS, CME

MedScape
Provided by SCP Communications

Address: *http://www.medscape.com*
Cost: No charge; registration.

MedScape, "The Online Resource for Better Patient Care," has approached the environment rather differently than some of the other health care sites. With its daily intellectual tickler (Today's [clinical] Question), tidy layout (in file folder graphics), and specifically constructed Topics (e.g., articles on AIDS, managed care, menopause, and oncology), it has foregone the directory approach and formulated a literature-based service. The full text of numerous journals, an *Exam Room* with PicTours, CME listings, and medical news from *Medical Tribune* rounds out the content. It is short on links to other health care sites, but long on innovative approaches to delivery of health care information. It also offers MedPulse, a weekly e-mail newsletter to registered members. Recently, MedScape added a free MEDLINE service. In addition, they offer an enhanced MEDLINE full-text service, whereby you retrieve the citations that come from a journal that has the entire article on-line. Additionally, MedScape offers a "Go to List of PreConfigured Keyword Searches" option that gives pre-executed searches on large topics, such as AIDS, cancer, and women's health (with subcategories) and returns citations from full-text journals. Although quite innovative in its approach to providing full text and MEDLINE, the addition of the various options discussed in the chapter on Networks, such as MeSH mapping, subheadings, and limiters needs to be addressed.

LINKS

Physicians' Guide to the Internet (PGI)
Provided by Eric Golanty

Address: *http://www.webcom.com/pgi/*
Cost: No charge; registration.

The green balls are soothing, and the content is nicely separated and logically delivered. There are six divisions plus "Etc." What wonderful links the site has; Physician Lifestyle includes jobs and grants, personal finance, and so on. Clinical Practice has HealthGate's (http://www.healthgate.com) MEDLINE, Patient Education, Hospitals on the Web, and more. There is CME, Medical Libraries, FunStuff, and New Physician minutiae, such as how to repay medical school loans. The economical but powerful "Other Medical Internet Gateways," hyperlinks to catalogs like Yahoo!, that in turn hyperlink to the voluminous world of health care resources. The Doctor's Key Club has private forums, discounts on CME tuition, medical books, and MEDLINE searches by a medical librarian. This is a class act.

Miscellaneous

ChronicIllnet
Provided by Viaticus and Caltype Biomedical

LINKS

Address: *http://www.calypte.com/ci_home.html*
Cost: No charge.

The creators of ChronicIllnet (CI) have a particular point of view regarding chronic illness that could make for spirited clinical discussions. CI provides information on chronic diseases such as AIDS, cancer, Persian Gulf War Syndrome, and chronic fatigue syndrome. *Online News,* written by two correspondents who report on clinical, governmental, and social aspects of the afore-mentioned illnesses, is an innovative approach to providing current information. A *Science Reading Room* gives both an independent comment and the original abstract of seminal clinical articles and *Stories from the Frontline* chronicles individual battles with chronic illness. The Research Bulletin Board lists the requests of people seeking information on chronic illness. Even more content (bibliographies and full text of articles, for instance) on the particular diseases would be welcomed.

Health Database Sampler
Provided by Information Access Company

Address: *http://www.iacnet.com/health/welcome.htm*
Cost: No charge.

A limited but useful resource, this database of pamphlets published by a variety of organiza-tions and associations is linked to a variety of diseases and conditions. There are pamphlets on everything from backache to gallstones. There is a browsable alphabetical list of topics or a table of contents designed to find a subject of interest. The full text of the pamphlet is available; the URL (although it does not hyperlink) for the authoring association is given. If the informa-tion is updated and augmented, it will represent a serviceable encyclopedia for health care pro-fessionals to share with their patients.

The Medical Reporter (TMR)
Provided by Information Access Company

LINKS

Address: *http://www.dash.com/netro/nwx/tmr/tmr.html*
Cost: No charge.

Monthly "issues" of *The Medical Reporter* (an exclusively Cyberspace publication) contain med-ically-related articles emphasizing preventive medicine, primary care, and patient advocacy. It also includes new treatments in medicine. The list of links is eclectic and quite thorough. If it has hit the newspapers and TV, there will likely be a story in the TMR.

Online Health Network
Provided by IVI Publishing

Address: *http://healthnet.ivi.com*
Cost: No charge.

The *Mayo Clinic Health Letter* from the Mayo Foundation is a well-written, well-received print publication. That newsletter and its on-line cousin, the *Mayo Online Health Magazine* (MOHM) furnish the main content of this informative site. The editors provide a Newsstand of "Hot Topics," from the latest treatment of an enlarged prostate to tips on summer-related health issues. Other features include "Housecall," a free monthly e-mail bulletin, hosted conversations with specialists to discuss various clinical issues, and a "Find It" search engine that searches past issues of MOHM, as well as back issues of the *Letter.* It shows the other sites how consumer-based information ought to be presented.

THE HISTORY OF MEDICINE

Introduction

This section represents a bit of a departure from our general discussions of Internet resources. Generally these sites, or the manuscripts, documents, instruments, illustrations, or other information that they "catalog," have been maintained by librarians, historians, archivists, and other information professionals who have for years endeavored to make their collections accessible to researchers. Usually a user must, through a lengthy process, correspond with the institution or travel to the institution to do research. The Internet allows for numerous variations on this theme.

First, institutions (universities, governments, and hospitals) have specified what is in their collections (by name of doctor, disease, or instrument) or articulated which on-line database within their establishment will help you find what you are looking for. This sort of preparatory site (preparing you to know who to ask, where to go, and in what section to find it) is invaluable to the novice or established researcher. The majority of such sites give practical information on the hours that the collections are open to the public, whether you can borrow or photocopy material, and the like.

Second, some institutions or sites actually offer documents on-line. The unusual Florence Nightingale site (see review) is one such example, in which the content could be used by a researcher in a study of 19th century health, economic, and religious concerns.
Third, there are essays or collections that chronicle an exhibit or centennial event (there have been a number lately) of a particular institution or procedure. These often encyclopedic overviews of a subject can be used as illustrations for teaching or as a springboard for further research.

Because our space is limited, we have chosen initially to list the five directories that will most likely lead you to the majority of the sites that have been reviewed or bookmarked. Also, because of the consistently high caliber of most of these sites, the reviews here are representative of the best; the remainder have been bookmarked. You will find some sites referred to within related reviews, so as to capture the diversity of the subject but not review each one in its entirety. These sites will lead you to a copy of the Hippocratic Oath, a 19th century set of trepanning tools, or an essay on the history of radiology. The history of the health sciences has found a vibrant home on the Internet.

Directories

LINKS

History of Biomedicine
Provided by MIC-KIBIC at the Karolinska Institute

Address: *http://www.mic.ki.se/History.html*
Cost: No charge.

Its unadorned table of contents is deceptive. There are 13 categories, from General (which includes museums, libraries, and special collections) to Ancient Egyptian Medicine, to Islamic Medicine, and the simple but enormous, Modern Period, 1601 to the present. In this History of Biomedicine, you choose one of the subjects, such as Early Modern Period, and then you can choose (among some 20-plus sites) to view 23 pages about the Black Death written by a professor at Boise State University. This site is about content (and international content at that). It does not link to the institution that might have the document or information; it links to the information (document, portrait, or collection) itself. Although there is no organization to the inclusion of documents (it is not alphabetical or by specialty, only by time period), it is a browser's dream. First, you can look at a portrait of Paracelsus at the New York Academy of Medicine Library (http://www.nyam.org:80/publish/malloch/paracel.html), then read a piece on Laennec and the stethoscope from the Museum of Beaux Arts in France (www.enst-bretagne.fr:3000/~calais/KEMPER/laennec_E.html), and top it off with information on the Blue Baby Operation (http://www.med.jhu.edu/medarchives/page1.html), which celebrated its 50th anniversary at Johns Hopkins Hospital. It is a powerful example of where this on-line medium can lead you. Bookmark this site and the collections it mentions, you will want to return again and again.

LINKS, SEARCH

MedWeb: History
Provided by Emory University Health Sciences Center Library

Address: *http://www.gen.emory.edu/medweb/medweb.history.html*
Cost: No charge.

MedWeb is fundamentally good at what it does, offering hyperlinks to numerous subject-specific sites. In this case, it is the history of the health sciences. The main title, History, has been delineated into numerous categories, including Bibliographies, Gastroenterology, Lists of Internet Resources, Medical Illustration, Medical Libraries, and so on. The largest area, Sites, is basically a reiteration of all the smaller entries. MedWeb's exceedingly brief or nonexistent annotations do not detract from the wealth of information providers they have gathered. It is a suitable place to commence your search for historical health science information.

Primary Care Internet Guide (PCIG): Medical History
Provided by Department of Public Health and Primary Health Care, University of Bergen, Norway

LINKS, SEARCH

Address: *http://www.uib.no/isf/guide/history.htm*
Cost: No charge.

Augment your MedWeb search with a visit to the PCIG. This Norwegian site has hyperlinks to more libraries and documents, and a few to museums that are absent in MedWeb. No annotations are included.

Some Electronic Resources in History of Science, Medicine and Technology
Provided by Johns Hopkins University, Department of the History of Science, Medicine and Technology

LINKS

Address: *http://www.welch.jhu.edu/history/IOHMelec.html#A1.4*
Cost: No charge.

If you're looking for a little more discussion and a sense of the range of history of medicine collections, try this helpful tome. Embedded in lengthy descriptions are the names of on-line databases, Gophers, Web sites, USENET groups, and the like that are useful to historians and other interested parties. "Published" in September 1995, its content has already been overshadowed by numerous sites, but its basic information remains valid and helpful. A similarly helpful but often dated essay is Peter Hirtle's "Surfing the Internet for the History of Medicine" (gopher://una.hh.lib.umic...sstacks/medhist%3ahirtle) that textually describes the myriad ways to find history of medicine information on the Internet.

WWW Virtual Library: History of Science, Technology and Medicine
Provided by Tim Sherratt, Australian Science Archives Project

LINKS, SEARCH

Address: *http://www.asap.unimelb.edu.au/hstm/hstm_spe.htm*
Cost: No charge.

The Medicine and Health section is just one of many in this exciting "catalog" that includes Biology, Computers, Physics, and Women Scientists. There are no annotations, but the WWW Virtual Library has a number of exhibit and commemorative history of medicine sites not reflected in other directories. Hyperlink to the Museum of Contraception (http:www.salon1999.com/07/features/contra.html), Milestones in Neuroscience Research (http://weber.u.wahington.edu/~chudler/hist.html), or the History of Brain Surgery (http://www.brain-surgery.com/history.html) without ever leaving your keyboard.

Guides

American Association for the History of Nursing
Provided by American Association of the History of Nursing (AAHN)

LINKS

Address: *http://users.aol.com/nsghistory/AAHN.html*
Cost: No charge.

The AAHN is a professional organization open to anyone interested in the history of nursing. Fulfilling its purpose to stimulate interest in the history of nursing, serve as a resource for information related to nursing history, and produce and distribute materials related to the history and heritage of the nursing profession, it has produced a serviceable Web site. It includes a fine bibliography for nursing history, an instructive bibliography for historical methodology, and a useful (but not hyperlinked) group of institutions where you might do research. There are hyperlinks to other Internet resources. The full text of its journal would be a welcome future addition.

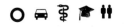

The Bakken Library and Museum
Provided by Eric S. Boyles, The Bakken Library and Museum

LINKS, SEARCH

Address: *http://www.tc.umn.edu/nlhome/m557/rhees001/blm/welcome.html*
Cost: No charge.

The Bakken is one heck of a place to visit, and that can be said of its Web site as well. The museum itself holds a unique collection of 10,000 rare books and 2,000 scientific instruments relating to the historical role of "electricity in life." The site offers the catalog (in chronological or alphabetical order) of thousands of bibliographic descriptions of the books (although not their content—now that would be a researcher's fantasy come true). There is no instrument catalog on-line, but you learn how to find out about the collection. There is information on the museum exhibits, the well-received K-12 educational resources, the medicinal garden, and on and on. Earl E. Bakken was the inventor of the first transistorized cardiac pacemaker. The museum was his vision. This site, like Bakken's instrument, successfully transfers "information" through an electronic source.

Ancient Medicine/Medicina Antiqua
Provided by Lee T. Pearcy, Episcopal Academy, Pennsylvania

LINKS

Address: *http://www.ea.pvt.k12.pa.us/medant/rsrcs.htm*
Cost: No charge.

Contained within this "resource for the study of Greco-Roman Medicine and medical thought from Mycenaean times until the fall of the Roman Empire," is a fine introductory bibliography to Greek and Roman medicine for graduate students. It also includes a gynecology bibliography from the impressive Diotima Project (http://www.uky.edu/ArtsSciences/Classics/gender.html) which is collecting materials on the study of women and gender in the ancient world. Pearcy offers hypertexts to several Hippocratic and Galenic works, reproduces all but the articles from a recent Society for Ancient Medicine Review (which includes lots of news relevant to ancient study), and has a serviceable list of other resources on the Internet.

Caduceus-L: History of the Health Sciences Forum

Provided by Moderator: Inci A. Bowman, The Moody Medical Library, The University of Texas Medical Branch, Galveston

Address: *http://www.utmb.edu/mml/cadu.htm*
Cost: No charge.

"Caduceus-L is a moderated electronic bulletin that provides a forum for exchanging information on any aspect of the history of the health sciences. It includes announcements, inquiries, and discussion on access to historical resources." Send an e-mail to Mailserv@Beach.UTMB.Edu and type in the message line: SUBSCRIBE CADUCEUS-L. It is open to anyone interested in the history of the biomedical sciences and health care. Caduceus-L can also be reached through the History of Medicine section of Medical Matrix (http://www.slackinc.com/matrix/basic/history.html).

Harvey Cushing/John Hay Whitney Medical Library

Provided by Toby A. Appel, Yale Medical Library

LINKS, SEARCH

Address: *http://info.med.yale.edu/library/historical/*
Cost: No charge.

There are many university-related sites that detail their history of medicine collections. Yale's site is straightforward and representative of many such sites like Harvard's Francis A. Countway Library of Medicine (http://www.med.harvard.edu/countway/) and Johns Hopkins' Alan Mason Chesney Medical Archives (http://www.med.jhu.edu/medarchives/overv.htm) where there is useful information in their history of medicine collections. The catalogs of these biographies, rare books, manuscripts, ephemera, artifacts, and the like are not always in on-line databases. They are generally in printed sources, like the National Union Catalog or in university-based systems like Yale's ORBIS and Harvard's HOLLIS. Because of the scope of their collections, these university sites are the perfect purveyors of content-rich Web sites as money and time allow. Yale is expecting the full text of five 17th and 18th century texts (including Nicholas Culpeper's 1652 *The English Physitian*) to be available in the near future. Until such similarly expensive, labor-intensive work is done, get your basic service information through such sites, and then contact or visit the institutions. The Cushing site also has a well-executed Selected Internet Resources, not only for the History of Science, Technology, and Medicine, but also for basic medical Internet Resources.

History of Women & Science, Health, and Technology: A Bibliographic Guide to the Professions and the Disciplines

Provided by Phyllis Holman Weisbard and Rima D. Apple, University of Wisconsin

LINKS, SEARCH

Address: *gopher://gopher.adp.wisc.edu/11/.browse/.METAGLSHW*

Cost: No charge.

This important book in the history of the health sciences has a valuable site for those interested in this subject. The table of contents is as it appears in the published text, but each section (e.g., Women in the Scientific Professions, Health and Biology, Home Economics-Domestic Science) is hyperlinked to the bibliographic journal and book entries (some are briefly annotated, some are not) on that subject. Books for Older Children and Young Adults, and an Author Index are included as well. A search engine allows you to find by entering, for example "breast feeding," a number of articles or texts that include pertinent information. From the seminal 1983 *Power & Profession of Obstetrics* by William R. Avery, to an article on the medicalization of menopause, these sources will stimulate research and discussion.

Michigan Digital Historical Initiative (MDHI)

Provided by University of Michigan-Historical Center for the Health Sciences

LINKS, SEARCH

Address: *http://http2.sils.umich.edu:80/HCHS/*

Cost: No charge.

MDHI illustrates the fortuitous result of a collaboration between a university, a philanthropic organization (W.K. Kellogg Foundation), and technical support from the University of Michigan's School of Information and Library Studies. This Web application contains guides to and access policies for archival, manuscript, and museum materials. It also includes images of documents, photographs, graphic art, exhibits on special topics, and on-line assistance for other repositories and individuals wishing to develop similar projects. Each hyperlink logo (e.g., Guide to Collections, Guide to Artifacts, Guide to Graphic Art) points to alphabetical and subject listings. Having chosen something to view, for example, an amputation scalpel, you see the picture and a description, then have the option of seeing related instruments or related materials. A related instrument was the amputation tenaculum (I, too, had to look it up). MDHI is also developing an index, both in Michigan and nationally, on repositories of historical medical significance. More than just telephone numbers and addresses, it seems that it will directly link you to that institution's archival holdings. Additionally, in a cooperative spirit, MDHI offers tips on how to catalog artifacts, copies of technical guidelines, information about historical and educational

CD-ROM products being developed, and links to additional Internet resources on health sciences and scientific instrumentation. So far, in the "Guide" category, it doesn't get much better than this.

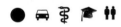

National Library of Medicine-History of Medicine Division
Provided by National Library of Medicine

Address: *http://www.nlm.nih.gov/about_nlm/organization/library_operations/history_of_medi cine/history_of_medicine.html*
Cost: No charge.

The NLM is a likely place to start or at least get consultation on a history of medicine research project. The size and breadth of its collection of books, exhibits, photographs, modern manuscripts, early Western manuscripts, oral histories, audiovisuals, and the like number in the thousands to hundreds of thousands. The items are not cataloged on the Internet. They will be found through NLM's on-line catalog, CATLINE (available through some other Internet sites), RLIN (Research Libraries Group, Inc.), and OCLC (Online Computer Library Center). This site also lists various specialized catalogs that may be useful as you do your research. The site and its content are quite sparse. It is included here because it is mentioned in most history of medicine Internet resources, and because the institution's collections are of such significance in the study of the health sciences.

NLM-Online Images from the History of Medicine
Provided by National Library of Medicine (NLM)

SEARCH

Address: *http://wwwoli.nlm.nih.gov/databases/olihmd/olihmd.html*
Cost: No charge.

Sixty thousand images! These reproduced photographs, artwork, and printed texts are drawn from the extensive (and much larger) collection of the History of Medicine Division at NLM. There are notes about usage and copyright, ordering high-resolution reproductions, technical limitations, and how to best view the illustrations. A search engine allows searching for images using text expressions, like "nurses and operations," or searching for images by frame number (if you have already found it once), or Browsing and retrieving 10 random frames. This is where the photo of Lincoln wearing his hat (viewing the graves of fallen soldiers) resides. Enjoy yourself. You might want to augment NLM's collection with IMMI, The Index of Medieval Medical Images in North America (http://www.mednet.ucla.e…urobio/immi/immihtml.htm). This NLM- and Ahmanson Foundation-supported project (through the on-line service of the Research Libraries Group, Inc., RLIN) describes and indexes the content of all medieval manuscript images (up to the year 1500) with medical components presently held in North American collections.

LINKS

Scientific and Medical Antique Collecting Guide
Provided by Tom E. Jones, Duke University

Address: *http://www.duke.edu/~tj/sci.ant.html*
Cost: No charge.

Collecting is one of the most common avocations among physicians and other health care professionals. This well-organized site will facilitate a broader understanding of the "how-to" aspects of this subject for the novice, as well as for seasoned collectors, dealers, and museum curators. In the Learning About Scientific/Medical Antiques section, there are hyperlinks to reference books, periodicals, organizations and societies, on-line virtual museums, and other Internet resources. Individually, and in their entirety, they produce a good overview on how to learn about and locate that surgical instrument, medical chest, or microscope you have been coveting. Even more pertinent is the Buying and Selling Scientific/Medical Antiques section, which includes such practical contributions as Conservation of Antiquities, on-line catalogs in which you can view and buy items over the Internet, and lists of dealers and markets. The helpful "Beware," gives tips on how you tell authentic instruments and artifacts from modern reproductions. Go out and collect something!

Documents or Exhibits

A Century of Obstetrics
Provided by University of Pennsylvania Medical Center

Address: *http://www.obgyn.upenn.edu/History/Index.html*
Cost: No charge.

The literature that accompanies an exhibit or anniversary celebration is a clever and instructive way to create or augment a Web site. Many such sites exist. "A Century of Obstetrics" is indicative of the various ones that have been bookmarked in this section. Following an introduction, the text covers the period 1890–1930 at the University Maternity Hospital and Maternity Life. There are hyperlinks to pictures of various parts of the hospital and equipment used in the facility. Next are hyperlinks to information on various practitioners (pictures and a short description) affiliated with the center. Finally, the era of Clinical Obstetrics, in the post-WWII era is discussed, with hyperlinks to brief descriptions or pictures on maternal mortality, Sprotte needles, fetal monitors, and the like. Although this sort of project (an exhibit and an initial Web site) does not lend itself to exhaustive information, extensive bibliographies or reprints of original articles would be a nice enhancement in future projects. Adventures With an Ice Pick: A Short History of Lobotomy (http://www.imsa.edu/~silence/lobotomy) and Deja Vu: AIDS in Historical Perspective (http://www.radio.cdc.ca/radio/programs/current/ideas/syphilis.html) are also fascinating sites.

Classic Works in Herbal Medicine
Provided by Southwest School of Botanical Medicine

Address: *http://sunsite.sut.ac.jp/arch/academic/medicine/alternative-healthcare/*
herbal-references/historical-references

Cost: No charge.

Here is a wonderful site—although you must have an Acrobat reader to see the complete work in a few cases. Currently, the site represents the writings of three luminaries in herbal medicine: John Uri Lloyd, Otto Mausert, and Benjamin Colby. The Classic Works hold great promise. Each example has a small biography followed by hyperlinks to some writings (such as Colby's 1848 *Guide to Health*) by the author. As the seemingly unabashed director Michael Moore writes, "These files are taken from the original publications, scanned and OCRed with OmniPage Pro…believe me I wouldn't have bothered if I didn't think they were worth sharing. I will add more as time permits." For anyone with the slightest interest in herbal medicine, sectarian practice, or the history of medical pharmacy, this is the place to watch.

History of Body Donation
Provided by John W. Evans, Willed Body Program, College of Medicine, University of California, Irvine

Address: *http://www.com.uci.edu/~anatomy/willed_body/history.htm*
Cost: No charge.

We applaud the variety on the Internet, especially when it teaches us something new. Here are some things we never knew. This site is one of the winners in the very informal "Unusual Content" category. You can find out all about the Uniform Anatomical Gift Act (how do medical schools get cadavers?), and you can learn about the history of cadaver dissection. Were dead criminals used for anatomical dissection? Is there currently a shortage of bodies for teaching institutions? Wow them at your next soirée or at your next grand rounds with the unusual but necessary details on some basic aspects of body donation.

Plague and Public Health in Renaissance Europe
Provided by Institute for Advanced Technology in the Humanities

Address: *http://jefferson.village.virginia.edu/osheim/intro.html*
Cost: No charge.

What promise this site doth hold. It can be used as a teaching tool, and it can be used as a springboard for further discussion. The Plague and Public Health project "involves the creation of a hypertext archive of narratives, medical consilia, governmental records, religious and spiritual writings and images documenting the arrival, impact and response to the problem of epidemic disease in Western Europe between 1348 and 1530. When completed, researchers will be able to follow themes and issues geographically across Europe in any given time period or chronologically from the first cases of bubonic plague in 1348 to the early sixteenth century." Currently an Introduction; Florence, 1348; Pistoia, 1348; and Lucca, 1348 are available. Completed at the end of 1994, we eagerly await additional text. Three cheers for the developers!

A Selection of Letters Written by Florence Nightingale

Provided by Kelly Brown, University of Kansas Medical Center, Clendening Medical Library

LINKS

Address: *http://www.kumc.edu/service/clendening/florence/florence.html*
Cost: No charge.

It's a Nightingale extravaganza; well, a fete, anyway. The name says it all—it is a very small selection of Nightingale's letters, in her own hand. Summaries of the letters run alongside an alphabetical listing (by recipient) and a chronological listing (both of which provide links to individual letters). Other Florence Nightingale resources in the History of Medicine Library, other Nightingale sites on the Internet, and a word about the recent exhibit are especially informative. How did they get those letters onto the Internet? These are only a pittance of the some 15,000 letters that she wrote, but how lovely that these are here for the reading.

MEDICAL LAW AND ETHICS

MCW Bioethics Database

Provided by Medical College of Wisconsin

LINKS, SEARCH

Address: *http://www.mcw.edu/bioethics/*
Cost: No charge.

Lots of information here! This site has tons of actual *content,* not just links. Although it is not as beautiful as some sites (this one is mostly text), if it is bioethics-related, you will find it at this scholarly site. The site is not difficult to use, but it is geared toward those with some background in bioethics. The MCW database, which alone makes this site worthwhile, consists not only of hundreds of detailed references on any topic, but also abstracts and/or commentaries that accompany each entry! The database includes chapters, books, book reviews, essays, court decisions, journal articles, laws and bills, and newspaper articles. *And,* it is so large that it has its own searchable index complete with a list of suggested key words! In addition to the database, there is information about the Wisconsin Ethics Committee Network and links to other big bioethics Web sites. You will want to become familiar with this one.

DeathNET

Provided by John Hofsess

LINKS

Address: *http://www.islandnet.com/deathnet/*

Cost: No charge.

Whether you agree with the right-to-die movement or not, this excellent site is worth visiting at least once. DeathNET, created by John Hofsess (executive director of The Right to Die Society of Canada) in collaboration with Derek Humphry (founder of the National Hemlock Society), is the definitive Internet resource on the issues of physician-assisted suicide and euthanasia and will instantly put your finger on the pulse of some of the most controversial subjects the medical field has seen in a long time. Topics available include ERGO! (Euthanasia and Research and Guidance Organization), the Senate Special Committee on Euthanasia and Assisted Suicide, and an extensive LAST RIGHTS Online library providing a listing of approximately 200 scholarly articles on physician-assisted suicide and euthanasia, as well as on-line newsletters and mailing lists. Although right-to-die issues dominate the site, the "Living Will" resources are worthy of mention, too. Great looking and well-organized, the site also provides numerous links.

MacLean Center for Clinical Medical Ethics

Provided by University of Chicago

LINKS, SEARCH

Address: *http://ccme-mac4.bsd.uchicago.edu/CCMEHomePage.html*

Cost: No charge.

The University of Chicago's MacLean Center for Clinical Medical Ethics, one of the most highly regarded ethics centers in the country, provides a wealth of information at its site. Although the site offers interesting information about the MacLean Center and its faculty, the real treat of this site is the *massive* listings of links it provides. The list of links is so comprehensive and well organized that it is an excellent place to begin when doing a search on any given topic in the area of medical ethics or health care law—especially for those who may not know where else to begin. Information is categorized in six major search areas: Bioethics Resources, End of Life Issues, Medical Resources, Law Resources, Health Care Reform, or Plague Sites. Under each of these headings, topics are extensively broken down. It is one of the most fun and easy sites to browse, yet it is quite sophisticated and scholarly. This site is superb.

Hooper's Forensic Psychiatry Resource Page

Provided by University of Alabama and Alabama Department of Mental Health and Mental Retardation

LINKS

Address: *http://ua1vm.ua.edu:80/~jhooper/*

Cost: No charge.

James F. Hooper, M.D., F.A.P.A., designed this site as "a place to start" for psychiatrists and attorneys looking for information on legal issues in psychiatry. Although some sections are hard to read because of the color schemes, the sections on Landmark Cases in Mental Health Law and U.S. Supreme Court Rulings Re: Mental Illness are an excellent resource. Dozens of famous and landmark cases are cited along with brief descriptions of each case. Other sections, not meant to be too scholarly, covering the insanity defense and incompetence might be of interest to beginners or the layperson. An interesting and fun site to browse.

Ethics in Science

Provided by Virginia Polytechnic Institute and State University, Department of Chemistry

LINKS, SEARCH

Address: *http://www.chem.vt.edu/ethics/ethics.html*
Cost: No charge.

This site is easy to use, covers what it is supposed to (ethics in science), and does it well. Although many aspects of this large topic are touched on, the emphasis is on *research* ethics in science. There is an extensive bibliography divided by type of science (e.g., human genome or engineering) and more general topics (e.g., plagiarism or science and our government), a list of links to other science ethics resources on the Net, and several general essays on the topic.

Shape Your Health Care Future with HEALTH CARE ADVANCE DIRECTIVES

Provided by American Association of Retired Persons, the American Bar Association Commission on Legal Problems of the Elderly, and the American Medical Association.

Address: *http://www.ama-assn.org/public/booklets/livgwill.htm*
Cost: No charge.

An *advance directive* is "…a document in which you give instructions about your health care if, in the future, you cannot speak for yourself." Although many people are aware of these documents, it is difficult to find easy-to-understand, accurate material describing them. Fortunately, the American Association of Retired Persons, the American Bar Association, and the American Medical Association provide an excellent resource on the subject. Their site provides basic "how-to" information, examples of advance directives, and clear and straightforward answers to commonly asked questions. This is a great site for any physician or patient interested in practical advice on this topic.

MEDICAL EDUCATION

MedWorld

Provided by Stanford Medical Alumni Association

Address: *http://www-med.stanford.edu/MedSchool/MedWorld/*
Cost: No charge.

Here's a real smorgasbord for medical students and for physicians who wish they still were medical students. This home page from a prestigious medical school has something for everybody—

ethics, humor, drama, and links to many other medical Web sites. Navigation is very easy with one click taking you to areas such as DocTalk, articles, fiction, research, and many more. If you're looking for a medical Web page that makes you feel like you are in a high-tech medical school of the future, this could be the one for you.

The Virtual Medical Student Lounge

Provided by Sween

LINKS

Address: *http://falcon.cc.ukans.edu.80/~nsween*

Cost: No charge.

A really cool page designed for medical students or pre-medical students. Everything from how to apply to how to survive medical school is here. Fun and education are mixed well. A strong point is the heavy career guidance, an area often neglected in medical school. For those struggling with a large debt, there is even financial aid information. Visually, the site is appealing, and it does a nice job of looking forward into residency. It has many opportunities to jump in and get involved.

MEd Guide

Provided by Martin Plattner

LINKS, JOURNALS

Address: *http://kernighan.imc.akh-wien.ac.at/stz/plattner/medallg.htm*

Cost: No charge.

This link page is encyclopedic in scope and general in its presentation. Anything you ever want for postgraduate medical education and on-line libraries can be found here. The site is useful but not terribly exciting. Large amounts of information are there, but visually they are not too impressive. This is a guide to medical education and related resources, such as libraries on the Internet. It offers links to medical specialties, medical education information, medical resource guides and indices, software information and file transfer protocol (FTP) archives, medical newsgroups, medical discussion forums, medical electronic journals, libraries on the Internet from all over the world, and information on universities, medical schools, and medical data banks. It is a good site if you want to find information, but you may not enjoy browsing unless you like to read catalogs.

Medical Education Page

Provided by Gregory Allen

Address: *http://www.scomm.net/~greg/med-ed/*

Cost: No charge.

A second year medical student has attempted to provide medical education resources to the masses in this site. The graphics are nice, the communication is friendly, and the resources are diverse and worldwide. The presentation may be incomplete and amateurish, but there is a lot of information here, and you can have some fun exploring.

Center for Advanced Instructional Media
Provided by Yale University

JOURNALS

Address: *http://info.med.yale.edu:80/caim/*
Cost: No charge.

This site is a rich repository of visual software in cardiology, human anatomy, nuclear medicine, avian anatomy, and other biomedical topics and a clearinghouse for available software, current research, publications, and a gallery of images. Much of the software comes from the Mosby-Year Book catalogue of CD-ROMS and other publications. The work of the Yale University Center for Advanced Instructional Media is highlighted. If you want medical images, this is a good source.

Radiology for Medical Students
Provided by Thomas Jefferson University

Address: *http://jeffline.tju.edu/CWIS/OAC/anatomy/Radiology/INDEX.HTML*
Cost: No charge.

A basic on-line introductory course on radiology geared toward the medical student (specifically designed for Thomas Jefferson University students, no doubt) can be found at this site. It is well executed and actually kind of cute. The information is not comprehensive, but it is only meant to be an introductory course.

Chapter 6: Rheumatology/Orthopedics
Provided by University of Iowa

Address: *http://indy.radiology.uiowa.edu/Providers/ClinRef/FPHandbook/06.html*
Cost: No charge.

This handbook from the Department of Family Practice at the University of Iowa Medical Center covers rheumatology, orthopedics, and musculoskeletal medicine at a level appropriate for medical students and residents. It is in outline form and conveys basic but useful medical information. This may particularly interest third or fourth year medical students, residents in pediatrics, medicine, family practice or orthopedics, or perhaps other health care professionals.

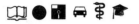

The Internet Pathology Laboratory for Medical Education
Provided by Edward C. Klatt, M.D., University of Utah Health Sciences Center

LINKS

Address: *http://www-medlib.med.utah.edu/WebPath/webpath.html#organ*
Cost: No charge.

An exhaustive file of classic images in pathology covers a wide variety of pathology topics. Images include items in general pathology, organ system pathology, clinical pathology, and diagnostic histopathology techniques. The high-quality images are suitable for teaching medical students, residents, and advanced levels of medical professionals. Images are available on CD-ROM at a reasonable price ($50 U.S. plus shipping and handling). Microscopic photos take a bit longer to load than do the gross photographs, but they are worth the wait.

Other useful items on this Web site include laboratory exercises, more than 1,500 multiple choice pathology questions for self-review, and mini-tutorials.

The laboratory exercises are in a problem-based format and written at the medical student level, but they would be useful for general review by residents of basic topics or for nonpathologists wishing to brush up on general pathology in their organ system of expertise. The examination questions are suited best for individuals preparing for United States Medical Licensing Examination Part I, but again, would be useful for general study at an advanced level. Examination questions are a little slow to load, but the "running tally" of number and percent correct is a handy feature. Mini-tutorials are excellent, but no mention is made of the availability of CME credit. A mirror site is now available at http://telpath2.med.utah.edu/WebPath/web path.html.

PROFESSIONAL ASSOCIATIONS AND SOCIETIES

JOURNALS

American College of Cardiology Home Page
Provided by the American College of Cardiology

Address: *http://www.acc.org/*
Cost: No charge.

This site is filled with excellent information for individuals dealing with diseases of the heart. The college presents an array of choices that range from training statements, practice guidelines, and position statements to a list of self-study publications, practice management techniques, and patient education tips. This site even offered visitors up-to-the-minute, on-line information straight from the annual meeting in March. Also worth checking out on this site is the on-line version of the *Journal of the American College of Cardiology.*

LINKS, JOURNALS

The American Academy of Dermatology
Provided by The American Academy of Dermatology (AAD)

Address: *http://www.aad.org*
Cost: No charge.

The *big kahuna* of dermatology Net sites! This site has by far the best and most comprehensive public and patient information. It has an attractive section on skin cancer and sun protection, a skin cancer quiz, and a risk profile that determines your risk for skin cancer based on things like your coloring and history of sun exposure. Quality informational brochures on 25 common skin problems are offered, along with disease-specific support and advocacy group information and links to university dermatology departments around the world. This is a wonderful resource for dermatologists, with its meetings calendar, e-mail list information, the skinny on the considerable CD-ROM products available, and valuable links to organizations such as the Centers for Disease Control and Prevention, the National Institutes of Health, and the National Library of Medicine. Easily accessible information about other dermatologic organizations, the doings of the AAD, upcoming meetings, and a What's New section on updates to the Web site are included here. This site links to valuable sites like the Cutaneous Reaction Database, Resources for laboratory testing available (with search engine), Dermatology Online Journal, Photobiology Online, Project Dermatologic Online Image Atlas, and the Contact Dermatitis Home Page that provides synonyms, uses, cross reactions, and references for a wide variety of contact allergens. This is every dermatologist's most important bookmark! The layout is very attractive.

American Association of Clinical Endocrinologists
Provided by the American Association of Clinical Endocrinologists and the American College of Endocrinology

LINKS, JOURNALS

Address: *http://www.aace.com*
Cost: No charge.

Although this site is designed for the endocrinology professional, it also includes a few features for those with an interest in the specialty. A number of areas on this site are password protected, most notably the "Tech Tips," the "Member Areas," and the "Postings." These areas are designed to appeal only to those people with a vested professional stake in this area. Not protected are clinical guidelines and a corporate sponsor list complete with links to firms with their own Web pages. Also helpful is the order vehicle for audio tapes, a member information guide, and the journal, *The First Messenger,* which can be read entirely on line.

American Gastroenterological Association
Provided by American Gastroenterological Association

LINKS

Address: *http://www.gastro.org*
Cost: No charge.

The physician-oriented home page of the American Gastroenterological Association has outstanding color and graphics and a well-structured menu that is not as helpful as you'd expect when you need to find anything of substance.

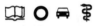

American Association of Immunologists Home Page
Provided by the University of California, San Diego

LINKS, JOURNALS

Address: *http://glamdring.ucsd.edu:80/others/aai*
Cost: No charge.

The site is exemplary as one of the several allergy and immunology professional organizational sites. It is well introduced by Association President Katherine Knight and provides questions and answers to and from immunologists, information about the association, and educational opportunities for immunologists.

The *Journal of Immunology* is one of several journals linked by this page. This site provides tables of contents, abstracts of full-length articles, and information for submissions to the *Journal of Immunology* .

The Questions and Answers section is a subpage where professionals and laypersons can ask questions of association members. Recently posted questions and responses ranged from basic questions to shop talk. A submission form is provided to address questions to the proper individuals and receive responses in an organized fashion.

Subpages include information about recent testimony before Congress, association bylaws, member lists, application information, an on-line newsletter, and a guest book.

Finally, several educational and professional opportunities are found at this site. A list of meetings, classes, courses, on-line journals, faculty and postdoctoral positions, and an "Automatic Grant Generator," as well as links to other biological sites are included.

The American Association of Immunologists Home Page is an excellent resource. This is a site where physicians and scientists may communicate freely about therapeutics and new developments in the field.

Clinical Immunology Society Home Page
Provided by Clinical Immunology Society

LINKS

Address: *http://www.globaldialog.com/~cis*
Cost: No charge.

This relatively young society was founded to promote excellence in the practice of clinical immunology. The site is divided into informational, membership, benefits, and links pages. Here individuals will learn about the society, how to become a member, and why membership is worthwhile. The "Other Links of Interest" page provides eight references to related medical organizations. This site is well organized and easy to navigate and will certainly grow as the society matures.

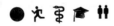

American Academy of Ophthalmology
Provided by American Academy of Ophthalmology

LINKS, SEARCH

Address: *http://www.eyenet.org/*
Cost: No charge.

A site that has it all, from basic information such as "What is an ophthalmologist?" to the latest news in ophthalmology, including U.S. Food and Drug Administration treatment approvals,

Medicare rules and regulations, and even listings of newly opened facilities. One section is devoted to a monthly questions and answer session on current ophthalmology topics. The ophthalmologist can benefit from the on-line forum about recent cases and the biweekly updated clinical pearls. There is also a section listing upcoming CME dates and registration information. This page has received praise from Infoseek and was listed in the top 5% of Web sites by Lycos. Filled with outstanding photos and graphics, this is definitely a site you do not want to miss. Included is a link to various search engines allowing access to virtually all sites devoted to ophthalmology. What more could you ask from the American Academy of Ophthalmology?

LINKS, JOURNALS

American Association for Pediatric Ophthalmology and Strabismus
Provided by American Association for Pediatric Ophthalmology and Strabismus

Address: *http://med-aapos.bu.edu/*
Cost: No charge.

It's simple but inviting; a well-organized site with many resources, including a collection of publications, a computer strabismus model, handouts for patients, a free MEDLINE link, and a place for e-mail feedback. The user-friendly layout makes for an easy informative session.

LINKS, SEARCH, CME, SPANISH

American Academy of Orthopaedic Surgeons On-Line System
Provided by the AAOS

Address: *http://www.aaos.org/*
Cost: No charge.

This site offers the "surfer" a plethora of information. It is designed to be a professional page, but the environment is as informative for patients as it is for physicians. The AAOS provides numerous fact sheets and brochures categorized by sport and injury. There is even a brochure on cast care offered in Spanish. For the professional, on-line member services are provided for use and convenience. Also provided are position and advisory statements, CME courses, research activities, discussion groups, annual meeting information, news releases, and international news. There is even a separate health policy page offering connections to the Health Care Financing Administration and the Social Security Administration. Also of note are the resource center, where anything from publications to self-study guides can be ordered, and the Orthopaedic Yellow pages, where you can search by company or product index code. This page is frequently updated, and to provide a responsive site, the AAOS incorporates an on-line survey for all visitors. This site definitely deserves a visit, but be careful, you may stay there awhile!

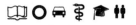

LINKS, JOURNALS, SPANISH

Association for Research in Otolaryngology
Provided by ARO

Address: *http://www.aro.org/showcase/aro/*
Cost: No charge.

If you want otolaryngology research happenings, this is the place. The site includes lists of current members of ARO, "what's new," abstracts, and various journal reproductions (some in Spanish). The *Virtual Library* covers many Internet sites relating to otolaryngology, including the home pages of some universities. The site is heavy in otology and neuro-otology at the expense of other otolaryngology topics. A strong point of this site is its frequent updates, often within a day or two. Video tapes are available on various issues. Most of these are at the professional level; however, some, such as "Passive Smoke," are public issues.

This site is a fine source to help those waiting for publication as well as those vying for research grants. It will predominantly be used by the serious otologic researcher.

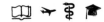

JOURNALS, CME, SPANISH

ICPS Home Page
Provided by International College of Physicians and Surgeons

Address: *http://www.users.interport.net/~icps*
Cost: No charge.

This site provides resources for Hispanic physicians practicing in the United States. It includes lots of facts and reports and the Centers for Disease Control and Prevention immunization module for CME credit.

American Pain Society
Provided by American Pain Society

Address: *http://cedar.cic.net/~aps/*
Cost: No charge.

APS is a chapter of the International Association for the Study of Pain, and this Web site will be most useful for members. The index to APS Bulletin is included and could be useful to non-members.

LINKS

International Association for the Study of Pain
Provided by International Association for the Study of Pain

Address: *http://weber.u.washington.edu/~crc/IASP.html*
Cost: No charge.

The most comprehensive of all pain sites meets the needs of members and non-members. The purposes of this Web site are to introduce health care professionals and scientists to IASP, to provide services to members, to increase awareness of the importance of pain to multidisciplinary inquiry, to communicate the importance of pain prevention and relief, and to extend the educational outreach of IASP. In addition to the typical organization of site information such as officers and calendar of meetings, this site has placed several reports of task forces on-line. For instance, there are two sets of guidelines on pain research with animals and humans. The purpose and an outline for each of five sets of core curricula in medicine, nursing, dentistry, pharmacy, and occupational and physical therapy are included and available from IASP. An annotated list of additional resources is included, as well as books available from IASP.

This site provides a moderate amount of information that could be useful to nonmembers. There are several interesting links. One includes a list of other Web sites of interest to pain researchers and clinicians. Another is a discussion group for oncology pain that is very active. A sample copy of the journal *PAIN* is available through registration on-line , as are authors guidelines.

American Academy of Pediatrics
Provided by The American Academy of Pediatrics

LINKS, JOURNALS

Address: *http://www.aap.org*
Cost: No charge.

Over time this site has evolved into a very professional on-line presence for the Academy. The home page is succinct, with links to information about the Academy and its membership. Links to resources for physicians and parents are under development. Notable is an excellent schedule of immunizations suitable for distribution to parents. Excerpts from recent issues of *Pediatrics* are available, as is the front cover of the publication. Links to the more notable Internet resources in pediatrics (some of which are profiled here) are provided. Although electronic contact with the academy is limited, pertinent phone numbers and mail addresses are presented.

American Society for Aesthetic Plastic Surgery Home Page
Provided by the American Society for Aesthetic Plastic Surgery

LINKS

Address: *http://surgery.org/*
Cost: No charge.

Most likely this will be the page that die-hard "surfers" will look to for information about plastic surgery. This patient-oriented page comes complete with all the basic information a patient wants when contemplating image-enhancing surgery. This page provides an introduction to plastic surgery, things to consider when choosing a qualified surgeon, and what the visitor should know before deciding on surgery. The explanations of the surgical procedures are detailed and enhanced with effective illustrations. Visitors are presented with three main reasons for surgery: minimizing effects on aging, redefining facial features, and body contouring. They are then invited to choose specific procedures, such as liposuction and blepharoplasty, for more details. This site is worth a visit, as many patients may arrive in your office with this information in tow.

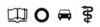

LINKS, SEARCH, SPANISH

American Academy of Child & Adolescent Psychiatry
Provided by American Academy of Child & Adolescent Psychiatry

Address: *http://www.aacap.org/web/aacap*
Cost: No charge.

This is a guild page, but much more than just an ego trip or a shill shop. There is an emphasis on the practical, with more than 50 "Facts for Families" (in English, Spanish, or French), a Report Card on the progress of the National Institute of Mental Health with child psychiatry research funding, sample letters to legislators, a glossary of legislative terms, and more.

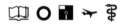

SEARCH, JOURNALS

American College of Radiology
Provided by American College of Radiology (ACR)

Address: *http://www.acr.org/*
Cost: Access to some areas limited to ACR members only.

Useful features include the WWW version of the ACR's Standards and Appropriateness Criteria, its "professional bureau" (i.e., job referral database), an on-line version of the *ACR Resource Guide,* and back issues of the *ACR Bulletin* (all issues from 1995 and 1996, text only with an on-line index). The site is reasonably well organized.

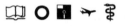

LINKS, SEARCH

RSNA Link
Provided by RSNA (Radiologic Society of North America)

Address: *http://www.rsna.org*
Cost: No charge.

The RSNA site is automatically important to any radiologist because of the status of RSNA as one of the world's premier radiologic organizations, host of the world's largest annual radiology convention, and publisher of *Radiology* (descriptively known as "The Gray Journal"), the most prestigious radiologic periodical around.

Ignoring status, RSNA Link is a genuinely useful site that can stand on its own merits. It is simple in appearance but thoughtfully organized. It offers useful services such as a good "hot list" of sites and vendors (RSNA Launchpad), detailed information about the annual RSNA convention (including an on-line registration option) and other conventions, a database of funding and grant opportunities, and classified advertisements. There is even talk of allowing submission of presentation abstracts to the convention via the WWW as early as next year.

LINKS, JOURNALS

American College of Rheumatology
Provided by American College of Rheumatology

Address: *http://www.rheumatology.org*
Cost: No charge.

This is the best rheumatology site on the Internet. This should not be surprising, as the ACR is the rheumatologist's professional organization. This site presents considerable organizational information, other rheumatologic information, journal listings, and tables of contents. The site is sufficiently diverse and lists enough other connections so that from here you can find virtually anything available that pertains to rheumatology. While still improving and developing, this is the best available source of rheumatologic information for physicians and nonphysicians.

GOVERNMENT AND INTERNATIONAL SOCIETIES AND AGENCIES

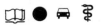

LINKS, SEARCH

Centers for Disease Control and Prevention Home Page
Provided by Centers for Disease Control and Prevention (CDC)

Address: *http://www.cdc.gov*
Cost: No charge.

This is the home page of "The Nation's Prevention Agency"—the Centers for Disease Control and Prevention. Now celebrating its 50th anniversary, this agency has a full-service graphic front page with references to health information, traveler's information, publications and products, data and statistics, training and employment, and other informational topics. This is a major governmental home page with mountains of data and information that is recent and updated regularly. Subscriptions, search engines, and links to other major sites complete the CDC home page as an excellent reference for health care providers and patients alike.

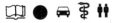

LINKS, SEARCH, MULTILINGUAL

Food and Drug Administration Home Page
Provided by United States Food and Drug Administration (FDA)

Address: *http://www.fda.gov*
Cost: No charge.

The FDA home page introduces the government consumer protection agency, which is concerned with quality assurance for consumables ranging from cosmetics to animal feeds. Subpages for each of the item classes are enhanced with savvy java scripting and colorful graphics. The site provides multilingual support and information for special audiences such as teens and health professionals. This is an excellent example of governmental success in multimedia education. The site is recently updated, thorough, and easy to navigate.

LINKS

Health Care Financing Administration
Provided by Health Care Financing Administration (HCFA)

Address: *http://www.hcfa.gov*
Cost: No charge.

This U.S. Department of Health and Human Services' branch is well known for its administration of Medicare and Medicaid support for some 40 million Americans. The front page of this site is literally and figuratively just the beginning. It boasts an attractive aerial view of the Baltimore location and a map to main subpages including *Information, Medicare, Medicaid, Press Information, Statistics and Data, Research, Regulations,* and *Government Services.* In addition, links to common forms, newly posted information, and customer service are provided.

The HCFA home page provides a simple, easy-to-use format with mountains of information for health care surfers. Although somewhat bland and "texty" beyond the initial home page, subpages are loaded with documents—which the HCFA is famous for. If you need the information, it is here somewhere!

The subpage of PUFs (public use data files) is particularly strong. Here, anyone can download documents that outline current and proposed payment rates and institutional provider information. Among the documents are the latest ICD-9-CM major diagnostic category (International Classification of Diseases, 9th Revision, Clinical Modification) and DRG (diagnosis related group) classifications.

This site is a winner as a resource for Internet surfers. Office staff and patients alike will certainly take interest in this site in future years as funding becomes more scarce and snail mail becomes less tolerable. Many will be happy to have quick access to this resource, its documents, and its support.

Health Volunteers Overseas
Provided by Health Volunteers Overseas

Address: *http://www.cybertech-mall.com/hvo1.html*
Cost: No charge.

This nonprofit organization provides education and relief to many people in different countries. The page is mainly text-based and informative about the organization, its goals, how to join, and, most important, how to finance the experience. This is a solid site with very good information to offer interested individuals. It is an excellent example of the power of on-line documents. No doubt this is an effective and inexpensive way for the organization to reach potential volunteers throughout the world.

International Service Agencies
Provided by International Service Agencies (ISA)

LINKS

Address: *http://www.charity.org*
Cost: No charge.

The home page of some 55 member agencies of the ISA. The home page is just the beginning! Within, individuals will find agencies with concerns ranging from medical care to education. Major programs such as CARE and UNICEF are found within along with mission statements and contact information. An excellent subreferencing system is included in these pages to assist with locating related agencies. This is a strong site with one-stop information about nearly every major service organization.

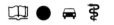

National Academy of Sciences Institute of Medicine Home Page
Provided by Institute of Medicine (IOM)

LINKS, SEARCH

Address: *http://www2.nas.edu/iom*
Cost: No charge.

This government agency aims to provide academic support for national and world health concerns. Most interesting is this page's section on recently released reports. Here, hard-bound versions of IOM documents can be ordered directly or summaries may be browsed on-line. Through this site, IOM members and laypersons may keep abreast of the Institute's latest news. Finally, a database search engine and links to other governmental agencies are provided. This a solid reference that is informative and easy to navigate.

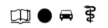

National Institutes of Health Home Page
Provided by National Institutes of Health (NIH)

LINKS

Address: *http://www.nih.gov*
Cost: No charge.

The front page is an excellent map leading to six main categories: *Welcome, News and Events, Health Information, Grants and Contracts, Scientific Resources,* and *Institutes and Offices.* Below the map there are graphics and descriptions of each of the categories.

The first two sections are excellent and provide general information about the Institutes themselves. Maps, personnel, recent activities, and employment information are among the lists. Subpages are well organized and easy to navigate. The next three sections are broad and thorough in their description of data and resources for scientists. The *Health Information* section is especially interesting because it provides links to other major health organizations, access to data from ongoing NIH studies, and practice guidelines for clinicians. The final section provides links to each of the individual Institute's home pages. Here individuals can delve into areas of interest to find yet more data and contacts. Surfing the NIH merely begins here!

This is a major site for health care workers as they look to one of the leading supporters of academic activity in the United States. Finding this government Web site to be fast, free of bureaucracy, and packed with information is a pleasant surprise.

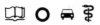

LINKS, SEARCH

Department of Health and Human Services Home Page
Provided by U.S. Department of Health and Human Services

Address: *http://www.os.dhhs.gov*
Cost: No charge.

The eye-pleasing wallpaper and navigational map of this home page lead to links about the Department and its agencies. Founded mainly to provide aid to those who cannot help themselves, this home page educates surfers about the government's resources allocated to this cause. Sections on consumer policy and employer information provide many of the facts, and search and "what's new" pages allow news to be located easily. The site is fast and easy to navigate.

LINKS

The USDOL OSHA Home Page
Provided by the U.S. Department of Labor, Occupational Safety and Health Administration

Address: *http://www.osha.gov*
Cost: No charge.

This agency, concerned mainly with protection of America's workers, set and maintain standards by providing consultation and technical assistance programs for businesses. The page opens with a graphic and text-based environment and references subpages about the organization, its offerings, and other related agencies. This solid site has a lot to offer the interested Net surfer. The load time is fast and the site is easy to navigate.

**LINKS, SEARCH,
MULTILINGUAL**

World Health Organization Home Page
Provided by World Health Organization (WHO)

Address: *http://www.who.ch*
Cost: No charge.

The World Health Organization, located in Geneva, Switzerland, supports research and documents epidemiology and etiology of diseases throughout the world. The subpages, 1995 and 1996 World Health Reports, Weekly Epidemiological Records, and WHOSIS (the WHO Statistical Information System) are interesting. A savvy double-window information system including publications, a library, terminology, and translation assistance is also available. This is a major medical site with mountains of information for any interested Web surfers.

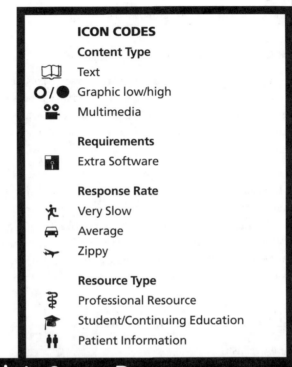

Chapter 10

ICON CODES

Content Type

📖 Text

O / ● Graphic low/high

🎥 Multimedia

Requirements

💾 Extra Software

Response Rate

🏃 Very Slow

🚗 Average

✈ Zippy

Resource Type

⚕ Professional Resource

🎓 Student/Continuing Education

👫 Patient Information

Other Health Care Resources

COMPUSERVE*

ALLIED HEALTH AND NURSING

⚕ 🎓 **UK Professionals Forum**

Keyword: *UKPROF*

Cost: No charge to CompuServe members.

This growing forum contains the only CompuServe hangouts specifically for dentists and pharmacists. A "leading medical journal" apparently listed the health care section as being voted one of the 10 best places on the Internet to discuss medical issues. You will find plenty of conversations in the dental, nursing, pharmacy, and other health-related areas. Not surprisingly, the most common threads center around clinical and technical issues, workplace issues, and improving health care provisions within each specialty.

Note: Premium services are abundant on CompuServe and are indicated on all menus and points of entry by a "$" symbol.

* Subscription and CompuServe software required.

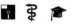

LINKS

Nurse*Forum

Provided by the American Nurses Association (ANA)

Keyword: *NURSE*

Cost: $10/month above usual connect charges.

If you're a nurse using CompuServe, this is the place to be. One of the best ways you can use the Internet is by trading information—and that's what people do here. Topics include job openings, workplace issues, specific procedures and techniques, education and certification, nurses in recovery, legal issues, and home care. For a professional area, the forum has a community feeling.

The libraries present a wide range of information about the ANA and state nurses associations, educational programs (including continuing education), certification dates and registration, and Internet resources and tips. In addition, there are announcements and transcripts from meetings and conferences, calls for papers and study participants, FAQs, a legislative library, catalogs, ANA brochures (plain ASCII text), and editorial guidelines for publications. The new newsletter, *HealthCare Online,* is available but requires Adobe Acrobat. Members are expected to their use real, full names and to create profiles of their professional selves.

GENERAL HEALTH INFORMATION

AMIA/MedSIG

Provided by American Medical Informatics Association (AMIA)

Keyword: *MEDSIG*

Cost: No charge to CompuServe members.

Both the AMIA and this forum center around medical computing, that is, the use of computers in a medical context. It is open to all health care professionals, not just AMIA members. This is a resource for any health care professionals (or students) interested in buying, using, or simply keeping up with related computer developments.

Discussion and library topics cover such computer-related issues as office computing and different kinds of hardware. Health care specialties include mental health, nursing, dental, and pharmacology. Other areas cover the usual health care interests such as policy and legal questions, research and bioethics, international resources, and education and employment.

The sysops recognize that other CompuServe members will ask health-related questions here. They try to confine these questions to a specific, public message area.

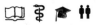

SEARCH, JOURNALS

Comprehensive Core Medical Library (CCML)

Provided by CCML and CD PLUS Technologies

Keyword: *CCML, CCMLAIDS*

Cost: Varies (searches $1 to $3; reprints up to $42).

This database information stretches back to 1982 and includes what was available in the CCML AIDS database. Sources of information include current major medical references and textbooks, plus "prominent general journals" such as the *New England Journal of Medicine, Lancet, Mayo Clinic Proceedings, Science,* and *Nature,* and the annual publication, *Year Book of Infectious Diseases.*

SEARCH, JOURNALS

Health Database Plus (HDB)

Provided by Information Access Company (IA)

Keyword: *HLTDB*

Cost: Varies ($1 to $1.50).

If you want to find information with some depth but that is not extensive, check out this site. Information in this database is divided into two categories, by source. "Health and Fitness Journals" contains the following diverse information from periodicals (updated weekly): articles from journals, reports, and consumer-oriented magazines; abstracts of articles from professional journals such as the *New England Journal of Medicine* and *The Lancet* (full text available only for *Journal of the American Medical Association);* and health-related articles from publications that do not necessarily focus on health.

"Health Reference Books and Pamphlets" contains information from nonmagazine sources: medical reference books, excerpted; and pamphlets and brochures produced by various organizations

Health Database Plus is really a topic-specific part of Magazine Database Plus.

HealthNet

Keyword: *HNT*

Cost: No charge to CompuServe members.

This resource comes in two parts: the HealthNet Reference Library and a Sports Medicine library. Despite the name, these areas are not in the standard forum "library" format. You can click through lists of topics (from general to more specific). The organization is easy to understand but has several layers. When you reach the information, though, the concepts and terms are explained clearly.

The Reference Library contains mainly basic information on major topics within these groups: diseases, symptoms, medication (prescribed, not over-the-counter), home care and first aid, obstetrics and gynecology, and ophthalmology.

The Sports Medicine area focuses on sports-related health information. It begins with a general discussion of exercise and nutrition. It also covers the more common recreational sports: running, swimming, aerobics, racquetball, tennis, and scuba diving.

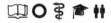

IQuest Medical InfoCenter
Provided by IQuest Medical Infocenter

SEARCH, JOURNALS, MULTILINGUAL

Keyword: *IQUEST*

Cost: Varies (searches $1 to $3, reprints up to $42).

IQuest, gives you access to multiple sources of information. The only drawback is that you must go looking for the single database (of 450) that you want to search. References to "articles, abstracts and citations from thousands of periodicals, newsletters, and newspapers are provided." You can sometimes obtain the full text, rather than a reference or abstract (depending on the database).

The databases are grouped by general subjects: consumer medicine, drugs, medical research, and nursing and allied health. Pricing varies widely among the databases and some are also available elsewhere in CompuServe, under fewer layers of menus.

At press time, IQuest was about to release a Windows-based, stand-alone product. This software will be available in the Reference Library of the Help Forum. On-line help is available from live search specialists by using the SOS command.

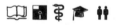

Knowledge Index
Provided jointly with Dialog Information Services, Inc.

SEARCH, JOURNALS, MULTILINGUAL

Keyword: *KI*

Cost: $21/hour above usual connect charges.

Knowledge Index (KI) is another of CompuServe's database of databases (over 100). Many of these contain specific health- and medicine-related information. For example, KI includes the *Merck Index Online,* current biotechnology abstracts (references only), Ageline, and mental health abstracts.

Other databases, which include about 40 newspapers from around the United States, legal resources, and food science and technology abstracts, will contain some health information and are worth using.

You must consider the time of day when using KI, because service is available only during local non–business-day hours (remember, you can check the hours and rates before entering any surcharge area).

KI requires that you use SmartSearch, special software that you can download for free from CompuServe. You can use SmartSearch to set up searches off-line, keeping your KI connect charges to a minimum.

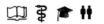

SEARCH, JOURNALS, MULTILINGUAL

PaperChase

Provided by Beth Israel Hospital

Keyword: *PCH*

Cost: $18-24 an hour. Average search about $6.

Accounts available for individuals, institutions, and groups.

PaperChase gives you access to references and abstracts of literally millions of journal articles, proceedings, reports, monographs, and books. You can print or download search results, and PaperChase saves your old search patterns. Other features let you verify references and order photocopies of complete articles (a translation service is available from the photocopy provider).

When you use PaperChase, you are searching four separate databases at once. This scope and efficiency helps offset the extra cost,. It also eliminates duplicate search results for you. PaperChase offers four excellent resources: MEDLINE; Health Planning and Administration (from the American Hospital Association), which contains 675,000 references to topics on the non-clinical side of health care delivery; AIDSLINE, which compiles more than 80,000 references on clinical, research, and health policy related specifically to AIDS; and CANCERLIT (from the National Cancer Institute), the major database for cancer-related resources with almost one million references and abstracts pertaining to cancer and cancer research.

Family Services

Family Services Forum

Keyword: *MYFAMILY*

Cost: No charge to CompuServe members.

Help and support for families is the key here. The focus is on couples starting families, parents and children, and siblings—not extended families. That still leaves plenty to talk about, as daily issues and major traumas affect all nuclear families no matter how well (or poorly) they function.

DISEASES, DISORDERS, AND DISABILITIES

Aging

Retirement Living forum

Keyword: *RETIREMENT*

Cost: No charge to CompuServe members.

This general forum retains good-sized areas for health and medical issues. Library topics are spun toward the elder set and include: general health and medicine, Medicare, nutrition and eating right, caregiving, fitness, and Alzheimer's. In the message areas, "Ask a Pharmacist" is a nifty feature (brought to you by the American Society of Consultant Pharmacist Research Foundation). Most messages elsewhere are socially oriented.

AIDS

LINKS

Pride! Health Forum

Keyword: *PRIDEHEALTH*

Cost: No charge to CompuServe members.

Looking for an area on CompuServe that talks about AIDS, rather than just listing references and abstracted articles? This is it. The list of AIDS-related Web resources is a cool Web page itself and contains dozens of links. The AIDS report covers the International AIDS conferences, complete with abstracts. The AIDS news clipping service works slightly better than Aids News Clips.

The list of general health-related Web links also has good stuff of interest to men and women, gay or not. "Shrink Rap"! features a resident therapist who takes e-mailed questions from forum members and composes replies into periodic mini-essays. Incidentally, the forum is open to all—even straight people. Respect for others is required, however.

Attention Deficit Disorder

MULTILINGUAL

Attention Deficit Disorder Forum

Provided by Thom Hartmann and Mythical Intelligence

Keyword: *ADD*

Cost: No charge to CompuServe members.

The ADD forum is dedicated to anyone interested in attention deficit disorder (ADD), especially adults who have children with ADD/ADHD or who have ADD themselves. Discussion ranges from defining ADD to how to deal with it to where to find more information. "Ask the Doctors" is a public place for questions. The International Library includes files in German, and there is an entire German-language message area.

Cancer

Cancer Forum

Keyword: *CANCER*

Cost: No charge to CompuServe members.

This forum attracts national and international participants. Various kinds of cancer, sorted by cancer type, draw the most attention. Other issues discussed are insurance and bereavement. The Coffee Shop is very popular. Research information is not available.

Physicians Data Query
Provided by National Cancer Institute (NCI)

SEARCH

Keyword: *PDQ*
Cost: Varies ($1 to $10).

A database with extensive information on cancer comprises four parts at this site. The Consumer Cancer Information File describes over 80 types of cancer for the layperson, from prognoses to treatment. The Professional Cancer Information File targets care providers, covering prognoses, stage, classes, and treatment. Bibliographies of additional information are also available. The Directory File lists basic contact information in two directories: one for individual cancer specialists and one for organizations with NCI cancer centers or approved programs. The Protocol File contains detailed information on approximately 1,000 treatment protocols for cancer. Information includes study providers (including the contact person).

Chronic Illness

Chronic Illness Forum

Keyword: *CIFORUM*
Cost: No charge to CompuServe members.

Weeks after opening in the spring of 1996, this forum boasted of having thousands of postings. It has a medical consulting staff that tries to check the validity of medical information, but of course they must disclaim any guarantee. The forum offers a private area (sysop permission required) for well friends, relatives , and caregivers of chronically ill people. Another private area (CV/resume required) is just for M.D.s and D.O.s. Both messages and libraries are grouped by illness or issue, for example CFS/CFIDS/ME and insurance.

Disabilities

Handicapped Users' Database
Provided by the Veterans Administration (VA)

SEARCH, JOURNALS

Keyword: *HANDICAPPED*
Cost: No charge to CompuServe members.

You can find hundreds of items on rehabilitation research and technologies here. The audience is people of all ages with disabilities, and their families and friends. The information covers such practical topics as work and housing, scientific topics, and computer access and technology (equipment and software).

Information is presented in subdirectories: lists of organizations, software and hardware reviews, a reference library, news items, and the IBM Special Needs exchange. Disabilities discussed include hearing, sight, speech, mental, learning, mobility and motor, developmental, brain injury, and epilepsy and other illnesses. Articles are available from the *Disability Rag* and *The Catalyst,* plus *The Journal of Rehabilitation Research and Development.*

Health and Fitness

Health & Fitness Forum

Keyword: *GOODHEALTH*
Cost: No charge to CompuServe members.

Here's a meeting place for people interested in various aspects of health and fitness. Some topics overlap with other forums, such as migraines—indeed, the Weight Management Forum (GO GOODDIET) grew out of one of this forum's most active areas. Less common yet interesting areas include martial arts, skating, and nutrition. Running and mental health are among the most popular topics.

Migraine

Migraine Forum

Keyword: *MIGRAINE*
Cost: No charge to CompuServe members.

People who have headaches can trade information, resources, and stories. Discussions cover the different kinds of headaches, why you get them, how to prevent and get rid of them, and where to find help. Regular open conferences provide real-time conversations, with transcripts available afterward.

Rare Disorders

National Organization for Rare Disorders (NORD)
Provided by the National Organization for Rare Disorders (NORD)

SEARCH, JOURNALS

Keyword: *NORD*
Cost: No charge to CompuServe members.

If you are interested in information about an "orphan" disease, you probably already know about NORD. Orphan diseases strike comparatively few people and therefore attract significantly less research and attention than more common ones. NORD aims to fulfill its stated missions of education (professionals and patients alike), service, and the support of research of orphaned diseases.

Here you can find out about NORD and how it works; look through the Rare Diseases Database for descriptions of the diseases and their symptoms, causes, and treatment; read newsletters from voluntary health agencies centered around specific or groups of orphan diseases; read articles on prevalent health issues from such government agencies as the National Institutes of Health, the Centers for Disease Control and Prevention, and the Food and Drug Administration; search the Orphan Drug Database for information on medications pronounced orphans by the FDA; or sign up for the NORD networking program, for those afflicted by a disorder (and their families) to mutually support one another.

Sexuality

 ### Human Sexuality Database and Forum

SEARCH, JOURNALS   **Keyword:** *HSX100 (open forum), HSX200 (adults only); HSXTOP (Databank), HSXKEY (keyword search of Databank)*
Cost: No charge to CompuServe members.

All aspects of human sexuality are addressed in this database and forum. The forum covers questions and answers, networking, support, and the like. This can mean anything from "Does my body look normal?" to talking with children about sex and sexuality, to age-related questions (for both younger and older persons). Daily conferences provide frequent real-time conversations and contact with other forum members.

The Databank archive includes articles, Q&A transcripts, manuals, and interviews. Also included are a dictionary of terms, a private Q&A hotline, an FAQ list, and AASECT information and member directory.

To maintain a comfortable atmosphere, the forum has strict rules regarding conduct to help ensure that everyone remains polite and respects one another. It seems to work.

Women's Health

Women's Wire/Health & Fitness area

Keyword: *WOMEN, WWFORUM*
Cost: No charge to CompuServe members.

Women's Wire focuses on topics directly related to and those often of interest to women. The Health & Fitness Department covers women's health, for example, reproductive health; health problems noted for affecting women, such as depression and heart disease; and more general topics, such as fitness.

You can find information in the form of articles, brochures, reports, and fact sheets. Sources are always credited, and no one is shy about pointers to more information—look especially for the resource lists in the Health News & Referrals section.

The Women's Wire Live forum sets up conferences, special guests, and topical discussions centered around monthly themes.

Agencies and Associations

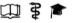

National Technical Information Service (NTIS)
Provided by the U.S. Department of Commerce

SEARCH

Keyword: *NTIS*
Cost: Varies (searches $1 to $3).

Use this database to look for reports on government-funded research, development, and engineering. Once you find a reference, you can usually view an abstract or even order the report from the NTIS. Additional help is available by using SOS to contact a search specialist (that is, a real live person) on-line.

PsycINFO
Provided by American Psychological Association (APA)

SEARCH, JOURNALS, MULTILINGUAL

Keyword: *PSYCINFO*
Cost: $1/search.

PsycINFO contains abstracted articles in psychology and the behavioral sciences. (You can order reprints.) In addition to the fields themselves, PsycINFO also touches on issues surrounding the raw data and theories, including such topics as social issues and education. Because the sources come from all over the world, you can find references to articles in various major languages.

Other CompuServe Resources		
Site Name	Keyword	What You Will Find
AARP	AARP	For members of American Association of Retired Persons (AARP)
A.D.A.M. Software	CDVENA	CD-ROM software you can order to help learn anatomy
AIDS News Clips	AIDSNEWS	CompuServe's own culling of the news services, getting stories that contain the word "AIDS" (so it includes some stories on "study aids" and other unrelated topics
Ample Living	AMPLE	Libraries include health, medical, and diet items
Chronic Hepatitis Forum	HEPA	For those with chronic hepatitis and other hepatic illnesses; refers to other Internet resources
Consumer Reports	CONSUMER	Reports ratings, and consumer information from the Consumers Union, especially for CompuServe
Consumer Reports Drug Refernce	DRUGS	Strictly for patients, this is a good place to start learning about the more common categories of over-the-counter drugs
Diabetes Forum	DIABETES	Very active forum with news, discussion, and support for those with diabetes and related disorders; also now on the Web
Disabilities Forum	DISABILITIES	All kinds of disabilities and resultant issues, including chronic pain, mobility, mental health, "comfort zone," and a new "mall"
Government Publications Online	GPO	Catalog of selection of governmental publications (mainly business oriented, e.g., OSHA); consumer information on food and nutrition

Other CompuServe Resources (cont'd)

Site Name	Keyword	What You Will Find
IBM Clinton Health Care Reform Plan	IBMHEALTH	In IBM's BookManager format, the entire text of President Clinton's 1994 proposed plan
IVI Publishing	CDVENA	Software publisher of CD-ROM titles, including the *Virtual Body, Prime Practice* (with the Mayo Clinic), and *Sign Language for Everyone*
Legal Research Center	LEGALRC	Seven databases, including Child Abuse and Neglect from the U.S. Department of Health and Human Services
Mind/Body Sciences Forum	MIND	How the brain works and affects the rest of the body; includes comparatively cutting-edge, non-Western topics such as smart drugs and neuro-linguistic programming (NLP)
Multiple Sclerosis Forum	MULTSCLER	For patients, friends, and relatives, and caregivers interested in MS and coping with it
Muscular Dystrophy Association Forum	MDAFORUM	Regular conferences, "Ask the Expert" board (Q&A via sysop), and many libraries about MDA, ALS, and surrounding issues
Natural Medicine Forum	HOLISTIC	"Alternative" health and medicine: homeopathy, etc.
New Age A & B Forums	NEWAGEA NEWAGEB	More on non-Western healing and medicine, among other favorite New Age subjects
Public Health Forum	PUBHLTH	Health prevention and promotion, administration, communicy, and news
Publications Online	PUBONL	Subscriptions to newsletters, including *International Health News* (digest of latest medical developments from 45 journals); requires Adobe Acrobat
Safetynet	SAFETYNET	Discussion of safety issues, including occupational health, emergency medical services, training, and associations; mainly for professionals
Syndicated Health Columns	COLUMNS	Her Health, His Health, and The Medical Adviser
Weight Management Forum	GOODDIET	New support and informative area that recently grew out of active discussions in the Health and Fitness Forum
Information USA	LESKO	Explains how and where to get information from the government. Includes Federal Database Finder.

AMERICA ONLINE (AOL)*

GENERAL HEALTH INFORMATION

SEARCH, LINKS, MULTILINGUAL

Better Health & Medical Forum

Provided by the Health ResponseAbility Systems, Inc.

Keyword: *HRS, Better Health, Health Focus*

Cost: No charge to AOL members.

This mega-forum for all other health care areas on AOL was started by two AOL community members. It boasts of having an area for most medical issues, from disease prevention to treatment and support. There is a "Health Professionals Network," more than 50 message centers or bulletin boards, and more than 200 monthly self-help and support group meetings. The area also has numerous links to almost all the major medical Web sites and a front-end for MEDLINE.

---

* Subscription and AOL software required.

Columbia/HCA Live Physician's Chat (America Online)
Provided by the Columbia/HCA Corporation

LINKS

Keyword: *Columbia Net, Columbia/HCA, One Source, Columbianet*
Cost: No charge to AOL members.

Like most other AOL medical areas, this one has an archive of medical and health-related information, complete with a way to search it, and several bulletin boards. What makes this one different is its forums, in which you can ask physicians and medical experts your questions through message posting or in a "live" chat setting. There are also many Web links in this forum, but most lead to sites related to Columbia/HCA and its aims.

Health Channel (America Online)
Provided by America Online

LINKS, SEARCH, JOURNALS

Keyword: *Cancer, Health, Medicine, Health News, Health Live, Health Reference, Health Web*
Cost: No charge to AOL members.

This umbrella forum features jumps to other AOL health and medical forums. There are links to health magazines, reference works, like an on-line medical dictionary, other medical forums, live programs and chats. It usually takes three or more clicks to find the forum you want from the AOL Health Channel; use it when you are exploring or just plain lost.

MEDLINE (America Online)
Provided by the Health ResponseAbility Systems, Inc.

LINKS, SEARCH

Keyword: *Medline*
Cost: No charge to AOL members.

From this single AOL screen, you can search the MEDLINE database three different ways: standard, advanced, and by using InfoStar. Remember, however, that the single button simplicity of this screen belies the fact that you must have the AOL Browser working to access the screens where you construct your search, then wait for the AOL server to submit the search. The results are good; the searches are easy to narrow and control, but there are often long waits for information to appear.

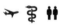

Merriam Webster Medical Dictionary (America Online)
Provided by Merriam Webster

SEARCH

Keyword: *Medical Dictionary*
Cost: No charge to AOL members.

Here is an easy way to look up those strange medical terms you encounter while reading in the AOL medical forums without ever leaving the service. You can enter an entire term or just the part of it you know. The dictionary returns a list of all definitions that contain the term. There are no graphics or links, so response is speedy. Queries, however, must be simple. Only "AND" statements can be used to narrow a search. The search engine only looks for matches in the list of terms, not in each term's definition.

Scientific American Medical Publications (America Online)
Provided by the Scientific American

LINKS, SEARCH, JOURNALS

Keyword: *SA Med (Cancer J Sciam, Cancer Journal for the Cancer Journal)*
Cost: No charge to AOL members.

Scientific American archives three publications in its AOL forum—the monthly *Medicine Bulletin,* the quarterly *Surgical Bulletin,* and the bimonthly *Cancer Journal of the Scientific American.* Not only can you search the back issues of all these publications, but you can also download most articles and any art associated with them. Occasionally, it takes a few more than three clicks and some waiting to find the information you want, but it is usually worth the wait.

DISEASES, DISORDERS, AND DISABILITIES

Cancer

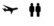

American Cancer Society (America Online)
Provided by the American Cancer Society (ACS) and Health ResponseAbility Systems' Better Health and Medical Forum

LINKS, SEARCH

Keyword: *ACS*
Cost: No charge to AOL members.

This forum features current reference materials from the society about the following subjects: what is cancer and who gets it; risk factors and prevention; early detection; types of cancer; research highlights; and smoking and tobacco.

Most information is aimed at patients and their families who need information after receiving a cancer diagnosis. There are plenty of referrals to organizations for cancer patients and off-line ACS services, as well as notes about ACS fundraising and cancer awareness activities. From this forum you can enter chat areas, link to the ACS Web site, and search all the reference information in the ACS archive by keyword.

Avon's Breast Cancer Awareness Crusade (America Online)

Provided by a collaboration between Avon's Breast Cancer Awareness Crusade and its partners, NABCO (National Association of Breast Cancer Organizations), the YWCA, NCI (National Cancer Institute), and the CDC (Centers for Disease Control and Prevention) as well as Woman's Day Online

LINKS

Keyword: *Crusade*

Cost: No charge to AOL members.

Avon devotes a portion of its presence on AOL to its crusade for greater breast cancer awareness. This forum hosts a message center where breast cancer survivors, family, and friends can trade information and support. It also is home to an information center, with current information about breast cancer screening and treatment and general information about Avon's crusade.

Bernie Siegel Online (America Online)

Provided by Bernie Siegel and other exceptional people

Keyword: *Bernie*

Cost: No charge to AOL members.

Bernie Siegel, founder of ECaP (Exceptional Cancer Patients) and author of several books about exceptional living in the face of medical challenges, has a home here. In addition to a mailbox where you can write Bernie, a thought for today, an exceptional story, and question of the week, this site has moderated chat room programs and special message centers.

Diabetes

American Diabetes Association(America Online)

Provided by the American Diabetes Association (ADA) and Health ResponseAbility Systems' Better Health and Medical Forum

SEARCH

Keyword: *DIABETES, AMERICAN DIABETES*

Cost: No charge to AOL members.

This site contains diabetes reference materials about the following subject areas: the disease and patient profiles, medical treatments of diabetes, nutrition and fitness, sex, pregnancy and parenting, living with diabetes, and complications and related concerns.

Because patients with diabetes and their families face living with the continual purchase of such items as insulin, blood glucose monitors, and special medical-identification products, this forum includes a special "Buyer's Guide to Diabetes Supplies." There is also information in the forum about diabetes research, legislation, and advocacy. From this forum you can enter chat areas, read and post messages to diabetes bulletin boards, and search all the reference information in the ADA archive by keyword.

Multiple Sclerosis

Multiple Sclerosis Online (America Online)
Provided by the Health Channel of America Online, Health ResponseAbility Systems (HRS), the National Multiple Sclerosis Society, and Real Living with MS Magazine

LINKS, JOURNALS

Keyword: *Multiple Sclerosis*
Cost: No charge to AOL members.

Through this single AOL keyword, you can access the National Multiple Sclerosis Society Forum, the HRS' MS message center, and *Real Living with MS,* a print publication that maintains an archive and subscription service on AOL. The National Multiple Sclerosis Society Forum addresses the following areas: the disease and patient profiles; signs, symptoms, and diagnosis; research and clinical trials; treatments for MS and its symptoms; rehabilitation and management; unorthodox therapies; book reviews; and updates and what's new? None of these areas are searchable.

Psychiatry and Mental Health

Issues in Mental Health (America Online)
Provided by the Health ResponseAbility Systems, Inc.

Keyword: *IMH, MH*
Cost: No charge to AOL members.

A special forum that houses all the mental health message boards from the Better Health & Medical Forum. These currently include discussion of daily living, relationships, parenting, and attention deficit disorder, among others. There is also a special software library with documents and applications related to mental health that you can download.

Psych Online (America Online)
Provided by Online Psychological Services, Inc.

LINKS

Keyword: *Online Psych, Psych Online*
Cost: No charge to AOL members.

This area has an extensive number of forums, covering everything from attention deficit disorder to suicide prevention. Each of the 20 or more forums has a "What Is It?" section where you can read a brief overview of the psychological issue and a big list of resources, such as books, Internet newsgroups, and Web sites. There are also chat rooms and message centers for psychological topics. This area is large. Most useful information is three or more clicks away and, lamentably, none of the archives are searchable.

Respiratory Disorders

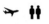

LINKS, SEARCH

American Lung Association (America Online)

Provided by the American Lung Association (ALA) and America Online

Keyword: *ALA*

Cost: No charge to AOL members.

This site contains current reference information for asthma, asthma and children, smoking and tobacco control, lung disease and related disorders, influenza (flu) and pneumonia, environmental health, medical and legislative news, and special events and Programs. The archived information is extensive and includes limited information about equipment used in the diagnosis and treatment of respiratory illness. From this forum you can enter chat rooms, link to lung and respiratory Web sites, and search all the reference information in the ALA archive by keyword.

Appendixes

1. Building a Web Site

2. Internet Providers and
   Obtaining Internet Software

3. Fun Internet Resources

4. Health Care Newsgroups

5. Further Reading

Building a Web Site

Hospitals, medical practices, and health professionals are increasingly establishing a presence on the World Wide Web. Many are flocking to this new self-publishing medium because it is dynamic multimedia and it is quick. Because the World Wide Web is fast becoming the medium of choice for health information, what better way is there to be a part of this burgeoning environment than to create your own Web site?

As the "Wild Wild Web" days give way to the productive development of cyberspace, the experience of early explorers shows us how to build health sites of real value. We can expand on this experience by adding our own contributions and providing value to our communities, both local and global.

DO IT YOURSELF OR OUTSOURCE?

You will need to decide whether to develop the site yourself or to outsource to one of the many Web page design companies. The advantage of outsourcing is that you will get a team experienced in hypertext markup language (HTML), design, and the latest Web technologies. On the other hand, the cost of development will be higher, and you will likely be dependent on them for updates, which may be $50/hour or more.

Software editing programs are available that allow creation of a site without learning the complexities of HTML. Among the programs enticing many to become self-publishers are Adobe PageMill, InContext Spider, HoTMetaL PRO, Quarterdeck WebAuthor, and Netscape Navigator Gold. Many of these companies have their own Web sites containing information about their programs. Visit their sites on the Web and compare.

The advantages of learning to create your own Web page include lower development costs, but more important, the ability to update frequently without an outsource charge. In addition, as these editing programs become more sophisticated, you will be able to create material in Web format directly and bypass the step of using a word processor. Eventually, the experience you gain with your first Web site will allow you to become your own publisher for many of the documents of your organization.

Whether you choose to outsource or to do it yourself, you are responsible for putting together the content. Although Web design services are usually capable, they will not understand as fully as you do, the medical content and the needs of your users. Anyone considering developing a Web site should understand the essential issues to be successful.

TEN STEPS TO A SUCCESSFUL WEB SITE

1. Define Your Mission

The first step to a successful Web site is to define your mission. Why are you building the site? Is your goal to present useful information about your hospital, clinic, practice, service, or laboratory? Or are you developing your own personal page? Are you building a health care information site that organizes available resources in a specific topic area? You will also need to define your audience. Will it be local, regional, global, or a combination?

Once you have determined why and for whom, create a short mission statement such as "to promote my clinic regionally and meet the health information needs of the members in my health plans" or "to provide information about stroke prevention and the services of my neurosurgical practice to the citizens of my state."

If you are creating a Web site for your practice or organization, look at what is currently on the Web. By doing this you will develop a sense of what works and what doesn't. You will get ideas from various sites that you can incorporate into your site. Remember that there is still much left to pioneer, so brainstorm with your colleagues about what may best meet the needs of your audience. If you can, ask your target audience; they may be your friends and neighbors.

If you are creating an information resource that organizes the links on the Web in a certain topic or field, you also must know what has already been developed. You can do this by using search engines for key words or by looking at sites like Yahoo! Health (http://www.yahoo.com/health) that contain large directories of medical sites. If a similar site already has been developed, ask yourself how your site will add value over that site.

Once you have decided on your mission, stay focused. There are thousands of sites out there. A key aspect of survival is to become the best that you can be for your specific mission. If you have another mission, consider creating a second Web site.

2. Select and Register Your Name

Selecting a name is a very important component of your Web presence. It defines your site. Ideally select a simple name, yet one that fits the content of the page. Because the name of your site may be incorporated into your Universal Resource Locator (URL), use a name that is memorable. InterNIC (http://www.internic.net), the domain name registration service, will register names up to 24 characters. If your name is longer, you can use an abbreviation or initials, although these may be more difficult to remember (unless, of course, you are CNN). Keep in mind that your site will be added to search engines, lists, and directories. So, the character of your name alone may determine whether someone comes to visit.

Once you have selected a name, determine whether it is already in use by using the Whois query on InterNIC. You may need to consider several names before finding one that has not been taken. Remember, you can create your own name. Humans have been creating language for thousands of years, and modern times are no exception. If you create your own, make it understandable. Many new names are created using "net," "Web," or "cyber" as prefixes or suffixes. Although many of these types of names are already in use, new root words are being created weekly, so keep an eye on the computer and Internet press for ideas. Because it may take up to 2 months to register your name with InterNIC, do it early. Initial registration is $100, and there is a $50 annual fee.

3. Organize Your Content

Content is the essential core of your site. Without good content, users will lose interest regardless of the graphics. What do you want to include in the site? Look at brochures or other previously developed print material about your organization for ideas; however, avoid simply putting your brochure on-line. Your Web site should be much more than an electronic business card.

As you assimilate your content, you should organize the material into major topic areas. Initially, limit the number of major topic areas to no more than five to seven. Select a name for each topic area and create a sequential list of the topics. These topic headings may become the titles of your individual page and become incorporated in your navigation tools (see No. 5). As it grows, make adjustments as needed, striving for a logical organization of content.

4. Create a Design

A good way to start designing your Web site is to develop your logo. This is an important element because it will not only be on the front page that welcomes your audience, but also on each subsequent page. Unless you have design experience, you may want some professional help with the logo. Together, you can decide on the size and shape of the logo. It should be prominent enough to clearly denote your site, yet not too large as to dominate the rest of the page or take too long to load. Surf the Web for ideas. When selecting the style or color(s) for your logo, you are making a decision that will affect the style and color scheme used for the rest of the site.

A common error seen on Web pages is the lack of a site identifier, such as a logo or the site's name, on each page of the site. The Web is a sharing community, and once your site is placed on a host computer, you have agreed to be linked by others. Indeed, to survive, you will want your site linked to as many other relevant sites as possible. However, those that link to material on your site may link directly to one of your interior pages, bypassing your front page. You should place your logo or your site's name on every page to prevent being unrecognized as the source of your information.

The layout of your pages should be consistent. This will make it easy for the user to understand and navigate your site. If you center your major topic heading on one page, do the same for the remaining pages. Organize your content on each page in as logical and as intuitive a fashion as the material allows. Then you can add graphic elements to best feature your content. The content drives the design, not vice versa. When incorporating graphic elements into your page(s), strive for consistency. Pages with too many different graphic elements, subserving similar functions, are confusing. You can, however, also have fun and bring spirit into the style of your page. The main issue is balance. Most of your graphic elements should be small. Keep in mind that many modems may still be 14.4 bps or less, and even those that are 28.8 bps handle complex graphics slowly. Repeat visitors come to your site for its content, don't let slow-to-load graphics cause them to surf to another site.

The background of your pages should be the same throughout your site unless you have areas of special emphasis. Be careful about using dark or unusual colors. Although this may make your site different from the rest, it can be difficult to read. This does not mean that your site must be dull. Well-placed design elements, small graphics, some open space, and a balance of colors can all give the site an attractive look.

Remember, your front page is your front door. Make it inviting and give your visitors a sense of what is inside. Avoid clutter, yet provide enough information to entice them to enter. Avoid "under construction" signs. It is better to describe your plans for the site; focus on what is coming instead of what is missing.

5. Determine the Navigation Scheme

Although a part of the design, navigation is so important that it should be discussed separately. Easy navigation is the key. Having to search for the pathway that leads to the information desired can be frustrating, and your users may choose a more friendly site. One commonly used and effective mechanism is a navigation bar. This is a series of links to your major topic areas. It should also include a link to your front page. This can be arranged across the top of the page under the logo or be placed vertically along the left or, more commonly, along the right margin. Once visitors have surfed deep into your site, they can easily go back to the front page or any of your topic pages by using the navigation bar. Adding another navigation bar at the bottom of the page allows users that have come to the end of the page an easy path to other pages in your site.

If your site grows to contain many pages, your users will need to dig deeper and deeper into your site to find the information they want. At this point, you may want to consider using an on-site search engine to help them find information quickly. Remember, however, that a search engine does not replace well-organized content that is easy to navigate. If the only way to get the information for your site is to do a search, would-be visitors may just use the global search services and not visit your site at all.

6. Encourage Interactivity

One of the fundamental differences between Web publishing and print publishing is interactivity. Authors of print publications are unlikely to get feedback except, perhaps, in the form of a letter. The Web allows easy feedback on the very day your material is published. Encourage your users to share their thoughts with you. This will help ensure that you are meeting their needs and will be a source of suggestions that may help your site grow and improve.

Feedback is often through e-mail. Feature your e-mail link prominently throughout your site. The e-mail address should contain your site name, such as info@health-site.com. Place this link in a consistent position on each page so your users will know where to find it. The link is commonly placed at the top or bottom of each page. Although you can use a small envelope icon, it may be more effective to provide an invitation to e-mail such as, "send your comments and suggestions to info@health-site.com" or, "if you want your site added to this page, send the name and URL to info@healthsite.com".

Other methods of interactivity are forms for users to input the information directly on the site. For example, if you are requesting suggestions for links, you can provide a form that includes space for the name of the site, the URL, and the contributor's name and e-mail address. Be careful about building lengthy forms. Although they are necessary for some purposes, such as entering orders, they can be cumbersome for routine feedback.

7. Host the Site

If you are interested in a lot of extra work, frustration, and worry, then set up your own Web server. Most who are focused on creation and organization of effective content will be happy to let others maintain a high-capacity, 24-hour-per-day server. You will need to find a host for your site. That is, a computer directly linked to the Internet. Many communities have small companies that will host sites, and generally they can be found in your local directory or on the Web. A service such as America Online will also host your site.

Your host will advise you about loading your Web site information on the server, usually using an FTP (File Transfer Protocol) program. Most will allow you to load information as often as you wish. Even if your host computer is located across the country, you can still load an updated page in seconds.

Once your site is on the server, get on-line and pull it up on your browser to test it. View your site through several of the popular browsers, such as Netscape and Microsoft Internet Explorer, because each presents the material somewhat differently. Confirm that your links are correct and active. Visitors finding inactive links will quickly lose interest.

8. Announce Your Site

Unfortunately, building a Web site does not necessarily mean that you will have visitors. With thousands of Web sites available, you must announce your site. The global search engines will allow you to post your site at no charge; just complete the forms provided by the search engine sites. These generally request your site's name and URL, your name and e-mail address, and a brief description of your site. Post your site with as many search engines as possible. You should check the search engines yourself in a few weeks to make sure that you were listed. You can also post an informational e-mail in an appropriate newsgroup or LISTSERV. However, this is not the place to advertise; you are simply announcing your presence on the Web. If your site contains links to other sites on the Web, send an e-mail message to those sites to notify them that they have been linked. This courtesy will be appreciated. Some of these services or individuals may create a reciprocal link to your site, increasing your visibility.

Newsletters, newspapers, and broadcast media are good ways to publicize your site. Some computer journals will accept a short vignette. You can also create a business card with the name of your site and its URL and e-mail address.

9. Stay Out of Trouble

If you post medical information, or if you link your users to other sites that contain medical information, make sure to post an effective disclaimer. For example:

> The medical information available on the World Wide Web comes from many sources. There are likely to be errors and omissions in this information. Neither HealthSite, its contributors, or … warrant that the information on HealthSite, or accessed through HealthSite, is accurate or complete. Please direct your medical questions to your health care provider.

Do not publish copyrighted material without permission. InterNIC does not check domain names for copyright violations. If you are building a site for your hospital, clinic, or practice, this will likely not be an issue. Otherwise, you should determine whether the information already has been copyrighted. For more information on US copyright law, visit the Copyright Clearance Center, Inc., Online (CCC Online) at http://www.copyright.com.

10. Provide a Service

Finally, realize that your site provides a service. Your users may become dependent on it as a source of information. Think of publishing on the Web as a form of broadcasting—some call it *cybercasting*. Keep your content current; the mantra of Web publishing is update, update, update. Is there new content, news about your organization, new hours, new staff, a new clinic, a new service, a new link? Your front page is a good place to feature your new additions. This allows your repeat users to know at a glance what is new without the need to surf through the entire site.

You must be willing to respond to your visitors questions and suggestions in a timely fashion. If you are unwilling to respond to certain types of questions, such as health advice, you may need to state that clearly on your site.

THE FUTURE

As your site becomes recognized, you will build a sense of community through interactivity and by the service you provide. Some users will become invaluable resources for improvement of your site. If appropriate, you may want to incorporate those individuals into your Web staff. For example, an information-rich site designed for global use may need representatives from various countries to contribute information. As you incorporate other individuals into your structure, make sure that you insist on a commitment to accuracy and to timely service.

As more sites develop with overlapping interests, it is likely that there will be an integration of sites. Millions of small individual sites will be hard to use and locate, despite the best search engines. Consequently, we will likely see a complex interdependence develop among sites with overlapping interests.

Work on developing a clear, content-rich site that is attractive and easy to navigate. Listen to your users, and let your site grow naturally to meet the needs as they evolve. Build effective Internet relationships and, most of all, keep it fun.

Internet Providers and Obtaining Internet Software

Boardwatch Magazine maintains an updated list of all ISPs (Internet service providers) in the United States at (http://www.boardwatch.com).

ON-LINE SERVICES

Compuserve
USA/Canada: (800) 848-8199
UK: (800) 289-378
Australia: (800) 025-240
New Zealand:
http://www.compuserve.com

WOW!
(800) 943-8969
http://www.wow.com

America Online (AOL)
(800) 827-6364
http://www.aol.com

Prodigy
(800) 776-3449
http://www.prodigy.com

Microsoft Network
(800) 386-5550
http://www.msn.com

Delphi
(800) 695-4005
http://www.delphi.com

The WELL
(800) 935-5882
http://www.well.com

INTERNET SERVICE PROVIDERS

Largest US ISPs

NetCom
(800) 353-6600
http://www.netcom.com

IDT Corp
(201) 928-1000
http://www.idt.com

Sprynet
(206) 957-8997
http://www.spry.com

Internet America
(214) 861-2999
http://www.airmail.net

GNN
(703) 918-1802
http://www.gnn.com

TIAC
(617) 276-7200
http://www.tiac.net

Earthlink
(818) 296-2400
http://www.earthlink.com

CRL Network
(415) 837-5300
http://www.crl.com

MindSpring
(404) 815-0082
http://www.mindspring.com

AT&T WorldNet
(800) 967-5363
http://www.att.com/worldnet/

Concentric
(517) 895-0500
http://www.cris.com

Canada

Delphi Internet
(800) 544-5300

IBM Global Network
(800) 426-2255

Hookup Communications
(800) 363-0400

Novalink
(800) 274-2814
http://www.novalink.com

United Kingdom

CityScape Internet Services
01223 566-950
http://www.cityscape.com

Demon
0181 371-1234
http://www.demon.net

Compulink Information eXchange (CIX)
0181 296 9666
http://www.compulink.co.uk

Sprynet
(800) 289-378
http://www.sprynet.co.uk

Australia

AusNet
(800) 806-755
http://www.world.net

OzEmail
(800) 805-874
http://www.ozemail.com.au

InterConnect
(800) 818-262
http://www.interconnect.com.au

New Zealand

Actrix Networks Limited
04 389-6316
http://www.actrix.gen.nz

Planet
04 499-7250
http://www.planet.org.nz

Internet Company of NZ (ICONZ)
09 358-1186
http://www.iconz.co.nz

XTRA
(800) 289-987
http://www.xtra.co.nz

International Providers

IBM Global Network
http://www.ibm.com/globalnetwork

SPRINTLINK
http://www.sprintlink.net

SPRYNET
http://www.spry.com

OBTAINING INTERNET SOFTWARE

Chapter 1. Equipment
SoftWindows, *http://www.insignia.com*
The Well Connected Mac (comprehensive Mac site), *http://www.macfaq.com/newindex.html*
Windows 95.com, *http://www.windows95.com*

Chapter 2. Getting Connected
MacTCP, *http://www.apple.com*
MacPPP, *ftp://ftp.merit.edu/internet.tools/ppp/mac*
Trumpet Winsock, *http://www.trumpet.com.au*

Chapter 3. Internet Basics

E-mail
cc:Mail, *http://www.lotus.com*
Pegasus Mail, *http://www.pegasus.usa.com*
Eudora Light/Pro, *http://www.qualcomm.com*

Web Browsers
Netscape Navigator, *http://www.netscape.com*
Microsoft Internet Explorer, *http://www.msie.com*
AOL Browser, *http://www.aol.com*
CompuServe Spry Mosaic, *http://www.compuserve.com*
DosLYNX, *http://www.shareware.com*

Usenet
Free Agent/AGENT, *http://www.forteinc.com*
MacSoup, *http://www.inx.de/~stk/macsoup.html*

Telnet
Ewan, *http://www.cwsapps.com*
Comet (Mac), *ftp://ftp.cit.cornell.edu/pub/mac/comm*

FTP (File Transfer Protocol)
WS-FTP, *ftp://papa.indstate.edu/winsock-1/ftp/ws_ftp.zip*

Gopher/VERONICA
TurboGopher (Mac), *ftp://boombox.micro.umn.edu/pub/gopher/Macintosh-TurboGopher/*

ARCHIE
WSArchie, *ftp://ftp.coast.net/SimTel/win3/winsock*
Archie Search Site, *http://hoohoo.nsca.viuc.edu/archie.html*

WAIS (Wide Area Information Server)
WAIS Software, *http://www.shareware.com*
WAIS Search Site, *http://www.ai.mit.edu/the-net/wais.html*
WAIS Servers list, *http://www.wais.com*

Internet Relay Chat (IRC)
mIRC, *http://www.shareware.com*
WS IRC, *ftp://papa.indstate.edu/winsock-1/winirc/*

Chapter 5. Optimizing Internet Software

MacOpener, *http://www.dataviz.com*
Word for Word (Document conversion),
 http://www.mastersoft.com
Access PC (Mac),
 http://www.insignia.com
VuePrint (Convert/view image files),
 http://www.hamrick.com
UULite (Mac), *ftp://ftp.hiwaay.net/
 pub/mac/utils*

Chapter 6. Searching the Web

WebCompass,
 http://www:quarterdeck.com/

Chapter 7. Rules of the Road

McAfee's Virus Scan,
 http://www.mcafee.com
Mpack/Munpack, *http://www.
 shareware.com*

Pkzip/Pkunzip, *http://www.pkware.com*
Stuffit/Stuffit Expander (Mac),
 http://www.aladdinsys.com
UnStuff (PC),
 http://www.aladdinsys.com
Wincode, *ftp://oak.oakland.edu/SimTel/
 win3/encode*
WinZip, *http://www.shareware.com*

Shareware Web Sites

C!net, *http://www.cnet.com*
Jumbo, *http://www.jumbo.com*
Shareware.com, *http://www.
 shareware.com*
Stroud's Consummate Winsock
 Applications,
 http://www.cwsapps.com
Simtel, *http://www.coast.net/SimTel*

Fun Internet Resources

The Internet is full of interesting and fun information in addition to the professionally relevant sites. Here's our list of Internet FUN STUFF we thought you may like. Take some time to explore these resources and discover what they have to offer. The information could come in handy.

ENTERTAINMENT

Firefly
Music and movie fan site.
http://www.ffly.com

"ER" Storyline Ideas
Tell the producers of the hit show "ER" about your nights in the ER, and maybe they'll use your story.
http://www.wp.com/bytebloc/ersubmit.html

The Internet Movie Database (IMDb)
Comprehensive free source of movie information
http://us.imdb.com/

TV Listings
U.S. television and cable listings.
http://www.jdpub.com/listings

About the BBC
British television listings.
http://bbcnc.org.uk/

PBS Online
http://www.pbs.org/

The Amazing Fish Cam!
http://home.netscape.com/fishcam/fishcam.html

THE SIMPSONS
The official site for Bart and family.
http://www.foxnetwork.com/simpindx.htm

The Dilbert Zone
Your beloved Dilbert comes to the Internet!
http://www.unitedmedia.com/comics/dilbert/

Starwave Sites
Everything—sports highlights, showbiz, news.
http://www.starwave.com/

The Discovery Channel Online
http://www.discovery.com/

NEWS

Leadstory
A business news service.
http://www.leadstory.com

Europe Online
News and happenings from European
countries.
http://www.europeonline.com

CNN Interactive
All CNN has to offer: U.S and world
news, weather, sports, sci-tech, style,
showbiz, and health.
http://www.cnn.com

The New York Times on the Web
Daily news coverage straight from the
pages.
http://www.nytimes.com

Newspapers on World Wide Web
Newspapers from countries A to Z are all
available here.
*http://www.gt.kth.se/publishing/
news.html#R*

CRAYON
Create you own newspaper
http://crayon.net

**Planet Earth Home Page: News and
Newspapers**
*http://www.nosc.mil/planet_earth/
news.html*

FOOD

Epicurious
Gourmet food stuff.
*http://www.epicurious.com./a_home/
a00_home/home.html*

The Internet Chef On-Line Magazine
For food lovers! Cooking ideas, tips, and
recipes.
http://ichef.cycor.ca/

HEALTH

**American Association for
Therapeutic Humor**
Everyone needs a laugh!
http://www.callamer.com/itc/aath

Gesundheit! Institute
*http://www.well.com/user/achoo/
index.html*

Connecting With Nature
http://www.pacificrim.net/~nature/

Your Health Daily
http://nytsyn.com/med/

INTERNET INFORMATION

The Scout Report
A weekly publication providing a fast and easy way to stay informed of valuable resources on the Internet.
http://rs.internic.net/scout/report

This Is the Worst
If it's really bad it's here.
http://mirsky.com/wow/

Bits of Life + A Day in the Life of Cyberspace
A portrait of life in the digital age describes how the digital media affect how we work, play, and live.
http://www.1010.org/

iGuide
Guide to the Internet with site reviews.
http://www.iguide.com

100 Hot Web Sites
http://www.100hot.com/

EDUCATION

The Human Languages Page
Comprehensive catalog of language-related Internet resources.
http://www.willamette.edu/~tjones/Language-Page.html

A.Word.A.Day
Learn a new word every day.
http://136.142.93.166/words/today.html

Carlos' Coloring Book Home
Bring out the artist in you. Great fun for kids!
http://www.ravenna.com/coloring/

Strunk and White's Elements of Style
http://www.columbia.edu/acis/bartleby/strunk

Everything You Need to Write a Great Speech
http://speeches.com/index.html

The Electronic Zoo
Consult a veterinarian for questions about your pet.
http://netvet.wustl.edu/e-zoo.htm

ROGET's Thesaurus
http://humanities.uchicago.edu/forms_unrest/ROGET.html

Writer's Resources on the Web
http://www.interlog.com/~ohi/www/writesource.html

TRAVEL

city.net
Guide to communities around the
world.
http://www.city.net/

**Xerox PARC Map Viewer: World
0.00N 0.00E (1.0X)**
Pick a point on the globe and look at it
in detail
*http://pubweb.parc.xerox.com:80/
map*

The GNN/Koblas Currency Center
http://bin.gnn.com/cgi-bin/gnn/currency

TRAVEL—Internet Travel Network
Public reservation system with access to
air, car, and hotel information.
*http://www.itn.net/cgi/get?itn/
index:XX-AIRLINES*

Gateway to Antarctica–Home Page
http://www.icair/iac.org.nz/

How Far Is It?
Pick two spots and find out the distance
between them.
http://www.indo.com/distance/

Subway Navigator
Find routes in subway systems in cities
from around the world.
*http://metro.jussieu.fr:10001/bin/
cities/english*

GOVERNMENT

Welcome to the White House
See what's going on inside.
*http://www.whitehouse.gov/
WH/Welcome.html*

**Villanova Center for Information
Law and Policy**
http://www.law.vill.edu/

**Office of the Director of Central
Intelligence**
http://www.odci.gov/

The NASA Homepage
*http://www.gsfc.nasa.gov/
NASA_homepage.html*

U.S. Government Printing Office
http://www.access.gpo.gov/

U.S. House of Representatives
http://www.house.gov/

LITERATURE

Portico
Information about the British Library on-line.
http://portico.bl.uk/

The On-Line Books Page
http://www.cs.cmu.edu/Web/books.html

Library of Congress World Wide Web (LC Web) Home Page
http://lcweb.loc.gov/

NYPL Home Page (New York Public Library)
http://www.nypl.org/

Publisher's Catalogues Home Page
Find listings from major domestic and international publishers.
http://www.lights.com/publisher/

Amazon.com.Books
You'll find more books than you can imagine at this bookstore.
http://www.amazon.com/

Cyber-Seuss!
Dr. Seuss, of course!
http://www.afn.org/~afn15301/ drseuss.html

Internet Public Library
http://ipl.sils.umich.edu/

GREETINGS AND OCCASIONS

Internet Greeting Cards
Pressed for time? Send a card through the Internet.
http://www.tenn.com/igc/ lettershort.html

Virtual Flowers
Send a virtual bouquet to someone special.
http://www.virtualflowers.com

The Electric Postcard
Pick a card, write a message and send it.
http://postcards.www.media.mit.edu/ Postcards

ALMANAC

The World Factbook 1995
http://www.odci.gov/cia/publications/
95fact/index.html

The Atomic Clock
gopher://time_a.timefreq.bldrdoc.
gov:13/0

World Population
http://sunsite.unc.edu/lunarbin/
worldpop

USPS ZIP Code Lookup and Address
Information
http://www.usps.gov/ncsc/

GAMES

Match 23
http://www.gold.net/users/fj17/
index.htm

Web Maze (Myst)
http://shrubbery.com/ingram/myst/

Web-a-Sketch
http://www.digitalstuff.com/
web-a-sketch/

Mr. Edible Starchy Tuber Head
http://winnie.acsu.buffalo.edu/potatoe/

Happy Puppy Games
http://www.happypuppy.com/

MISCELLANEOUS

Scott Pakin's Automatic Complaint-
Letter Generator
Got a gripe? Here's the place.
http://www-csag.cs.uiuc.edu/
individual/pakin/complaint

TranceNet
Criticism of transcendental meditation
and other psychological phenomena.
http://www.trancenet.org/

Beakman Place and Jax Place's Place
Miscellaneous really cool stuff!
http://www.nbn.com/youcan/index.html

Health Care Newsgroups

KEY

Slow = less than 10 messages a day

Medium = 10 to 20 messages a day

Busy = 20 to 100 messages a day

High = >100 messages a day (avg. number)

Newsgroup	Description	Daily Message Traffic
alt.health.ayurveda	Really old medicine from India.	Slow
alt.health.oxygen-therapy	Discussion of oxygen and ozone therapy.	Slow
alt.image.medical	Medical image exchange discussions	Slow
alt.med.ems	Use misc.emerg-services instead.	Slow
alt.med.equipment	Discussion of medical equipment.	Slow
alt.medical.sales.jobs.offered	Jobs for medical industry salespeople.	Slow
alt.medical.sales.jobs.resumes	Resumes of medical industry salespeople.	Slow
alt.support	Support for dealing with emotional situations and experiences.	Slow
alt.support.cancer.prostate	Help for men with prostate cancer.	Slow
alt.support.cerebral-palsy	Cerebral palsy support.	Slow
alt.support.chronic-pain	Support group for those with chronic pain.	Slow
alt.support.diabetes.kids	Support for kids with diabetes and their families.	Slow
alt.support.endometriosis	Endometriosis support group.	Slow
alt.support.food-allergies	Discussion group for people with food allergies.	Slow
alt.support.glaucoma	Support for and by people with glaucoma.	Slow
alt.support.hearing-loss	Support group for hearing impaired.	Slow
alt.support.herpes	Discussion of herpes.	Slow
alt.support.inter-cystitis	Support for those with urinary interstitial cystitis.	Slow
alt.support.kidney-failure	Help for people dealing with kidney problems.	Slow
alt.support.musc-dystrophy	Discussion of muscular dystrophy.	Slow
alt.support.ostomy	Support and resources for people with ostomies.	Slow
alt.support.prostate.prostatitis	For individuals with prostatitis.	Slow
alt.support.psoriasis	For individuals with psoriasis.	Slow
alt.support.sinusitis	Inflammation of the sinuses support.	Slow
alt.support.skin-diseases	Support for those with psoriasis and other common skin afflictions.	Slow
alt.support.social-phobia	Help for xenophobes.	Slow

KEY

Slow = less than 10 messages a day

Medium = 10 to 20 messages a day

Busy = 20 to 100 messages a day

High = >100 messages a day (avg. number)

Newsgroup	Description	Daily Message Traffic
alt.support.spina-bifida	Support for people dealing with spina bifida.	Slow
alt.support.stuttering	Support for people who stutter.	Slow
alt.support.thyroid	Help for people with thyroid gland problems.	Slow
bionet.immunology	Discussions about research in immunology.	Slow
bit.listserv.medforum	Medical students' discussions. (Moderated: medforum@listserv.arizona.edu)	Slow
can.med.misc	Miscellaneous medical information related to Canada.	Slow
misc.handicap	Discussions of interest to persons with disabilities.	Slow
misc.health	Miscellaneous health issues.	Slow
misc.health.injuries.rsi.misc	All about repetitive strain injuries (RSI).	Slow
misc.health.injuries.rsi.moderated	Experts answer questions about RSI. (Moderated: rsi@usc.edu)	Slow
misc.health.therapy.occupational	All areas of occupational therapy.	Slow
sci.med.diseases.als	Amyotrophic lateral sclerosis research and care.	Slow
sci.med.diseases.hepatitis	Hepatitis diseases.	Slow
sci.med.diseases.osteoporosis	Osteoporosis information exchange.	Slow
sci.med.laboratory	All aspects of laboratory medicine and management.	Slow
sci.med.midwifery	The practice of obstetrics by midwives. (Moderated: midwifery@gsf.de)	Slow
sci.med.occupational	RSI and job injury issues.	Slow
sci.med.orthopedics	Orthopedic surgery, related issues, and management. (Moderated: bones@unixg.ubc.ca)	Slow
sci.med.pathology	Pathology and laboratory medicine.	Slow
sci.med.physics	Issues of physics in medical testing/care.	Slow
sci.med.prostate.bph	Benign prostatic hypertrophy.	Slow
sci.med.prostate.cancer	Prostate cancer.	Slow
sci.med.radiology	All aspects of radiology.	Slow
sci.med.radiology.interventional	Vascular and interventional radiology.	Slow
sci.med.telemedicine	Hospital/physician networks. No diagnosis questions.	Slow
sci.psychology.announce	Psychology-related announcements. (Moderated: psy-announce@psy.psych.nova.edu)	Slow
alt.health.cfids-action	Chronic Fatigue Syndrome Action Group. (Moderated: cfids-l@american.edu)	Medium
alt.med.allergy	Help for people with allergies.	Medium
alt.psychology	Use sci.psychology.misc instead.	Medium
alt.society.mental-health	General information about mental health.	Medium
alt.support.abortion	For pro-choice advocates.	Medium

Newsgroup	Description	Daily Message Traffic
lt.support.arthritis	Help for people with stiff joints.	Medium
alt.support.ataxia	Help for people who can't control muscle movements.	Medium
alt.support.cancer	Emotional aid for people with cancer.	Medium
alt.support.depression.manic	Support for those with extremely serious depression problems.	Medium
alt.support.epilepsy	Epilepsy support.	Medium
alt.support.menopause	Help for women during menopause.	Medium
alt.support.schizophrenia	Mutual support for schizophrenics.	Medium
alt.support.skin-diseases.psoriasis	For individuals with psoriasis.	Medium
alt.support.tinnitus	For coping with ringing ears and other head noises.	Medium
alt.support.tourette	Support for folks with Tourette's Syndrome.	Medium
bionet.neuroscience	Research issues in the neurosciences.	Medium
bit.med.resp-care.world	Respiratory Care World.	Medium
misc.health.arthritis	Arthritis and related disorders.	Medium
misc.health.infertility	Treatment and support of infertility.	Medium
sci.med.aids	AIDS: treatment, pathology/biology of HIV, prevention. (Moderated: aids@wubios.wustl.edu)	Medium
sci.med.cardiology	All aspects of cardiovascular diseases.	Medium
sci.med.immunology	Medical/scientific aspects of immune illness.	Medium
sci.med.informatics	Computer applications in medical care.	Medium
sci.med.psychobiology	Dialogue and news in psychiatry and psychobiology.	Medium
alt.abuse.recovery	Help for victims of abuse to recover.	Busy
alt.med.cfs	Chronic fatigue syndrome discussions. (Moderated: cfs-l@list.nih.gov)	Busy
alt.support.asthma	Support for dealing with labored breathing.	Busy
alt.support.breastfeeding	Discussion and support for breastfeeding.	Busy
alt.support.crohns-colitis	Support for sufferers of ulcerative colitis.	Busy
alt.support.diet	For those seeking enlightenment through weight loss.	Busy
alt.support.eating-disord	People over the edge about weight loss.	Busy
alt.support.grief	Support group for the grieving.	Busy
alt.support.headaches.migraine	Discussion of migraines and headaches.	Busy
alt.support.mult-sclerosis	Support for those with multiple sclerosis.	Busy
alt.support.post-polio	Postpolio syndrome discussion group.	Busy
alt.support.sleep-disorder	For all types of sleep disorders.	Busy
bit.listserv.autism	Autism list.	Busy

KEY

Slow = less than 10 messages a day

Medium = 10 to 20 messages a day

Busy = 20 to 100 messages a day

High = >100 messages a day (avg. number)

Newsgroup	Description	Daily Message Traffic
bit.listserv.medlib-l	Medical libraries discussion list.	Busy
bit.listserv.snurse-l	International nursing student group.	Busy
bit.listserv.transplant	Transplant recipients list.	Busy
misc.education.medical	Issues related to medical education.	Busy
misc.emerg-services	Forum for paramedics and other first responders.	Busy
misc.health.aids	AIDS issues and support.	Busy
misc.health.alternative	Alternative, complementary, and holistic health care.	Busy
misc.health.diabetes	Discussion of diabetes management.	Busy
misc.kids.health	Children's health.	Busy
sci.med	Medicine and its related products and regulations.	Busy
sci.med.dentistry	Dental-related topics; all about teeth.	Busy
sci.med.diseases.cancer	Diagnosis, treatment, and prevention of cancer.	Busy
sci.med.diseases.lyme	Lyme disease: patient support, research and information.	Busy
sci.med.nursing	Nursing questions and discussion.	Busy
sci.med.nutrition	Physiologic impacts of diet.	Busy
sci.med.pharmacy	The teaching and practice of pharmacy.	Busy
sci.med.prostate.prostatitis	Prostatitis.	Busy
sci.med.transcription	Information for and about medical transcriptionists.	Busy
sci.med.vision	Human vision, visual correction, and visual science.	Busy
talk.politics.medicine	The politics and ethics of health care.	Busy
alt.infertility	Discussion of infertility causes and treatments.	High (100)
alt.med.fibromyalgia	Fibromyalgia fibrositis list.	High (160)
alt.support.attn-deficit	Attention deficit disorder.	High (100)
alt.support.depression	Depression and mood disorders.	High (240)
misc.kids.pregnancy	Prepregnancy planning, pregnancy, and childbirth.	High (130)

KEY

Slow = less than 10 messages a day

Medium = 10 to 20 messages a day

Busy = 20 to 100 messages a day

High = >100 messages a day (avg. number)

Note: A number of moderated groups exist. These are groups that usually have one or more individuals (acting as editors and/or moderators) who must approve articles before they are published to the newsgroup. It is impossible to post directly to a moderated list. Instead send your message to the e-mail submission address given after the "Moderated" tag. Usually it takes a day or so for the message to appear. If the moderator believes your article is inappropriate for the newsgroup, it will be returned to you with an explanation.

Further Reading

The following books were consulted during the preparation of this book. If you're looking for additional information, they're excellent resources.

The Macintosh Bible, ed 5
Darcy DiNucci, Elizabeth Castro, Aileen Abernathy, David Blatner, Connie Guglielmo, John Kadyk, and Bob Weibel
(Peachpit Press, Berkeley, Calif, 1995)
The number one book for learning about the Mac, with almost a million copies in print. Thousands of useful tips and shortcuts.

Windows 95 Secrets, ed 3
Brian Livingston and Davis Straub
(IDG Books Worldwide, Foster City, Calif, 1995)
Brian Livingston is widely recognized as the authority on Windows. This is the book that explains all the undocumented features and how to best configure Windows 95 for optimum performance.

Windows 3.1 Configuration Secrets
Valda Hilley and James M. Blakely
(IDG Books Worldwide, Foster City, Calif, 1994)
An excellent all around reference to installing and configuring Windows 3.1 and Windows for Workgroups, with particular attention to customizing .ini files, and optimizing system memory.

Using the Internet with Your Mac
Mary Ann Pike and Scott Berkun
(Que Corporation, Indianapolis, Ind, 1995)
This is a complete reference to accessing the Internet for Mac users of all experience levels. Has an accompanying CD-ROM with more than 100 Internet programs.

Build a Web Site: The Programmer's Guide to Creating, Building, and Maintaining a Web Presence
Genesis and Devra Hall
(Prima Publishing, Rocklin, Calif, 1995)
The best guide to becoming a webmaster, with all you needed to know about HTML, CGI (common gateway interface), and other Web mysteries.

The Whole Internet for Windows 95: User's Guide & Catalog
Ed Krol and Paula Ferguson
(O'Reilly & Associates, Inc., Sebastopol, Calif, 1995)
The Windows 95 version of the classic Internet book.

A

AAHP Online, 153
AAPD Online, 225
AARP (CompuServe service), 272
Ability Home Page, 131
Access logs on web browsers, 106
Access PC, 293
Access speed
    definition, 3
Achoo (health care information site directory),
    97—98, 230
    WWW site, 97, 231
Actrix Networks Limited (Internet service provider),
    291
    WWW site, 291
Acupuncture.com , 148—149
A.D.A.M. Software (CompuServe service), 272
ADA Online, 225
Addresses
    definition, 4
    and errors messages from URLs, 44
Advances in therapy - Skin infections , 171
Adventures With an Ice Pick: A Short History of
    Lobotomy , 245
Aesclepian Chronicles , 151
AIDS and HIV WWW sites, 156–157, 268
AIDS News Clips (CompuServe service), 272
Airnews, 79
Alan Mason Chesney Medical Archives , 242
Alexander Technique, 149
Algy's Herb Page, 149–150
Allergy WWW sites, 157
Alliance of Genetic Support Groups , 182
AltaVista (search engine), 96
    Usenet index on, 79
    WWW site, 96
Alternative and complimentary therapies,
        WWW sites141–152
The Alternative Medicine Homepage, 142–143
Alzheimer's Association, 157–158
Alzheimer's Disease Resource Page, 158
Alzheimer's Disease Review , 158
Alzheimer's Disease WWW sites, 157–159
Alzheimer Web Home Page, 157

American Academy of Child & Adolescent
    Psychiatry, 258
The American Academy of Dermatology , 252–253
American Academy of Ophthalmology , 254–255
American Academy of Orthopaedic Surgeons On-
    Line System, 255
American Academy of Physician Assistants,
    223–224
American Association for Pediatric Ophthalmology
    and Strabismus, 255
American Association for the History of
    Nursing 241
American Association of Clinical Endocrinologists,
    253
American Association of Critical Care Nurses, 141
American Association of Immunologists Home
    Page, 253–254
American Cancer Society (America Online
    service), 275
American Cancer Society, 162
American Chiropractic Association Chiropractic
    Online, 218
American College of Cardiology Home Page, 252
American College of Clinical Pharmacy Home
    Page, 229
The American College of Nurse-Midwives, 223
American College of Radiology, 258
American College of Rheumatology, 258–259
American Diabetes Association (America Online
    service), 276
American Diabetes Association, 173
American Gastroenterological Association, 253
American Liver Foundation Homepage, 186–187
American Lung Association (America Online
    service), 278
American Lyme Disease Foundation, 188
American Pain Society, 256
American Physical Therapy Association, 129
American Psychiatric Press, Inc.-The Prime Site for `
    Insight, 207
American Society for Aesthetic Plastic Surgery
    Home Page, 257
American Society for Microbiology, 135

Note: Italicized entries are World Wide Web sites.

American Society of Health Systems Pharmacists Webpage, 228–229
American Society of Parasitologists, 199
American Standard Code for Information Interchange (ASCII)
  definition, 6
America Online (AOL), 63–64, 289
  alternate browsers with, 76–77
  e-mail on, 34–35, 77–78
  Global Network Navigator (GNN), 65
  international connections on, 64
  special services offered subscribers, 273–277
  usenet newsgroups on, 50
  WWW site, 287
AMIA/MedSIG (CompuServe service), 264
Ample Living (CompuServe service), 272
AMSO Bio, 153
AMSO Capitation: An Open Forum, 153
Ancient Medicine/Medicina Antiqua, 241–242
Anesthesia WWW sites, 159
The ANNDEE Homepage, 155
Anxiety WWW sites, 160
AOL (America Online). See America Online (AOL)
Archie, 56
  definition, 5
Arizona Health Science Library, 99
Arkansas Children's Eye Clinic, 192
Armed Forces Institute of Pathology Home Page, 199–200
Arthritis Diagnosis, Differentiation, and Classification, 160
Arthritis Foundation, 160
Arthritis WWW sites, 160–161
Article
  definition, 5
ASCII (American Standard Code for Information Interchange)
  definition, 6
Ask the Dietitian, 229–230
Association for Research in Otolaryngology, 255–256
Association of Operating Room Nurses, 141
Atlanta Reproductive Health Center, 91
Atlanta Reproductive Health Centre; Infertility, IVF, Endometriosis Homepage, 184–185
Atlas of Liver Pathology, 187
Attention Deficit Disorder Forum (CompuServe service), 268
AT&T WorldNet (Internet service provider), 290
  WWW site, 290
AusNet (Internet service provider), 291
  WWW site, 291
Avon's Breast Cancer Awareness Crusade (America Online service), 276

B

Backup of computer programs and files
  definition, 7
  devices for, 10–11
The Bakken Library and Museum, 241
Bandwidth
  definition, 8
Baud
  definition, 9
BBS (Bulletin Board Service)
  definition, 10
Bernie Siegel Online (America Online service), 276
Better Health & Medical Forum (America Online service), 273
Biomedical Imaging Conferences, 175
BioMedNet, 233
Birthmarks aka Port Wine Stains, 170
Birthmarks WWW sites, 170
Blue Baby Operation, 239
Boardwatch Magazine, 287
"Bones are Us", 194–195
Bookmarks in web browsers, 43
Boolean operators and logic, 88–90
  definition, 11
BPS (Bits Per Second). See Baud
Brain WWW sites, 161
Breast Cancer Information Clearinghouse, 164
Breast Lecture, 161
Breast WWW sites, 161
  cancer, 164–165
Brian's Chronic Hepatitis Home Page, 183
Brigham RAD, 175
Bug
  definition, 12
Bulletin board service (BBS)
  definition, 10
Business and politics of health care WWW sites, 152–154

C

Cache files, 105
Caduceus-L: History of the Health Sciences Forum, 242
California College of Podiatric Medicine, 221
Cancer Forum (CompuServe service), 268
Cancer WWW sites, 162–166, 268–269, 275–276
  breast, 164–165, 276
  gynecologic, 165
  pediatric, 166
  skin, 166
Cardiology Compass, 166–167

Cardiology WWW sites, 166–167
CC:Mail (e-mail software), 33
   WWW site, 290
CDA Online, 226
Center for Advanced Instructional Media, 251
Centers for Disease Control and Prevention Home
     Page, 259
A Century of Obstetrics, 245
CGI (Common Gateway Interface)
   definition, 13
Chat
   definition, 14
The Children's Hospital Online Information
     Resource, 201
Children with DIABETES, 173
Chiropractic Health for Washington State, 219
Chiropractic Resources Referral Directory, 218
Chiropractic WWW sites, 218–219
Chiroweb, 218
Chronic Hepatitis Forum (CompuServe service), 272
Chronic Illness Forum (CompuServe service), 269
ChronicIllnet, 237
CINet, 95–96
Citation
   definition, 15
CityScape Internet Services (Internet service
     provider), 291
   WWW site, 291
Classic Works in Herbal Medicine, 246
Clinical Immunology Society Home Page, 254
Clinical Reviews in Depth, 180
Clinical Trials: Osteoporosis/Specific Disease
     Category Listing, 195
Cnet, 291
Colgate-Palmolive Company, 226–227
Collaborative Hypertext of Radiology, 175
Columbia/HCA Live Physician's Chat (America
     Online service), 274
Common gateway interface (CGI)
   definition, 13
Communications software, 21–22
Community of Science
   (medical information network), 126
   WWW site, 126
Comprehensive Core Medical Library, CHAP 9
Compression
   definition, 16
Compulink Information eXchange (CIX), 291
   WWW site, 291
CompuServe (Internet on-line service provider),
     60–62, 289
   accessing via Telnet, 52
   downloading files in, 76
   e-mail on, 33–34

   external newsreader with, 74–75
   Netscape with, 73–74
   special services offered subscribers, 263–273
   Sprynet, 65
   usenet newsgroups on, 50
   WOW!, 65
   WWW site, 289
Computers
   backup devices for, 10–11
   basic Macintosh (Apple) system, 5
   basic PC (IBM compatible) system, 4–5
   considerations when buying, 11–12
   laptops, 5
   Mac vs. PC, 8–10
   operating systems, 6–8
   PC vs. Mac, 8–10
   selecting the correct, 3–12
Concentric (Internet service provider), 290
   WWW site, 290
Connection
   definition, 17
Consumer Reports (CompuServe service), 272
Consumer Reports Drug Reference (CompuServe
     service), 272
Contact Lens Council, 219
Controlled language
   definition, 18
Cookie files, 104
Copyright Clearance Center Online, 286
Crash
   definition, 19
Credit card numbers, security of, 107
CRL (Internet service provider), 290
   WWW site, 290
Crohn's disease WWW sites, 167
Cutaneous disease and reactions WWW sites,
     170–171
Cutaneous Drug Reaction Database, 171
Cyberspace
   definition, 20
Cyberspace Hospital Ophthalmology Department,
     192–193
Cyberspace Telemedical Office, 234
Cystic Fibrosis, 167–168
Cystic fibrosis WWW sites, 167–168

D

Database
   definition, 21
Deaf Gopher, 134
DeathNet, 248
DejaNews (search engine), 96
   WWW site, 79, 96

Deja Vu: AIDS in Historical Perspective, 245
Delphi Internet (Internet service provider), 289
Delphi (Internet on-line service provider), 67, 289
Demon (Internet service provider), 291
    WWW site, 291
Dentistry On-Line, 227
Dentistry WWW sites, 225–227
Department of Health and Human Services Home
        Page, 262
Dept. of Dermatology - University of Iowa, 168
Dermatology in the Cinema, 168
Dermatology-Mie University School of Medicine
        HomePage, 168
Dermatology WWW sites, 168–170
Diabetes Forum (CompuServe service), 272
Diabetes Monitor, 173–174
Diabetes WWW sites, 173–174, 276
Diagnostics, drugs, and devices WWW sites,
        154–156
Diagnostic Test Information Server, 155
Digestive diseases WWW sites, 178
Digital Journal of Ophthalmology, 193
Digital Urology Journal, 215
Diotima Project, 242
Disabilities Forum (CompuServe service), 272
Diseases, Disorders, and Related Topics, 231
Diseases of the Liver, 187
Division of Rheumatology, University of Colorado
        Health Sciences Center, 160–161
Dr. Bob's Mental Health Links, 207
Dr. Bower's Complementary Home Page, 143
Dr. Greenson's Gastrointestinal and Liver Pathology
        Homepage Extravaganza, 187
Dr. Pribut's Running Injuries Page, 130
Drs4Kids, 201
Doctor's Guide to the Internet, 235
Doctor's Home Page, 234
Document
    definition, 22
Document delivery
    definition, 23
DOE Office of Human Radiation Experiments,
        209
DOS operating system, 6–8
Download
    definition, 24
Drugs, devices, and diagnostics WWW sites,
        154–156
Duquesne University, Study of Rheumatoid
        Arthritis, 161
Dysphagia Resource Center, 178–179
Dysphagia WWW sites, 178–179

E

Earthlink (Internet service provider), 290
    WWW site, 290
E-mail, 26–36
    addresses, 29–30
    America Online (AOL), 34–35
    attaching files to, 32–33
    cc:Mail, 33
    CompuServe, 33–34
    definition, 25
    Eudora, 33
    managing and organizing, 31–32
    in Microsoft Internet Explorer (MSIE), 70
    Netscape, 33
    Pegasus, 33
    returned, 35–36
    software for, 33–35
    verification of identities of senders of, 106–107
Emergency medical services WWW sites, 127–128
The Emergency Medicine and Primary Care Home
        Page, 179
Emergency medicine WWW sites, 179–180
Emerging Infectious Diseases WWW sites, 180
Emerginet, 127
Emulation
    definition, 26
Ethics in Science, 249
Ethics WWW sites, 247–249
Eudora (e-mail software), 33
    WWW site, 292
Excite (search engine), 90, 96, 97
    WWW site, 96

F

Family Health, 181
Family medicine WWW sites, 181
Family Services Forum (CompuServe service), 267
FAQ (Frequently Asked Question)
    definition, 27
FDA Center for Food Safety and Nutrition,
        230
Federal Emergency Management Agency, 128
Fibromyalgia WWW sites, 181–182
Files
    compressed, 83–84
    downloading in CompuServe, 76
    transferring between PC and Mac, 84
File Transfer Protocol (FTP). See FTP
        (File Transfer Protocol)
Finding the Path, 179

Firewall
    definition, 27
Flame
    definition, 28
Food and Drug Administration Home Page, 259
Food and Nutrition Information Center, 230
Foot and Ankle Web Index, 221
A Foot Talk Place on the Net, 220
Francis A Countway Library of Medicine, 242
Free Agent, 292
Frequently asked question. See FAQ (Frequently
        Asked Question)
FTP (File Transfer Protocol), 55
    definition, 29
Functionality
    definition, 30
Fun resources on the Internet, 295–300

G

GASNet, 159
Gateway
    definition, 31
Genetics WWW sites, 182–183
Get Well, 150
Global Emergency Medicine Archives, 180
Global Network Navigator (GNN), 65, 288
    WWW site, 288
Goals of Midwives Alliance of North America, 222
Gopher, 55–56
    definition, 32
Gopherspace, 56
    definition, 33
Government agencies WWW sites, 259–262
Government Publications Online (CompuServe
        service), 272
Grand Rounds Archive, 197
Graphical user interface. See GUI (Graphical User
        Interface)
The Gray Lab CancerWeb, 162
Guide to Poisonous and Toxic Plants, 205
GUI (Graphical User Interface), 6, 7
    definition, 34
Gynecologic cancer WWW sites, 165
Gynecologic Oncology, 165

H

Hacker
    definition, 35
Handicapped Users' Database (CompuServe
        service), 269–270
Hans Popper Hepatopathology Library, 188
*Harvey Cushing/John Hay Whitney Medical
        Library, 242–243*
Health Action Network Society, 143–144

Health & Fitness Forum (CompuServe service),
        270
Health Care Financing Administration, 259–260
*HealthCare Information Resources: Alternative
        Medicine, 144*
Health care newsgroups on the Internet, 301–304
Health Channel (America Online service), 274
Health Database Plus (CompuServe service), 265
Health Database Sampler, 237
HealthGate (medical information network),
        112–115
    WWW site, 112
HealthNet (CompuServe service), 265–266
Health Policy Central, 154
Health Trek, 147
Health Volunteers Overseas, 266
HealthWeb: Radiology, 176
HealthWorld Online (medical information
        network), 115–118
    WWW site, 115
Heartweb, 167
Hepatitis B Foundation Home Page, 183
Hepatitis C Info and Support, 184
Hepatitis Weekly, 184
Hepatitis WWW sites, 183–184
History files on web browsers, 106
History of Biomedicine, 239
History of Body Donation, 246
History of Brain Surgery, 241
History of medicine WWW sites, 238–247
*History of Women & Science, Health, and
        Technology: A Bibliographic Guide to the
        Professions and the Disciplines, 243*
HIVNALIVE, 156
HIVNET, 157
HKDA Online, 226
HOLA Information System, 234–235
Holistic Internet Community, 145
Homeopathic Education Services, 150–151
Homeopathic Internet Resources List, 151
Homeopathy Home Page, 151
Home page
    definition, 36
*Homepage of The American Academy of
        Pediatrics, 257*
Hookup Communications (Internet service
        provider), 290
*Hooper's Forensic Psychiatry Resource Page,
        248–249*
Hospital Web, 231
Host
    definition, 37
HotBot (search engine), 96
    WWW site, 96

HSTAT: Health Services/Technology Assessment Text, 131
HTML (Hypertext Markup Language), 42–43
    definition, 37
    using WWW documents to learn, 43
HTTP (Hypertext Transport Protocol)
    definition, 38
Human Sexuality Database and Forum (CompuServe service),271
Hypersensitivity WWW sites, 171–172
Hypertension, Dialysis, and Clinical Nephrology (HDCN): Renal Disease Electronic Journal , 185
Hypertext
    definition, 39
The Hypertextbook of Pediatric Critical Care, 201–202
Hypertext Markup Language (HTML). See HTML (Hypertext Markup Language)
Hypertext Transport Protocol (HTTP)
    definition, 38

I

IBM Clinton Health Care Reform Plan (CompuServe service), 272
IBM Global Network (Internet service provider), 290, 291
    WWW site, 291
ICPS Home Page, 256
Idea Nurse, 138
IDT Corp. (Internet service provider), 290
    WWW site, 290
Impotence WWW sites, 184
Index of Medieval Medical Images in North America, 244
Indiana University Department of Radiology, 176
Infections WWW sites, 171
Infertility WWW sites, 184–185
Information for Genetic Professionals, 182
Information USA (CompuServe service), 273
Infoseek (search engine), 96
    WWW site, 96
Infotrieve (medical information network), 126
    WWW site, 126
Inktomi (search engine), 96
    WWW site, 96
Integrated services digital network (ISDN). See ISDN (Integrated Services Digital Network)
InterConnect (Internet service provider), 291
    WWW site, 291
Intergovernmental Health Policy Report, 154
International agencies and societies WWW sites, 259–262

International Association for the Study of Pain, 256–257
International Lung Sounds Association, 210
International Service Agencies, 260–261
Internet
    connecting to, 13–24
    credit card numbers on, 107
    definition, 40
    fun resources on, 295–300
    medical networks on, 111–126
    on-line service providers, 289. See also Internet on-line service providers (ISPs)
    on-line services on, 15–17. See also Internet on-line service providers (ISPs)
    optimizing your use of, 69–84
    security on, 103–107
    service providers, 290
    software for, 292–293
    viruses on, 108
Internet America (Internet service provider), 288
    WWW site, 290
Internet and On-line Resources, 144–145
Internet Company of NZ (Iconz), 291
    WWW site, 291
Internet Grateful Med (medical information network), 118–120
    WWW site, 118
Internet mailing lists. See Listserves
Internet Mental Health, 207
Internet on-line service providers (ISPs), 289
    America Online (AOL), 60, 63–64, 289. See also America Online (AOL)
    choosing, 59–68
    CompuServe, 61–62, 289. See also CompuServe (Internet on-line service provider)
    definition, 43
    Delphi, 67, 289
    Microsoft Network, 66, 289
    Prodigy, 60, 66, 289
    The WELL, 67, 289
    WOW!, 69, 289
The Internet Pathology Laboratory for Medical Education, 251–252
Internet relay chat (IRC), 58
    definition, 41
Inter Nurse, 139
An Introduction to Osteopathic Manual Therapy: Diagnosis and Treatment of Axial Skeleton, 227
IQuest Medical InfoCenter (CompuServe service), 266

IRC (Internet Relay Chat),58
   definition, 41
The Irish National Virology Reference Laboratory Home Page, 216
ISDN (Integrated Services Digital Network), 19–20
   definition, 42
ISP (Internet Service Provider)
   connecting to, 13–17
   definition, 43
Issues in Mental Health (America Online service), 277
IVI Publishing (CompuServe service), 272

J

JAVA (programming language), 37
JHU Center for Hearing and Balance, 197
The Johns Hopkins Hospital Virtual Children's Center, 202
Jonathan Tward's Multimedia Reference Library, 233
Journal of Emergency Medical Services, 128
Journal of Family Practice Online, 181
Jughead, 56
   definition, 43
Jumbo, 293

K

Keywords
   definition, 89
Kidney disease WWW sites, 185–186
KKH Web Server - The International Obstetrics and Gynecology Resources, 217
Knowledge Finder (medical information network), 126
   WWW site, 126
Knowledge Index (CompuServe service), 266

L

The Language of Dermatology, 169
LAN (Local Area Network)
   definition, 44
Laparoscopy.com, 212
Legal Research Center (CompuServe service), 273
Lifesphere, 133
Life Time Online - Breast Cancer, 165
Limit and Limiters
   definition, 45
List of Poison Information Resources, 205
Listserves, 52–54
   professional information on, 53–54
   subscribing to, 53

Liver disease WWW sites, 186–188
Local area network (LAN)
   definition, 44
Login
   definition, 46
Lupus Home Page, 188
Lupus WWW sites, 188
Lycos (search engine), 97
   WWW site, 97
Lyme disease WWW sites, 188

M

MacLean Center for Clinical Medical Ethics, 248
MacNursing Home Page, 140
MacOpener, 293
MacPPP, 292
MacSoup, 50–51
   WWW site, 293
MacTCP, 292
Magellan (search engine), 97
   WWW site, 97
Mailing list
   definition, 47
Mapping
   definition, 48
Marfan syndrome WWW sites, 189
Marilyn's Midwifery Page, 221–222
MARRTC Fibromyalgia, 181
Massage Therapy, 151
Mass General Hospital Department of Neurosurgery, 189–190
Matrix Dermatology Resources, 169
McAfee's Virus Scan, 293
McGill General Surgery Home Page, 213
MCW Bioethics Database, 247
M.D. Anderson Cancer Center, 163
The MedAccess Site, 202
Medconnect-Information Services for the Medical Community, 234
Medconnect, 128
MEd Guide, 250
Medical, Clinical, and Occupational Toxicology, 213
Medical Acupuncture Web Page, 149
Medical associations and societies WWW sites, 251–258
Medical Education Page, 250–251
Medical Herpetology, Snakebite and Wilderness Med, 206
Medical law and ethics WWW sites, 247–249
Medical Matrix History of Medicine, 242
Medical Matrix Pulmonology, 210
Medical Matrix –Rheumatology, 211
Medical Matrix, 232

Medical Mycology Research Center, Galveston, Texas, 171
Medical networks on the Internet, 111–126
    Community of Science, 126
    HealthGate, 112–115
    HealthWorld Online, 115–118
    Infotrieve, 126
    Internet Grateful Med, 118–120
    Knowledge Finder, 126
    Ovid, 120–123
    Physicians' Home Page (PHP), 123–125
    Plymouth Area Communities Medical
        Access, 126
The Medical Radiography Home Page, 176
The Medical Reporter, 237
Medical Source, 152
Medical subject headings (MeSH)
    definition, 49
Medical technology WWW sites, 134–135
Medicine On Line, 162
MEDLINE
    definition, 50
    need of on medical information network, 111
MEDLINE (America Online service), 274
MEDLINE, 234, 236
MEDMarket Virtual Industrial Park, 155
Med Nexus, 235
MedScape, 236
Med TechNet, 135
MedWeb: Alternative Medicine, 146
MedWeb: History, 239–240
MedWeb Toxicology, 213
MedWeb, 232
MedWorld, 249–250
Melanoma Research Project, 166
Mental health and psychiatry WWW sites,
    207–209
Mental Health Infosource, 208
Merriam Webster Medical Dictionary (America
        Online service), 274–275
MeSH (Medical subject headings), 51, 114
    definition, 49
MetaCrawler, 97
Metathesaurus
    definition, 51
MGH/Child Neurology, 192
MGH Neurology, 189
Michigan Digital Historical Initiative, 243–244
Microbial Underground, 134
Microsoft Internet Explorer (MSIE), 70–71
    "cookie" file on, 104
    WWW site, 292

Microsoft Network (MSN), 66, 287
MIDIRS, 222
Midwifery WWW sites, 221–223
Migraine Forum (CompuServe service), 270
Milestones in Neuroscience Research, 241
MIME (Multipurpose Internet Mail Extensions),
    32, 83
    definition, 52
Mind/Body Sciences Forum (CompuServe
        service), 273
MindSpring (Internet service provider), 290
    WWW site, 290
MIRC, 292
Modem (MOdulator-DEModulator)
    cable, 20
    definition, 53
    external, 19
    internal, 19
    selecting, 18–21
    troubleshooting problems, 20–21
The Mole Hill, 166
Most Commonly Ingested Plants, 206
Mother Nature's General Store, 145
Mpack/Munpack, 293
MRI (Magnetic Resonance Imaging) WWW
        sites, 174
MRI Patient Information, 174
Multiple Sclerosis Forum (CompuServe service), 273
Multiple Sclerosis Online (America Online
        service), 277
Multitasking
    definition, 54
Muscular Dystrophy Association Forum
        (CompuServe service), 273
Museum of Beaux Arts in France, 239
Museum of Contraception, 241
Music Therapy, 151–152

N

*National Academy of Sciences Institute for Medicine
        Home Page, 261*
National Association of EMTs, 128
National Cancer Institute, 163
*National Center for Human Genome Research,
        182–183*
National Eye Institute, 193
*National Fibromyalgia Research Association,
        181–182*
National Information Center on Deafness, 133
*National Information Center on Health Services
        Research, 152*

National Institute of Arthritis and Musculoskeletal and Skin Diseases, 211
National Institute of Dental Research, 225–226
National Institutes of Health Home Page, 261
National Library of Medicine-History of Medicine Division, 244
National Library of Medicine (NLM)
    definition, 55
    UMLS project, 51
National Marfan Foundation, 189
National Organization for Rare Disorders
        (CompuServe service), 270
National Osteoporosis Foundation, 195
The National PA Page, 224
National Parkinson Foundation, 199
The National PA Student Page, 224
The National Psoriasis Foundation, 172
The National Rehabilitation Information Center Home Page, 130
National Skin Centre, Singapore, 169
National Technical Information Service
        (CompuServe service), 272
National Vitiligo Foundation, Inc., 172
Natural Medicine, Complementary Health Care and Alternative Therapies/IBIS, 146–147
Natural Medicine Forum (CompuServe service), 273
NetCom (Internet service provider), 290
    WWW site, 290
Net Connections for Communication Disorders and Sciences, 134
Netiquette, 101–103
    definition, 56
Netscape Navigator (Web browser)
    configuring for multiple users, 71–72
    "cookie" file on, 104
    e-mail with, 33
    reading newsgroups with, 51
    using with CompuServe, 73–74
    WWW site, 292
Network
    definition, 57
Neurology, neuroscience, and neurosurgery WWW sites, 189–192
    pediatric, 192
Neurosciences on the Internet, 190
Neurosource, 190–191
NEUROSURGERY://ON-CALL, 191
New Age A & B Forums (CompuServe service), 273
New Jersey Chiropractic Page, 219
Newsgroups. See Usenet newsgroups
NewsPage - Health Insurance and Managed Care, 154
New York Academy of Medicine Library, 239
NIDDK Home Page, 174

Nightingale, Florence WWW sites, 139, 247
NIH Grants and Contracts, 152–153
NLightN, 97, 116
NLM (National Library of Medicine). See National Library of Medicine (NLM)
Noodles' Panic-Anxiety Page, 160
Novalink (Internet service provider), 290
    WWW site, 290
NurseForum (CompuServe service), 264
Nurses' Call, 139
Nursing and Allied Health Internet Directory, 137
Nursing and Health Care Resources on the Net, 138
Nursing and the NCLEX, 138
Nursing HealthWeb, 139
Nursing Network Forum, 136
Nursing Net, 136
Nursing Related Web Servers, 137
Nursing WWW sites, 136–141
    historical, 241
Nutrition WWW sites, 99, 229–230

O

Obstetric Ultrasound, 177–178
Occupational Therapy Talk Back, 132
Occupational therapy WWW sites, 132
Off-line
    definition, 59
Omni, 232–233
Oncolink, 163–164
Oncology Online, 164
On-line
    definition, 59
Online Birth Center Midwifery, Pregnancy, Birth and Breastfeeding, 222
Online Health Network, 238
On-line identities, verification of, 106–107
Online Mendelian Inheritance in Man, 183
On-line services. See Internet on-line service providers (ISPs)
OpenText (search engine), 97
    WWW site, 97
Open Text, 89
Operating system
    definition, 60
Ophthalmology WWW sites, 192–194
    pediatric, 192
Optometric Computing, 220
Optometry WWW sites, 219–220
Orthopedics WWW sites, 194–195
    for medical students, 251
OS/2 operating system, 7
Osteometer HomePage, 196
Osteopathy WWW sites, 227–228

Osteoporosis - Doctor's Guide to the Internet, 196
Osteoporosis WWW sites, 195–196
Osteovision, 196
O.T. Internet World, 132
O.T. Online, 132
Otolaryngology WWW sites, 197–198
Otology Online, 197–198
Outbreak, 180
Ovid (medical information network), 120–123
    WWW site, 120
OzEmail (Internet service provider), 291
    WWW site, 291

P

Packet
    definition, 61
Paediapedia: An Imaging Encyclopedia of Pediatric
        Disease, 202
Page
    definition, 62
Pain and pain management WWW sites, 198–199
Pain Net, 198
PanAmerican Society for Pigment Cell
        Research, 170
PaperChase (CompuServe service), 267
Parasites WWW sites, 199
Parellel port
    definition, 62
Parkinson's disease WWW sites, 199
Pathology WWW sites, 199–201
    for medical students, 251–252
Patient Info Documents on Digestive Diseases, 178
PEDBASE Homepage, 203
Pediatric Points of Interest, 203
Pediatric Rheumatology Home Page, 212
Pediatrics WWW sites, 201–204
    cancer, 166
    dentistry, 225
    neurology, 192
    ophthalmology, 192–193
    rheumatology, 212
PEDINFO: A Pediatrics Web Server, 203–204
Pegasus Mail (e-mail software), 33
    WWW site, 292
The People's Plague Online, 215
PEYRONIE DISEASE, 216
Peyronie's Disease, 216
Pfizer/Zyrtec Allergy Information Page, 157
Pharmaceutical Information Network Home-
        page, 156
Pharmacy WWW sites, 228–229
Physical therapy and rehabilitation WWW sites,
    129–131

Physician assistants WWW sites, 223–224
Physicians Data Query (CompuServe service), 269
Physicians' Guide to the Internet, 236
Physicians' Home Page (medical information net-
        work), 123–125
    WWW site, 123
Physiotherapy Global-Links Home Page, 129
Pkzip/Pkunzip, 293
Plague and Public Health in Renaissance Europe,
        246
Planet (Internet service provider), 291
    WWW site, 291
Plastic and reconstructive surgery WWW sites,
        204–205
Plastic Surgery Info Service, 204
Plink, 205
Plug and play
    definition, 64
Plymouth Area Communities Medical Access
        (medical information network), 126
    WWW site, 126
Podiatric Medical Educational Network, 220–221
Podiatry Online, 220
Podiatry Quick Reference, 221
Podiatry WWW sites, 220–221
Point of presence (POP)
    definition, 65
Poison Ivy, western poison oak, poison sumac, 206
Poisons WWW sites, 205–206
Polio Survivors Page, 206
Polio WWW sites, 206
Politics and business of health care WWW sites,
        152–154
POP (Point of Presence)
    definition, 65
A Potpourri of WWW Sites of Interest to
        Midwives, 222–223
Prevline: Preventions Online, 208
Pride! Health Forum (CompuServe service), 268
Primary Care Internet Guide (PCGI): Medical
        History, 240
Prodigy (Internet on-line service provider),
        60, 66, 289
Professional medical associations and societies
        WWW sites, 252–259
Project Dermatology x Atlas, 169
Proprietary
    definition, 66
Prosthetics Research Study WWW Home Page, 131
Proxy server
    definition, 67
Proxy services
    definition, 68

Psoriasis WWW sites, 172
Psych Central, 208
Psychiatry and mental health WWW sites,
    207–208
Psych Online (America Online service), 277
Psychopharmacology Tips, 209
Psychopharmacology WWW sites, 209
PsycINFO (CompuServe service), 272
PT at Northeastern University, 129
Publications Online (CompuServe service), 273
Public Health Forum (CompuServe service), 273

R

Radiation Oncology, 135–136
Radiation WWW sites, 209
Radiologic therapy WWW sites, 135
Radiology for Medical Students, 251
Radiology Web Server, 176–177
Radiology WWW sites, 175–177
    for medical students, 251
RC-WEB, 133
RENALNET, 185–186
Research Clearing House, 130
Research on Alzheimer's Disease, 158–159
Respiratory Care Home Page, 133
Respiratory Disorders, 210
Respiratory disorders WWW sites, 210, 278
Respiratory on the Web, 132
Respiratory therapy WWW sites, 132–133
Retirement Living forum (CompuServe
        service), 267–268
Rheumatology, Criteria and Other Resources, 211
Rheumatology/Orthopedics, 250–251
Rheumatology Resources, 211–212
Rheumatology WWW sites, 210–212
    for medical students, 251
    pediatric, 212
Robert's Neurology Listings on the Web, 191
The Rollin' Rat, 207
RSNA Link, 258
RX list, The Internet Drug list, 229

S

Safetynet (CompuServe service), 273
Scientific American Medical Publications (America
        Online service), 275
Scientific and Medical Antique Collecting
        Guide, 245
SCSI (Small Computer Systems Interface)
    definition, 69
SDI (Selected Dissemination of Information)
    definition, 70

Search capabilities
    definition, 71
Search engines, 85–100
    Achoo, 97–98
    AltaVista, 96
    and Boolean logic, 88–90
    case sensitivity of, 90
    clNet, 95–96
    concept searches on, 90
    definition, 72
    DejaNews, 96
    differences in searches on different, 91–92
    Excite, 90, 96, 97
    HotBot, 96
    ideal, 95, 100
    Infoseek, 96
    Inktomi, 96
    limiting hits on, 94–95
    Lycos, 97
    Magellan, 97
    maximizing hits on, 92–94
    MetaCrawler, 95
    nesting of limiters on, 90–91
    NLightN, 98, 116
    Open Text, 89
    OpenText, 97
    relevance ranking by, 91
    sophisticated techniques for using, 99–100
    stemming of keywords on, 89
    truncating of keywords on, 89–90
    using, 86
    WebCrawler, 97
    Yahoo!, 97
Search history
    definition, 73
Search strategy, 78
    definition, 74
Security of information on the Internet, 103–108
Selected Cases in Toxicology from the Rocky
        Mountain Poison Control, 214
Selected dissemination of information. See SDI
        (Selected Dissemination of Information)
A Selection of Letters Written by Florence
        Nightingale, 247
Self Breast Examination and Mammography, 165
Serial line Internet protocol/Point to point protocol.
        See SLIP/PPP (Serial Line Internet
        Protocol/Point to Point Protocol)
Server
    definition, 75
Services
    definition, 82
Set building
    definition, 76

Shape Your Health Care Future with HEALTH CARE ADVANCE DIRECTIVES, 249

ShareGuide, 147

Shareware
definition, 77
sources of on WWW, 293

Shareware.com, 293

Shell account
definition, 78

Sheri's Fibro Page, 182

Simtel, 293

The Skin Channel, 171–172

Skin Deep, 170

Skin WWW sites
cancer, 166
diseases, 170
psoriasis, 172
reactions, 171
vitiligo, 172–173

SLIP/PPP (Serial Line Internet Protocol/Point to Point Protocol), 23–24
definition, 79

Small computer systems interface. See SCSI (Small Computer Systems Interface)

Software for Internet
sources, 292–293

SoftWindows, 292

Some Electronic Resources in History of Science, Medicine and Technology, 238–247

The Source: The Osteopathic Medical Student Web Site, 227

Sources Index, 212

Southampton University Massage Club, 151

Southern California Orthopedic Institute Home Page, 195

SPAM
definition, 80

Speech, language, and hearing WWW sites, 133–134

Spermatology Home Page, 185

SPRINTLINK (Internet service provider), 291
WWW site, 291

SPRYNET (Internet service provider), 64, 290–291
WWW site, 290–291

St. Jude Children's Research Hospital, 166

Starting Point for Nephrology, Renal Pathology, and Transplantation Home Pages, 186

Stroud's Consummate Winsock, 293

Student education information WWW sites, 249–251

Stuffit/Stuffit Expander, 293

Subheadings
definition, 81

Successfully Treating Impotence, 184

Surgery WWW sites, 212–213

The Swiss Anaesthesia Server, 159

Syndicated Health Columns (CompuServe service), 273

Systemic Lupus Erythematosus, 188

Systems
definition, 82

T

T1/T3 line
definition, 85

Talarian Index, 198–199

TCP/IP (Transport Control Protocol/Internet Protocol), 22–23
definition, 85

TeleSCAN: Telematics Services in Cancer, 164

Telnet, 51–52
definition, 87

Terms
definition, 89

Text-based
definition, 91

Textword
definition, 93

TIAC (Internet service provider), 290
WWW site, 290

Topics in Primary Care: Nephrolithiasis, 186

Toxicology WWW sites, 213–214

Toxikon: Medical Toxicology On-Line, 214

Transport control protocol/Internet protocol. See TCP/IP (Transport \\Control Protocol/Internet Protocol)

The Transporter, 230

Trauma Org, 214

Trauma WWW sites, 214

Trumpet Winsock, 292

Tuberculosis WWW sites, 215

TurboGopher, 292

U

UK Professionals Forum (CompuServe service), 263

Ultrasound WWW sites, 177–178

The UNC-Chapel Hill Division of Neurosurgery, 190

Unified Medical Language System (UMLS), 51

Universal Resource Locator. See URL (Universal Resource Locator)

University of Alberta Department of Laboratory Medicine and Pathology, 200

University of California-San Diego Shiley Eye Center, 193

University of Kentucky College of Pharmacy Home Page, 154–155

University of Michigan Pathology Handbook, 200

University of Missouri-Columbia Department of Ophthalmology, 194
University of Texas Health Sciences Center - San Antonio Trauma Page, 214
University of Washington Department of Pathology WWW Server, 201
UNIX operating system, 7–8
UnStuff, 293
URL (Universal Resource Locator), 39–40
  case sensitivity of, 40
  definition, 97
  and error messages, 44
Urology WWW sites, 215–216
The USDOL OSHA Home Page, 262
Usenet newsgroups, 45–51
  accessing, 49
  Agent (newsreader), 50
  definition, 99
  on America Online (AOL), 50
  on CompuServe, 50
  locating, 45–46
  MacSoup, 50–51
  medical, 299–302
  moderated vs unmoderated, 49
  Netscape, 51
  participating in, 46–47
  posting to, 48–49
  reliable news feeds from, 78–79
  software for, 49–51
  value of FAQs (Frequently asked questions), 48–49

V

Vanderbilt Pediatric Interactive Digital Library, 204
VERONICA (Very Easy Rodent-Oriented Netwide Index to Computer Archives), 56
  definition, 101
The Vestibular Disorders Association, 198
V.I.P.-the Vitiligo Information Pages, 172–173
Virology WWW sites, 216–217
Virtual Diabetes, 174
Virtual Hospital, 177
The "Virtual" Medical Center Pathology and Virology Center, 217
The Virtual Medical Student Lounge, 250
Virtual Nursing Center, 140
Virus
  definition, 102
Viruses (computer), 108
The Visible Human Project, 177
Vitiligo WWW sites, 172–173
VuePrint, 293

W

WAIS (Wide Area Information Servers), 57
  definition, 103
Web. See World Wide Web (WWW)
Web browsers, 37
  access logs on, 106
  bookmarks in, 43
  cache files on, 105
  definition, 104
  history files on, 106
  toolbar buttons on, 41
WebCompass, 98
  WWW site, 293
WebCrawler (search engine), 97
  WWW site, 97
Webmaster
  definition, 105
The WEBster - The Fine Art of Nursing, 140
Weight Management Forum (CompuServe service), 273
Welcome to the Crohns Disease Ulcerative Colitis Inflammatory Bowel Disease Pages, 167
Welcome to the Department of Neurosurgery at NYU, 192
The Well Connected Mac, 292
The WELL (Internet on-line service provider), 67, 289
Wellness Zone, 146
The Whole Brain Atlas, 161
WholeNurse, 137
WHO Midwifery Board, 223
Wide area information server. See WAIS (Wide Area Information Server)
Wilmer Eye Institute, 194
Wincode, 293
Windows 95.com, 292
Windows operating system, 6–8
WinZip, 293
Women's health WWW sites, 217
  historical, 243
Women's Medical Health Page, 217
Women's Wire/Health & Fitness area (CompuServe service), 271
Word for Word, 293
World Health Organization Home Page, 262
World Wide Web
  building a site for, 281–287
World Wide Web Virtual Library-Pharmacy, 228–229

World Wide Web (WWW), 36–45
    browsers, 37–38. See also Web browsers
    definition, 106
    hypertext links in documents, 41–42
    searching on, 85–100. See also Search engines
    Telnet, 51–52
    usenet newsgroups, 45–51
WorldWide Wellness, 148
WOW! (CompuServe on-line information service),
        65, 289
WPIC Library Mental Health Resources, 208
WS-Archie, 292
WS-FTP, 292
WS IRC, 292
WWW. See World Wide Web
WWW Virtual Library: History of Science,
        Technology and Medicine, 240–241

X

The X-ray Century, 178
X-ray WWW sites, 178

Y

Yahoo! (search engine), 97
    WWW site, 97, 148
Yale Dermatology Home Page, 170
Y-Me National Breast Cancer Organization, 165

Z

Zippo, 79